Elsevier's Integrated
Neuroscience

Elsevier's Integrated
Neuroscience

John Nolte PhD

Arizona Health Sciences Center
Department of Cell Biology and Anatomy
Tucson, Arizona

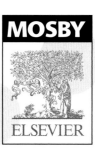

1600 John F. Kennedy Blvd
Suite 1800
Philadelphia, PA 19103-2899

ELSEVIER'S INTEGRATED NEUROSCIENCE   ISBN-13: 978-0-323-03409-8

Notice

Knowledge and best practice in this field are constantly changing. As new research and experience broaden our knowledge, changes in practice, treatment and drug therapy may become necessary or appropriate. Readers are advised to check the most current information provided (i) on procedures featured or (ii) by the manufacturer of each product to be administered, to verify the recommended dose or formula, the method and duration of administration, and contraindications. It is the responsibility of the practitioner, relying on their own experience and knowledge of the patient, to make diagnoses, to determine dosages and the best treatment for each individual patient, and to take all appropriate safety precautions. To the fullest extent of the law, neither the Publisher nor the Author assumes any liability for any injury and/or damage to persons or property arising out of or related to any use of the material contained in this book.

The Publisher

Library of Congress Cataloging-in-Publication Data

Nolte, John.
  Elsevier's integrated neuroscience / John Nolte—1st ed.
    p. ; cm. — (Elsevier's integrated series)
  Includes index.
  ISBN 978-0-323-03409-8
  1. Neurosciences. 2. Nervous system—Diseases. I. Title.
II. Title: Integrated neuroscience. III. Series.
  [DNLM: 1. Nervous System. 2. Nervous System Physiology. WL 100 N798e 2007]
RC341.N6558 2007
612.89—dc22

                                                        2007006745

Acquisitions Editor: Alex Stibbe
Developmental Editor: Andrew Hall

Printed in China

Last digit is the print number: 9 8 7 6 5 4 3 2 1

Preface

Authors often try to regale potential readers with accounts of the importance of their disciplines, but the nervous system truly is of unique importance. Thomas Edison once commented that "[T]he chief function of the body is to carry the brain around," alluding to the critical role of the nervous system in mental experience. Joints, kidneys, and even hearts can be bypassed or replaced without altering a person in fundamental ways, but the essence of a person is lost when activity of the nervous system ceases. This has made the nervous system a source of endless fascination for me for decades, fanned by the explosive growth in recent years of knowledge of its molecular workings. I hope I have been able to convey some of the fascination in this book.

The book is meant to be an overview of those aspects of the nervous system, particularly the central nervous system, most germane to students of the health sciences. I tried to develop topics systematically, with each chapter building on those preceding it. Material from multiple chapters is integrated in a series of clinically based questions at the end of the book.

Despite its unique role, the nervous system obviously collaborates in a functional sense with the rest of the body.

These interdependencies are underscored by the integration boxes distributed throughout the book, pointing to related topics in other books of the series.

This overview of the structure and function of the nervous system would never have come about without the help of many friends and colleagues, to whom I owe a great debt of gratitude. Thanks to Ed French, Ted Glattke, Chris Leadem, Nate McMullen, Naomi Rance, Scott Sherman, Cristian Stefan, Marc Tischler, Todd Vanderah, and Steve Wright for their helpful suggestions on the content of the book and comments on the manuscript. Thanks to Ray Carmody and Elena Plante for the images in Chapter 8. Thanks to Jay Angevine for the whole-brain section used in Figure 1-4 and for use of the sections that are the basis for the drawings in many other figures. Thanks to my students for helping me figure out what works and what doesn't. Thanks to Andy Hall and others at Elsevier for their patience and support. My love and special thanks to Kathy, who came back into my life and held it together throughout the writing of this book.

John Nolte, PhD

Editorial Review Board

Contents

Series Preface

How to Use This Book

The idea for Elsevier's Integrated Series came about at a seminar on the USMLE Step 1 exam at an American Medical Student Association (AMSA) meeting. We noticed that the discussion between faculty and students focused on how the exams were becoming increasingly integrated—with case scenarios and questions often combining two or three science disciplines. The students were clearly concerned about how they could best integrate their basic science knowledge.

One faculty member gave some interesting advice: "read through your textbook in, say, biochemistry, and every time you come across a section that mentions a concept or piece of information relating to another basic science—for example, immunology—highlight that section in the book. Then go to your immunology textbook and look up this information, and make sure you have a good understanding of it. When you have, go back to your biochemistry textbook and carry on reading."

This was a great suggestion—if only students had the time, and all of the books necessary at hand, to do it! At Elsevier we thought long and hard about a way of simplifying this process, and eventually the idea for Elsevier's Integrated Series was born.

The series centers on the concept of the *integration box*. These boxes occur throughout the text whenever a link to another basic science is relevant. They're easy to spot in the text—with their color-coded headings and logos. Each box contains a title for the integration topic and then a brief summary of the topic. The information is complete in itself—you probably won't have to go to any other sources—and you have the basic knowledge to use as a foundation if you want to expand your knowledge of the topic.

You can use this book in two ways. First, as a review book . . .
When you are using the book for review, the integration boxes will jog your memory on topics you have already covered. You'll be able to reassure yourself that you can identify the link, and you can quickly compare your knowledge of the topic with the summary in the box. The integration boxes might highlight gaps in your knowledge, and then you can use them to determine what topics you need to cover in more detail.

Second, the book can be used as a short text to have at hand while you are taking your course . . .
You may come across an integration box that deals with a topic you haven't covered yet, and this will ensure that you're one step ahead in identifying the links to other subjects (especially useful if you're working on a PBL exercise). On a simpler level, the links in the boxes to other sciences and to clinical medicine will help you see clearly the relevance of the basic science topic you are studying. You may already be confident in the subject matter of many of the integration boxes, so they will serve as helpful reminders.

At the back of the book we have included case study questions relating to each chapter so that you can test yourself as you work your way through the book.

Online Version

An online version of the book is available on our Student Consult site. Use of this site is free to anyone who has bought the printed book. Please see the inside front cover for full details on the Student Consult and how to access the electronic version of this book.

In addition to containing USMLE test questions, fully searchable text, and an image bank, the Student Consult site offers additional integration links, both to the other books in Elsevier's Integrated Series and to other key Elsevier textbooks.

Books in Elsevier's Integrated Series

The nine books in the series cover all of the basic sciences. The more books you buy in the series, the more links that are made accessible across the series, both in print and online.

 Anatomy and Embryology

 Histology

 Neuroscience

 Biochemistry

 Physiology

 Pathology

 Immunology and Microbiology

 Pharmacology

 Genetics

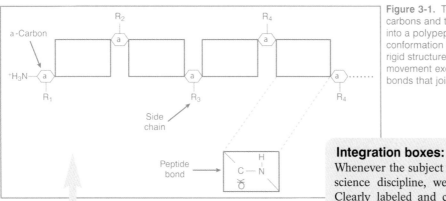

Figure 3-1. The peptide bond linking α-carbons and their side chains together into a polypeptide. The *trans* conformation is favored, producing a rigid structure that restricts freedom of movement except for rotation around bonds that join to the α-carbons.

Artwork:
The books are packed with 4-color illustrations and photographs. When a concept can be better explained with a picture, we've drawn one. Where possible, the pictures tell a dynamic story that will help you remember the information far more effectively than a paragraph of text.

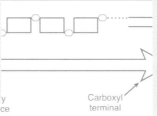

Integration boxes:
Whenever the subject matter can be related to another science discipline, we've put in an Integration Box. Clearly labeled and color-coded, these boxes include nuggets of information on topics that require an integrated knowledge of the sciences to be fully understood. The material in these boxes is complete in itself, and you can use them as a way of reminding yourself of information you already know and reinforcing key links between the sciences. Or the boxes may contain information you have not come across before, in which case you can use them as a springboard for further research or simply to appreciate the relevance of the subject matter of the book to the study of medicine.

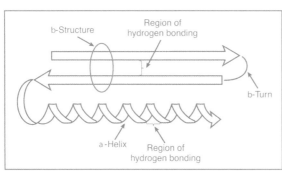

Figure 3-3. Secondary structure includes α-helix and β-pleated sheet (β-sheet).

MICROBIOLOGY

Prion Diseases

Prions (PrP^{Sc}) are formed from otherwise normal neurologic proteins (PrP) and are responsible for encephalopathies in humans (Creutzfeldt-Jakob disease, kuru), scrapie in sheep, and bovine spongiform encephalopathy. Contact between the normal PrP and PrP^{Sc} results in conversion of the secondary structure of PrP from predominantly α-helical to predominantly β-pleated sheet. The altered structure of the protein forms long, filamentous aggregates that gradually damage neuronal tissue. The harmful PrP^{Sc} form is highly resistant to heat, UV irradiation, and protease enzymes.

Since proline has no free hydrogen to contribute to helix stability, it is referred to as a "helix breaker." The α-helix is found in most globular proteins and in some fibrous proteins (e.g., α-keratin).

Text:
Succinct, clearly written text, focusing on the core information you need to know and no more. It's the same level as a carefully prepared course syllabus or lecture notes.

rmation
-structure) consists of

tabilized by hydrogen
f adjacent sequences.

(parallel) or opposite (antiparallel) direction. β-Structures are found in 80% of all globular proteins and in silk fibroin.

Supersecondary Structure and Domains

Supersecondary structures, or *motifs*, are characteristic combinations of secondary structure 10–40 residues in length that recur in different proteins. They bridge the gap between the less specific regularity of secondary structure and the highly specific folding of tertiary structure. The same motif can perform similar functions in different proteins.

- The four-helix bundle motif provides a cavity for enzymes to bind prosthetic groups or cofactors.
- The β-barrel motif can bind hydrophobic molecules such as retinol in the interior of the barrel.
- Motifs may also be mixtures of both α and β conformations.

Credits

The figures listed below are modified from the following books.

Figures 5-26, 10-8, 10-9: Drake R, Vogl W, Mitchell A: *Gray's Anatomy for Students*, Philadelphia, Churchill Livingstone, 2004.

Figures 3-2, 4-1, 4-2, 4-6, 4-10, 4-12, 8-5, 11-3, 11-4, 11-5, 12-2, 12-7, 12-15, 20-7: Nolte J: *The Human Brain: An Introduction to Its Functional Anatomy*, 5th ed. Philadelphia, Mosby, 2002.

Figure 1-9: Pollard TD, Earnshaw WC: *Cell Biology*, 2nd ed. (Updated). Philadelphia, Saunders, 2004.

Figure 20-2: Sanes DH, Reh TA, Harris WA: *Development of the Nervous System*, 2nd ed. San Diego, Academic Press, 2005.

Figures 6-1, 9-4, 10-10A, 10-11, 10-15: Standring S: *Gray's Anatomy: The Anatomical Basis of Clinical Practice*, 39th ed. London, Churchill Livingstone, 2004.

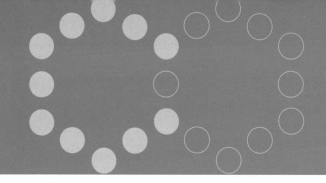

Cells of the Nervous System　　1

The functions of the mind are what distinguish us most as humans, and mental processes are tightly coupled to operations of the brain. We understand quite a bit about how the brain analyzes sensory inputs and programs movements, and we are beginning to understand how the brain is involved in more complex mental activities. Although we may never quite understand how activity in parts of the brain can result in something like self-awareness, it is clear that the mind ceases when brain function ceases. Our brains, unlike our limbs,

kidneys, and other organs, are the physical substrate of our humanness.

Despite its complexity, the nervous system contains only two functional classes of cells: nerve cells (neurons), which are the principal information-processing cells (Fig. 1-1), and glial cells, which play a variety of critical supporting roles. All neurons have a cell body (or soma). Most have numerous dendrites radiating from the cell body, often in distinctive patterns, and a single axon that ends as a series of axon terminals. Although there are numerous variations, the dendrites are the major information-gathering sites of neurons, locations where the axon terminals of other neurons form junctions called synapses; the axon, in contrast, conveys signals to other neurons.

●●● PERIPHERAL AND CENTRAL NERVOUS SYSTEMS

One broad way to subdivide the nervous system is into peripheral (peripheral nervous system, PNS) and central (central nervous system, CNS) parts. There is a series of fairly precise transition points between the two—the sites where the glial cells described later in this chapter change from PNS

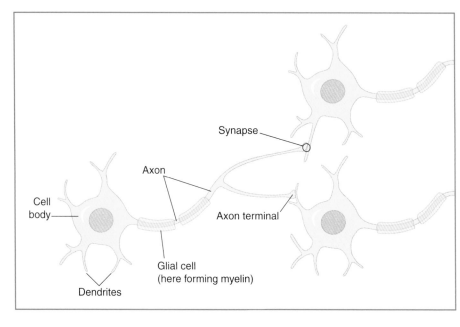

Figure 1-1. A stereotypical neuron and one example of a glial cell. Real neurons actually come in a wide variety of sizes and shapes, and there are several varieties of glial cell (see Figs. 1-10 and 1-12 to 1-15).

Synapse

Axon

Axon terminal

Cell body

Glial cell (here forming myelin)

Dendrites

types to CNS types—but to a first approximation the CNS is the part encased in the skull and vertebral column, and the PNS is the collection of neurons, dendrites, and axons involved in conveying information to and from the CNS (Fig. 1-2).

Parts of the Peripheral Nervous System

The PNS includes some neurons that live entirely outside the CNS, some with cell bodies in the PNS and processes in both the PNS and CNS, and the axons of other neurons with cell bodies in the CNS, all of which can be seen nicely in peripheral nerves associated with the spinal cord (Fig. 1-3 and

TABLE 1-1. Ori ns and Terminations of Fibers in Spinal Nerves

Functional Category	Location of Cell Body	Location of Synapses
Somatic afferent	Sensory ganglion (dorsal root ganglion)	Spinal cord and brainstem gray matter
Somatic efferent	Spinal cord gray matter	Skeletal muscle
Visceral afferent	Sensory ganglion (dorsal root ganglion)	Spinal cord gray matter
Visceral efferent	Spinal cord gray matter Autonomic ganglion	Autonomic ganglion Smooth or cardiac muscle, glands

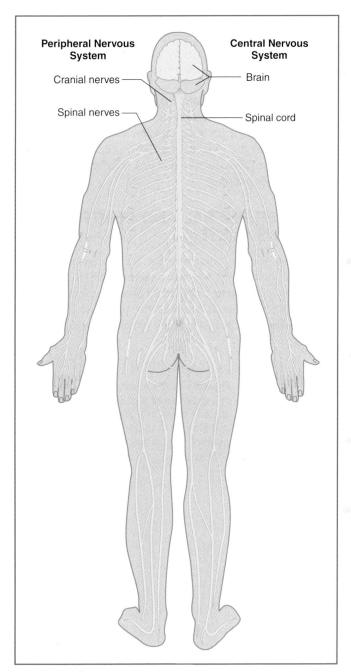

Peripheral Nervous System

Cranial nerves

Spinal nerves

Central Nervous System

Brain

Spinal cord

Figure 1-2. Central and peripheral nervous systems.

Table 1-1). Neuronal cell bodies in the PNS are clustered at various locations along the peripheral nerves that convey their axons, forming ganglia ("swellings"). Some of these neurons and their axons deal with somatic functions—those having to do with skin, muscles, and joints, involving events of which we are consciously aware or over which we have conscious control. Others deal with visceral functions, those having to do with smooth muscle, cardiac muscle, and glands. Hence, there are four different functional categories of nerve fibers in spinal nerves: somatic and visceral afferent and somatic and visceral efferent.[1] (There are also special senses involving the head, using information conveyed by cranial nerves, but the general ideas described here often apply to them as well.)

Sensory information, whether somatic or visceral, is conveyed to the CNS by primary sensory neurons (also called primary afferents), neurons with a cell body in a sensory ganglion, a peripheral process that picks up information from someplace in the body, and a central process that enters and terminates in the CNS (see Fig. 1-3). Somatic and visceral efferents, in contrast, are distinctly different from one another (see Fig. 1-3). The cell bodies of motor neurons for skeletal muscles reside in the CNS; each sends a long axon through the PNS to reach its target muscle. Getting messages to smooth muscle, cardiac muscle, and glands, on the other hand, involves a sequence of two autonomic motor neurons—the cell body of the first (a preganglionic neuron) in the CNS and that of the second (a postganglionic neuron) in an autonomic ganglion.

---

[1] Afferent and efferent are relative terms, simply meaning "carry to" and "carry from," respectively. In this case, they are used relative to the CNS (e.g., PNS afferents convey signals to the CNS), but these are general terms used elsewhere in the nervous system (e.g., CNS neurons receive afferent inputs from other CNS neurons).

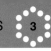

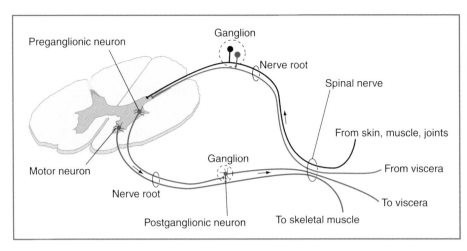

Figure 1-3. Schematic view of the origins and terminations of the fibers found in spinal nerves. Cranial nerves have some additional components, as described in Chapter 5.

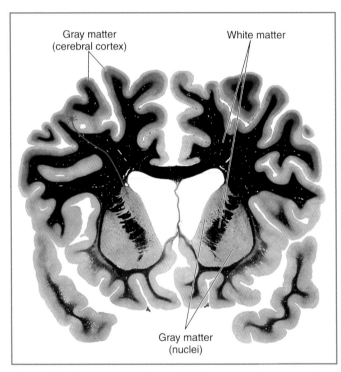

Figure 1-4. Segregation of the CNS into areas of gray matter and areas of white matter, shown in a coronal section of a human brain at about the level of the tips of the temporal lobes. The Weigert stain used on this section makes areas with abundant myelin appear dark. (Courtesy of Dr. Jay B. Angevine, Jr., University of Arizona College of Medicine.)

Parts of the Central Nervous System

Gray Matter and White Matter
The CNS is largely segregated into areas of gray matter, where neuronal cell bodies, their dendrites, and synaptic contacts are concentrated, and areas of white matter, where axons travel from one area of gray matter to another (Fig. 1-4). This segregation is not absolute, because axons for part of their course must travel among neuronal cell bodies to find the ones they are looking for.

A discrete area of gray matter, particularly when its neurons are functionally related to one another, is usually called a nucleus, although other names are possible. For example, an area of gray matter that forms a layered covering on the surface of some part of the CNS is called a cortex. Some areas of gray matter retain older, descriptive names based on their appearances, locations, or configurations (e.g., the substantia nigra, named for the dark pigment contained in its neurons).

A collection of functionally related CNS axons is most commonly referred to as a tract. Tracts typically have two-part names that specify their origins and terminations, respectively. For example, a spinocerebellar tract is a collection of axons that originate from neurons in the spinal cord and are on their way to terminations in the cerebellum. Here again, though, some older, descriptive names are still in use, such as fasciculus ("little bundle"), lemniscus ("ribbon," used for a bundle that is flattened out in cross-section), and peduncle ("little foot," a site where fanned-out axons converge into a compact bundle).

Central Nervous System Subdivisions
The CNS (Fig. 1-5) consists of the brain and spinal cord. The brain, by far the larger of the two, has three major parts: the cerebrum, brainstem, and cerebellum. The cerebrum accounts for nearly 90% of the weight of a human brain and is itself composed of two massive cerebral hemispheres, separated from each other by a deep longitudinal fissure, and a diencephalon buried between them (diencephalon means "in-between brain," referring to its location between the cerebral hemispheres and the brainstem). Each cerebral hemisphere includes a surface covering of cerebral cortex, together with subcortical nuclei and white matter. The diencephalon includes the thalamus, a collection of nuclei that are a major source of inputs to the cerebral cortex, and the hypothalamus, another collection of nuclei that control many aspects of autonomic and hormonal function. The brainstem extends from the diencephalon to the spinal cord and is subdivided into the midbrain, pons, and medulla. The cerebellum straddles the back of the pons and medulla, tethered there by a series of cerebellar peduncles.

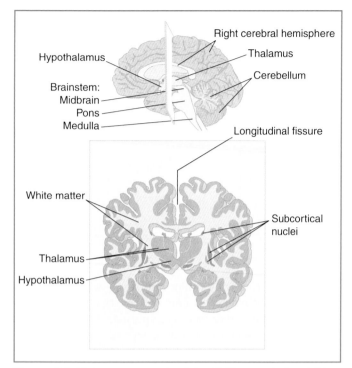

Figure 1-5. Major components of the CNS, seen in the right half of a hemisected brain (*upper*) and in a coronally sectioned brain (*lower*).

●●● NEURONS

Neurons come in a much wider variety of sizes and shapes than do cells in other tissues, but they nevertheless use variations of the same organelles and physiologic processes in ways similar to those of other cells. This makes the remarkably complex mental capabilities of humans even more mysterious. Two simple but fundamentally important facts help explain how this can happen in terms of the actions of arrays of basically similar neurons.

1. Human brains have an enormous number of neurons, probably about 100 billion. This is a big number: if someone could count one neuron per second and took no breaks for anything, it would take more than 3000 years to count them all! And this is only the beginning of the complexity, because each neuron receives numerous synaptic inputs—sometimes thousands—and in turn projects to many other neurons.

2. Individual neurons are precisely connected to particular other neurons (or to other parts of the body), conferring specific functions on different neuronal networks. One way this shows up is as a modular construction of different CNS areas. For example, all areas of cerebellar cortex look the same, but the details of where the inputs come from and where the outputs go to make some areas important for limb movements and others for eye movements.

So just as millions of transistors, all similar to one another, can be connected to form the basis of a desktop computer, billions of similar neurons hooked up in billions of neuronal circuits somehow form the physical substrate for the human mind.

Functional Parts of Neurons

Neurons are in the information-handling business, which involves (1) *collecting* information from someplace, either other neurons, internal organs, or the outside world; (2) doing some kind of *information processing*; (3) *conducting* the processed information to another location, nearby or far away, and (4) *transmitting* the information to other neurons or to a muscle or gland. They do all of this by a combination of electrical and chemical signaling mechanisms detailed in Chapters 2 to 4: for the most part, electrical signals are used to convey information rapidly from one part of a neuron to another, whereas chemical messengers (e.g., neurotransmitters) are typically used to carry signals between neurons. Hence, there are anatomically specialized zones for receiving, processing, conducting, and passing on information (Fig. 1-6). Although here too there are many variations, the branching, tapering dendrites emanating from a neuronal cell body are the principal sites for receiving information from other neurons (via synaptic inputs); the relatively long, cylindrical axon conducts information away from the cell body; and axon terminals transmit information onward. The information processing functions are shared by the dendrites, the cell body, and the part of the axon just emerging from the cell body (the initial segment), in ways described further in Chapter 2. This means that neurons are anatomically and functionally polarized, with electrical signals traveling in only one direction under ordinary physiologic circumstances. (The underpinning of this anatomic and functional polarization is the precise placement of different molecules in particular parts of the neuronal membrane.)

Convergence and Divergence

Although neurons are commonly drawn as having a few inputs and a few axon terminals (as in Fig. 1-6), this is the exception rather than the rule. The usual situation is one in which a very large number of synaptic inputs, often thousands, from a variety of places converge on a given neuron, and in which each axon diverges to provide axon terminals to a large number of other neurons (see Figs. 2-24 and 2-25 for a simple example).

Organelles

The cell body supports the metabolic and synthetic needs of the rest of the neuron and contains the usual organelles, with some in relative abundance (Fig. 1-7). The cell body and proximal dendrites contain only a small fraction of the total volume of a typical neuron, but they synthesize most of the protein and membrane components for the entire neuron. As a result, there is a prominent Golgi apparatus and a lot of rough endoplasmic reticulum (rER)—so much that aggregations of rER and free ribosomes can be stained and visualized in the light microscope as Nissl bodies. Synthesizing macro-

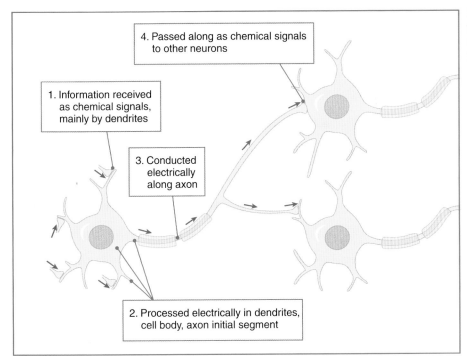

Figure 1-6. Spread of electrical signals within a neuron, and the use of chemical signals to transfer information from one neuron to another.

4. Passed along as chemical signals to other neurons

1. Information received as chemical signals, mainly by dendrites

3. Conducted electrically along axon

2. Processed electrically in dendrites, cell body, axon initial segment

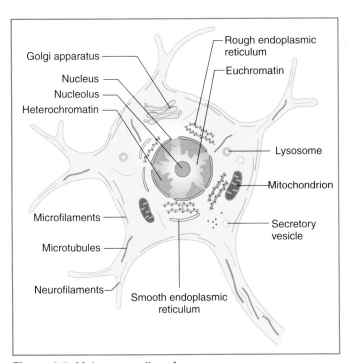

Figure 1-7. Major organelles of neurons.

Golgi apparatus

Nucleus

Nucleolus

Heterochromatin

Microfilaments

Microtubules

Neurofilaments

Smooth endoplasmic reticulum

Rough endoplasmic reticulum

Euchromatin

Lysosome

Mitochondrion

Secretory vesicle

molecules and pumping ions across the membrane (see Chapter 2) require energy, so mitochondria are also numerous.

Their elongated anatomy makes neurons effective at moving information around, but it also creates some logistical problems. Cells are delicate structures consisting mostly of watery cytoplasm enclosed by a thin lipid membrane, and the elaborate shapes of neurons carry this delicacy to an extreme. To maintain their structural integrity, neurons require an extensive system of mechanical support. Part of it, as described in

Chapter 7, is provided by the suspension of the CNS within a watery bath. A second major part is provided by an internal cytoskeleton consisting of a network of filamentous proteins (Fig. 1-8)—microtubules, neurofilaments, and microfilaments—similar to those used by other cells.

Microtubules, the thickest and longest of the three types of filament (about 25 nm in diameter and often tens of micrometers long), are cylindrical assemblies of 13 strands of a globular protein called tubulin. Tubulin itself has an α- and a β-subunit, and the strands are arranged so that all the α-subunits point toward one end of the microtubule (called the minus end) and all the β-subunits point toward the other end (the plus end). Microtubules are scattered through the cytoplasm, crisscrossing each other, but funnel into longitudinally oriented bundles in the axons and dendrites. As in most cells, axonal microtubules are oriented with their plus ends directed away from

PATHOLOGY

Cytoskeletal Proteins and Neurologic Disease

Cytoskeletal proteins figure prominently in the neuronal inclusions characteristic of a variety of neurodegenerative conditions (although it is seldom clear whether they play a causative role in the disorder or are a byproduct of some other pathology). For example, tau (τ), a microtubule-associated protein involved in the formation of cross-links between microtubules, is a major component of the neurofibrillary tangles seen in the neurons of patients with Alzheimer's disease. The Hirano bodies common in Alzheimer's disease, Pick's disease, and some other conditions contain not only tau but also neurofilament and microfilament proteins.

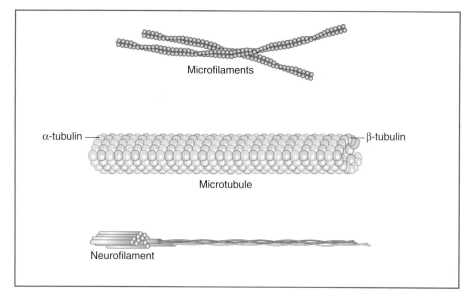

Figure 1-8. Microtubules, neurofilaments, and microfilaments, the major components of the cytoskeleton.

Microfilaments

α-tubulin — β-tubulin

Microtubule

Neurofilament

the nucleus. In contrast, some dendritic microtubules are oriented in both directions. In addition to imparting some structural support, microtubules help solve another problem—that of moving things around within neurons. Axons are long enough that it would typically take months or years for substances to move along their length by simple diffusion, but communication between the cell body and axonal terminals or distant dendrites has to be much faster than this. As a consequence, active processes of axonal (and dendritic) transport (Fig. 1-9) are required for normal neuronal function, both to move newly synthesized molecules out of the cell body (movement in an anterograde or orthograde direction) and to return "used" components or convey signals to the cell body (movement in a retrograde direction). Organelles, membrane components, and molecules enclosed in membrane vesicles move hundreds of millimeters per day in a process of fast transport in which motor molecules drag them along using microtubules as "railroad tracks." Some things move

preferentially down axons in the anterograde direction, with kinesin as the motor, while others move in the retrograde direction, with cytoplasmic dynein as the motor. The orientation of microtubules is an important factor in the differential distribution of organelles into axons and dendrites. Since dendrites have microtubules oriented in both directions, anything can move in either direction between cell body and dendrites. However, the uniform orientation of axonal microtubules means that things conveyed by dynein cannot move in an anterograde direction from the cell body down an axon.

Cytoplasmic molecules synthesized in the cell body (e.g., soluble enzymes, cytoskeletal components) move a few millimeters per day down the axon, mostly or entirely in the anterograde direction, by slow transport. The mechanism of slow transport is not understood, but it may involve some of the same motor molecules as fast transport.

Neurofilaments, ropelike assemblies about 10 nm in diameter, are the neuronal versions of the intermediate filaments

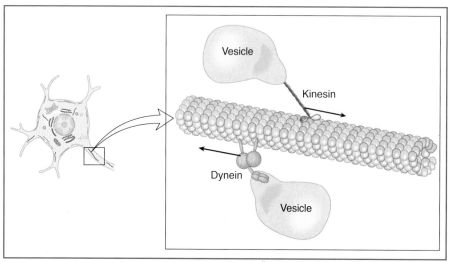

Figure 1-9. Fast anterograde and retrograde transport along microtubules.

Vesicle

Kinesin

Dynein

Vesicle

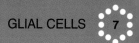

found in almost all cells. Unlike microtubules and microfilaments, they are not polarized and are not involved in any obvious way in transport functions. Their principal role appears to be one of structural support.

Microfilaments, the thinnest and shortest of the three types of filament (about 6 nm in diameter and less than a micrometer long), are twisted pairs of actin filaments. They are concentrated in the cytoplasm just beneath the neuronal cell membrane, where they are important for anchoring various membrane proteins in particular functional areas. In collaboration with neuronal myosin, they are also involved in another transport system, one that moves things to and from the surface membrane. Microfilaments also underlie the movement of growth cones (the tips of growing neuronal processes).

Categories of Neurons

Despite the basic similarity of neurons to one another, there is wide variability in the details of their shapes and sizes (Fig. 1-10). Cell bodies range from about 5 to 100 μm in diameter. Many axons are short, only a millimeter or so in length, but some, like those which extend from the cerebral cortex to the sacral spinal cord, measure a meter or more. There is also wide variability in the shape and extent of dendritic trees, many of them having elaborate and characteristic configurations. The pattern of dendritic and axonal projections is used to classify neurons as unipolar, bipolar, and multipolar. True unipolar neurons are common in invertebrates but rare in vertebrates (the pseudounipolar neurons found in vertebrate sensory ganglia have a unipolar appearance but actually start out as bipolar neurons). Bipolar neurons are most prominent in some sensory epithelia, such as the retina and olfactory epithelium. Multipolar neurons, by far the most numerous type, are widely distributed in the nervous system.

The length and destination of a neuron's axon gives rise to a functional classification (Fig. 1-11). Sensory neurons (primary afferents) convey information to the CNS. Motor neurons have axons that end directly on muscles, glands, or ganglionic neurons in the PNS. The vast majority of neurons are interneurons, neurons that are wholly contained within the CNS and interconnect other neurons. Some are small local-circuit interneurons with axons that extend a few millimeters or less. Others are projection interneurons with long axons. Some of these are tract cells, whose axons convey information from one part of the CNS to another (e.g., corticospinal neurons, spinothalamic neurons), while others project more diffusely to widespread CNS areas, helping modulate the background level of excitability of large numbers of neurons.

● ● ● GLIAL CELLS

Glial cells occupy nearly all the spaces between neurons and neuronal processes, both in the PNS and the CNS. Once thought to be a kind of cellular background matrix (*glia* is Greek for "glue") that stabilizes the shape and position of neurons, they are now known to do that and much more.

Glial Cells of the Peripheral Nervous System

PNS glial cells are all forms of Schwann cells. Some PNS axons (unmyelinated axons) are simply embedded in indentations in Schwann cells (Fig. 1-12); for these, the Schwann

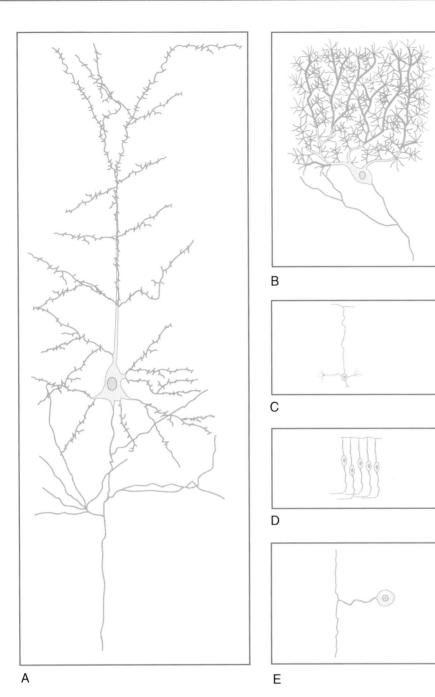

A

B

C

D

E

Figure 1-10. Range of sizes and shapes of neurons (all are drawn to the same scale). **A**, Large multipolar neuron in the cerebral cortex (pyramidal cell). **B**, Large multipolar cerebellar neuron with an elaborate dendritic tree (Purkinje cell). **C**, Small multipolar neuron in cerebellar cortex (granule cell). **D**, Bipolar neurons (olfactory receptor cell). **E**, Unipolar (pseudounipolar) neuron in a sensory ganglion.

cells help regulate the composition of the extracellular fluid but offer little in the way of electrical insulation. Other axons are myelinated (Fig. 1-13), covered by a succession of Schwann cells, each wrapped spirally around a length of the axon until the whole structure looks like a string of sausages. The constrictions between the "sausages" correspond to nodes of Ranvier, sites between adjacent Schwann cells where the axonal membrane is exposed to extracellular fluids. Myelin is an insulating covering that was a great evolutionary advance, because it allows axons that are relatively thin to nevertheless conduct action potentials rapidly. Current flows nearly instantaneously and unchanged through the myelinated portions of such an axon, and the action potential only needs to be regenerated periodically at the nodes (see Fig. 2-20).

Glial Cells of the Central Nervous System

In contrast to the PNS situation, there are several kinds of CNS glial cells: ependymal cells, oligodendrocytes, astrocytes, and microglia.

A single layer of ependymal cells lines the ventricles, the cavities in the CNS that reflect its derivation from an epithelial tube (see Chapter 6). In certain critical locations, this layer is specialized as a secretory epithelium that

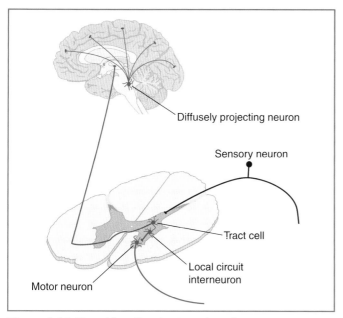

Figure 1-11. Broad functional categories of neurons.

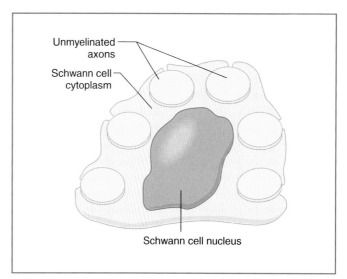

Figure 1-12. Schwann cell and unmyelinated PNS axons.

Figure 1-13. Schwann cell and myelinated PNS axon.

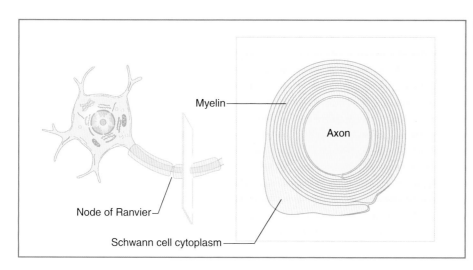

produces most of the cerebrospinal fluid filling the ventricles and the spaces surrounding the CNS (see Chapter 7).

Oligodendrocytes form myelin sheaths in the CNS (Fig. 1-14). Unlike Schwann cells, however, each oligodendrocyte forms myelin segments on multiple axons, sometimes dozens (the name means a cell resembling a "tree with a few branches").

Astrocytes ("star-shaped cells") are the most numerous of the CNS glia. They play a variety of roles, some suggested by their shape and configuration (Fig. 1-15). As their name implies, astrocytes have numerous processes radiating from their cell bodies, collectively filling up most of the spaces between neurons and their axons and dendrites. Some astrocytic processes have expanded end-feet that pave the surfaces of CNS capillaries, allowing astrocytes to provide metabolic support functions for neurons. Other processes cover neuronal cell bodies, synapses, and exposed areas of axons (e.g., nodes

of Ranvier), restricting the volume of extracellular fluid and allowing astrocytes to regulate its composition in several ways. For example, changes in pH and K$^+$ concentration resulting from neuronal activity are buffered by astrocytes, and uptake by astrocytes is an important mechanism for clearing neurotransmitters from the extracellular spaces around synapses. In addition, astrocytes modulate the signaling functions of neurons in other ways that are just beginning to be understood.

Microglia are small cells that are distributed throughout the CNS, essentially serving as an outpost of the immune system. They sit there quietly in normal, healthy brain, waving their processes around and monitoring their surroundings; in response to disease or injury they proliferate, transform into macrophage-like cells, and clean up cellular debris or invading microorganisms.

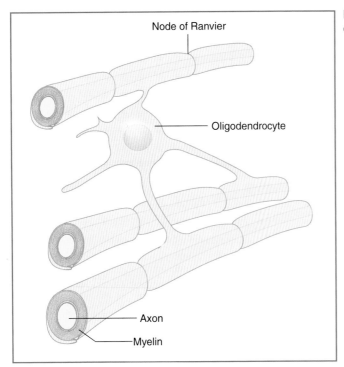

Figure 1-14. Formation of CNS myelin sheath by an oligodendrocyte.

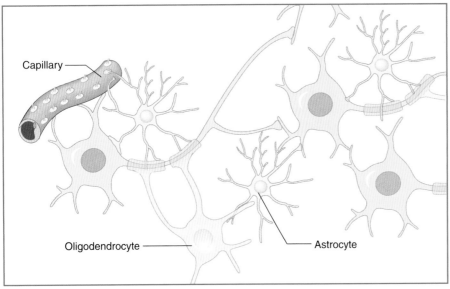

Figure 1-15. Astrocytes with processes abutting capillaries, neurons, and synapses.

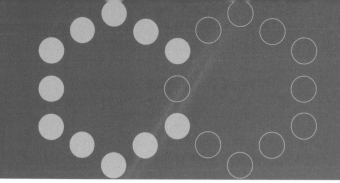

Electrical Signaling by Nerve Cells

2

Neurons develop and maintain their specialized structure through creative uses of the same organelles found in other cells (see Chapter 1). As described in this and the next chapter, they also produce, process, and exchange signals by adapting the electrical and secretory mechanisms used by other cells.

●●● SIGNALING IN THE NERVOUS SYSTEM

Two general kinds of signaling mechanisms are used in the nervous system: electrical signals move along the surface membrane of individual neurons, and chemical signals are transferred back and forth between neurons. Neither of these is exclusive. Some chemical messengers are also transported within neurons, and there are some instances of electrical signals passing from one neuron to another. However, *intra*neuronal information flow is primarily electrical, and *inter*neuronal information flow is primarily chemical.

Like all other cells, neurons are electrically polarized, with the inside negative to the outside. (By convention, the voltage in extracellular fluids is the reference point, so if the inside of

a cell is negative relative to the outside, the voltage across the membrane is some negative value.) The electrical signals produced within neurons are simply local alterations in this resting membrane potential. These electrical signals fall into two general categories (Fig. 2-1). Graded potentials, graded in both duration and amplitude, are produced in postsynaptic membranes and in the receptive membrane areas of sensory receptors. Some last only a few milliseconds, and others last many seconds. Their amplitudes vary, depending on factors such as the strength of a synaptic input or the intensity of a stimulus. Graded potentials spread passively from their site of initiation, like ripples spreading from the location where a pebble is dropped into a pool of water, and typically dissipate completely within a millimeter or so. Because most neurons are much larger than this in at least one dimension, a second kind of electrical signal is required by all but the shortest neurons. Action potentials are large, brief (about a millisecond) signals that propagate actively, undiminished in amplitude, along axons and some dendrites.

Neurons have also adapted the secretory mechanisms used by other cells, in this case as the basis for chemical signaling between neurons. Chemical synapses, described in Chapter 3, are sites at which electrical changes in one neuron cause the release of neurotransmitter molecules, which diffuse to a second neuron and cause electrical changes in it (see Fig. 2-1).

●●● MEMBRANE POTENTIAL

Cell membranes are lipid bilayers with an assortment of proteins embedded in them. Both the lipid and some of the proteins play critical roles in the electrical properties of neurons and other cells. Various inorganic ions are unequally distributed across the membrane (Table 2-1) and, in the absence of a membrane, would diffuse down their concentration gradients (Fig. 2-2A). The lipid bilayer prevents water and hydrophilic particles (such as the inorganic ions dissolved in extracellular and intracellular water) from diffusing between the inside and outside of the cell. On its own, this would prevent the development of any ionic concentration changes or charge separation across the membrane; with no charge separation, the voltage across the membrane would be zero (see Fig. 2-2B). This is where some of the membrane proteins

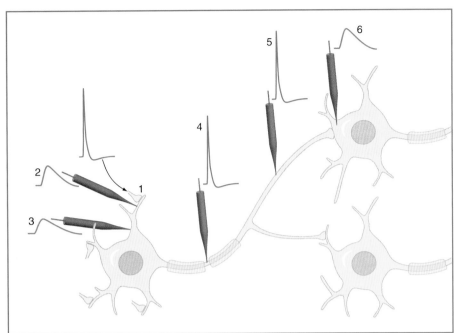

Figure 2-1. Chemical and electrical signaling by neurons. Chemical signals (neurotransmitters) released from presynaptic terminals (1) cause local production of graded potentials in postsynaptic sites (2); these become smaller and slower (3) as they spread from their site of production. Action potentials are used to convey large, constant-amplitude signals (4, 5) over long distances; these in turn invade axon terminals and cause transmitter release, resulting in graded potentials in other neurons (6).

come into the picture: by endowing the membrane with a selective permeability to some ions, they allow the development of an unequal charge distribution and hence a voltage across the membrane. For the resting membrane potential, the most important permeability and concentration gradient is that related to K^+.

Ion Channels and Concentration Gradients

Some membrane proteins are attached to its inner or outer surface, but others are transmembrane proteins (Fig. 2-3) that provide the only route for hydrophilic particles to cross the membrane in appreciable numbers. Some transmembrane proteins are energy-consuming molecular pumps that move particles *against* their concentration gradients, and others permit or facilitate the movement of such particles *down* their concentration gradients. Prominent among the latter are ion channels, which are most directly involved in establishing the resting membrane potential and producing its moment-to-moment variations.

Ion channels are proteins that zigzag across the membrane multiple times, with the membrane-spanning segments surrounding a central aqueous pore. The dimensions of a pore and the charges on the protein segments that line it make a

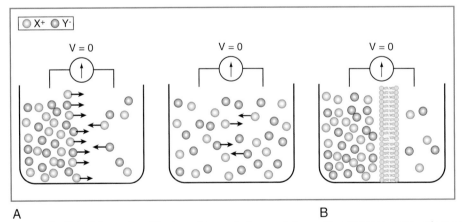

Figure 2-2. Consequences of a lipid bilayer for diffusion of ions. **A,** In a solution with adjoining areas of unequal ionic concentration, ions would diffuse down their concentration gradients (A1) until the gradients dissipated (A2). There would be no voltage between different parts of the solution in either the initial or the final state, because in any given area of the solution there would be equal concentrations of cations and anions (i.e., no net charge separation between different parts of the solution). **B,** Diffusion would be prevented by a lipid bilayer impermeable to ions, essentially maintaining state A1. The total number of positive charges on a given side of the bilayer would continue to equal the total number of negative charges. In the absence of charge separation, there would be no voltage across the membrane.

TABLE 2-1. Typical Ionic Concentrations Inside and Outside Mammalian Neurons

Ion	Extracellular Concentration (mmol/L)	Intracellular Concentration (mmol/L)
Na^+	140	15
K^+	4	130
Ca^{++}	2.5	0.0001*
Cl^-	120	5†

*Refers to free, ionized Ca^{++}. The intracellular Ca^{++} concentration is actually considerably greater than this, but most of it is bound or sequestered.
†The apparent paucity of intracellular negative charges is made up for by negatively charged proteins and organic anions.

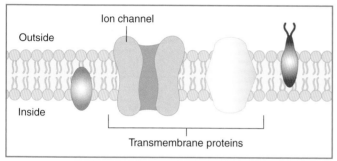

Figure 2-3. The lipid bilayer of a neuronal cell membrane, with some representative membrane proteins embedded in it.

channel more or less selective for particular ions. There are, for example, channels that allow Na^+ to pass through them much more readily than K^+ (and vice versa), relatively nonselective monovalent cation channels that do not discriminate much between Na^+ and K^+, and channels specific for other ions such as Ca^{++} or Cl^-. In addition, most or all channels can exist in at least two conformations: one in which the pore is unobstructed ("open"), and another in which part of the protein moves in such a way that the pore is occluded ("closed"). Channels switch back and forth between the open and closed states, and the amount of time different channels spend in one or the other state can be influenced by changes

in membrane potential (voltage-gated channels), by binding substances such as neurotransmitters (ligand-gated channels), by intracellular changes such as phosphorylation of the channel (Fig. 2-4), or in the case of some sensory receptors by mechanical deformation or temperature changes.

The number of ions of any given type that *can* move across a membrane at some point in time is determined by the number of channels open at that time. Although individual channels at any given instant are either open or closed, treatments that change the probability of channels being open (e.g., voltage changes, transmitter release) change the permeability of the membrane to that ion (Fig. 2-5). The net number of ions that actually *do* move across a membrane per second is a function of both the permeability to that ion and its electrochemical driving force (Fig. 2-6); ions can be driven across a permeable membrane by either a concentration gradient or a voltage gradient.

Equilibrium Potentials

Consider what would happen if the K^+ concentration inside a neuron were higher than that outside (which is in fact the case—see Table 2-1) and the membrane were permeable only to K^+ (i.e., the membrane contained only channels that were perfectly selective for K^+, some of which were open). K^+ ions would start to leak out, down their concentration gradient (Fig. 2-7A). However, this would make the inside of the cell negative relative to the outside, attracting K^+ ions back in. Before long, an equilibrium would be reached in which just as many K^+ ions would leak out as would return (see Fig. 2-7B). This equilibrium condition would not require any energy to maintain, because the equal and opposite movement of K^+ ions would not change the concentration gradient. Only a vanishingly small number of K^+ ions need to move before this condition is reached (hence no concentration changes) because a small number of anions and cations lined up just inside and outside the membrane is enough to create a steep voltage gradient across the very thin lipid bilayer. (In electrical terms, this small amount of charge separation is enough to charge the membrane capacitance.)

At such an equilibrium, the concentration gradient of an ion is exactly counterbalanced by the membrane potential, which is therefore termed the equilibrium potential for that

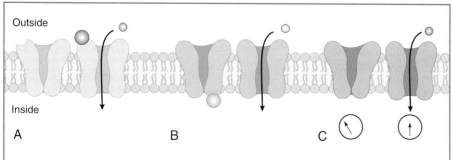

Figure 2-4. Examples of factors that can affect the probability of different types of channels being open or closed. **A**, Changes in the extracellular domain of the channel; in this case, binding a ligand. **B**, Changes in the intracellular domain of the channel; in this case, dephosphorylation. **C**, Changes in the voltage across the membrane; in this case, making the cytoplasm less negative.

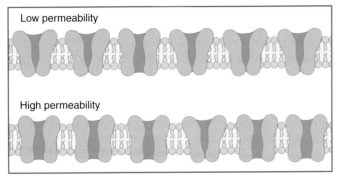

Figure 2-5. Channels flip back and forth between open and closed states, with the probability of being in one or the other state influenced by factors such as binding of a ligand. The permeability of the membrane at some point in time is a function of the total number of channels open at that time. Hence, the permeability of the membrane as a whole can change smoothly over time even though each individual channel is either open or closed.

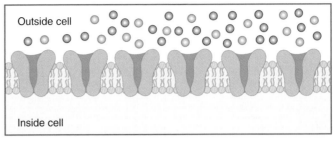

A

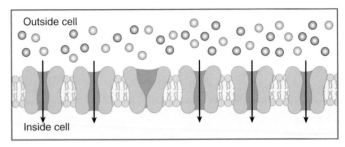

B

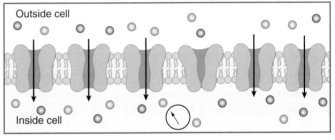

C

Figure 2-6. Net movement of a given ionic species across a membrane requires both open channels (lacking in **A**) and an electrochemical driving force—some combination of a concentration gradient (**B**) and an electrical gradient (**C**).

ion. This equilibrium potential can be expressed mathematically by the Nernst equation:

$$V_x = \frac{RT}{zF} \ln \frac{[X]_1}{[X]_2} \qquad (2\text{-}1)$$

where V_x is the equilibrium potential for ion x, R is the gas constant, z is the valence of ion x, T is temperature in °K, F is Faraday's number (the charge in one mole of monovalent cations), and $[X]_1$ and $[X]_2$ are the extracellular and intracellular concentrations of ion x.

Combining the constants, converting natural logs to $\log_{10}$, and solving this equation for typical K^+ concentrations and a body temperature of 37°C (310°K) yields

$$V_K = 62 \log_{10} \frac{[K^+]_o}{[K^+]_i} = 62 \log_{10} \frac{4}{130} = -92 \, \text{mV} \qquad (2\text{-}2)$$

Similar calculations for the major inorganic ions distributed unequally across typical neuronal membranes yield the values shown in Table 2-2.

Steady-state Potentials

The Nernst equation specifies the value of the membrane potential when the membrane is permeable to only one ion. However, things are never that simple. No individual channels are perfectly selective for just one ion, and real membranes have embedded in them multiple populations of channels with different ionic selectivities. The result is that real membranes are significantly permeable not just to K^+ but also to Na^+ (and to Cl^-), and the Nernst equation cannot specify the membrane potential.

The normal Na^+ concentration gradient is just the opposite of the K^+ gradient—$[Na^+]$ is higher *outside* than *inside*. Consider now what adding a small Na^+ permeability would do to the hypothetical K^+-based resting membrane potential. Na^+ ions would move into the neuron, not only because of the concentration gradient but also because they are positively charged and the inside of the neuron is negative. Because the Na^+ permeability is small, only a few ions would move, but this would be enough to make the neuronal interior less negative once a steady state was reached (Fig. 2-8A)—still negative to the outside but not so negative as if the membrane were permeable only to K^+. So changes in the membrane's

TABLE 2-2. Equilibrium Potentials*

Ion	Equilibrium Potential (mV)[†]
Na^+	+60
K^+	−94
Ca^{++}	+136
Cl^-	−86

*Calculated by the Nernst equation and the concentration values given in Table 2-1.
[†]Relative to an extracellular potential of 0.

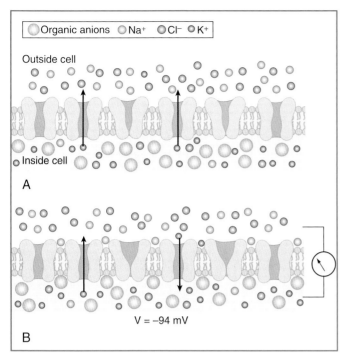

Figure 2-7. Development of an equilibrium membrane potential as a result of a concentration gradient across a semipermeable membrane. **A,** In response to a greater intracellular concentration of K$^+$, K$^+$ ions begin to move outward across the membrane. **B,** After a small number of K$^+$ ions have left, the resulting intracellular negativity draws K$^+$ ions back in (down the voltage gradient) as quickly as they leave (down the concentration gradient). The voltage gradient is developed abruptly across the membrane, where small numbers of negative and positive charges line up across from each other on opposite sides of the lipid bilayer.

permeability to particular ions can cause changes in the membrane potential. Moment-to-moment permeability changes are the basis of electrical signaling by neurons. Depending on how the permeability changes, the membrane potential can move in a positive (depolarizing) or negative (hyperpolarizing) direction.

A second consequence of adding permeabilities to a neuronal membrane is that now it is no longer at equilibrium. In this case, there is no electrical or chemical gradient to move Na$^+$ ions back out. In addition, the depolarization caused by adding some Na$^+$ permeability causes a few extra K$^+$ ions to leave. Left to their own devices, Na$^+$ ions would continue to leak in, extra K$^+$ ions would continue to leak out, and the Na$^+$ and K$^+$ concentration gradients, along with the membrane potential, would slowly fade away. This is avoided by the activity of an energy-expending molecular pump—a Na$^+$/K$^+$-ATPase that uses the energy derived from hydrolyzing ATP to move Na$^+$ out and K$^+$ in (see Fig. 2-8B). The Na$^+$/K$^+$-ATPase, together with other pumps with different ionic specificities, is responsible for maintaining the concentration gradients of various ions across the membrane.

Because of these multiple permeabilities, the membrane potential of real-world neurons is a weighted average of the equilibrium potentials for K$^+$, Na$^+$, and Cl$^-$, with the weighting

PHARMACOLOGY & PHYSIOLOGY

Therapeutically Inhibiting the Na$^+$ Pump

Cardiac glycosides such as digoxin inhibit the Na$^+$/K$^+$-ATPase, resulting in a smaller than normal Na$^+$ concentration gradient across cell membranes if administered in controlled doses. Because the Na$^+$ gradient is the energy source used to extrude Ca^{++} from cardiac muscle, digoxin causes an increase in Ca^{++} concentration in these cells and increased cardiac contractility results.

factor for each ion being the membrane's relative permeability to it. All of this can be expressed quantitatively by the Goldman-Hodgkin-Katz equation (often referred to simply as the Goldman equation):

$$V_m = 62 \log_{10} \frac{P_K [K^+]_o + P_{Na} [Na^+]_o + P_{Cl} [Cl^-]_i}{P_K [K^+]_i + P_{Na} [Na^+]_i + P_{Cl} [Cl^-]_o} \quad (2\text{-}3)$$

Although initially intimidating, this is simply a combined series of Nernst equations with relative permeabilities added

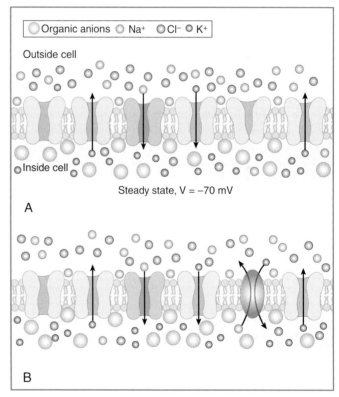

Figure 2-8. Development of a steady-state membrane potential. **A,** Addition of some Na$^+$ permeability to the membrane in Figure 2-7 results in inward movement of Na$^+$ ions, driven by both a concentration gradient and an electrical gradient. The inward movement of Na$^+$ ions makes the inside of the cell a little less negative, letting a little more K$^+$ escape, and before long a steady state is reached. This steady state by itself is unstable, because the net inward Na$^+$ movement and outward K$^+$ movement would dissipate the concentration gradients. **B,** This result is avoided by the activity of Na$^+$/K$^+$-ATPase, which pumps Na$^+$ back out and K$^+$ back in.

as weighting factors. If the permeability to two of the three ions becomes zero, this equation reduces to the Nernst equation for the remaining ion. The Goldman-Hodgkin-Katz equation specifies the limiting values for the membrane potential, which cannot be more negative than the most negative of the three equilibrium potentials (usually V_K) and cannot be more positive than the most positive of the three equilibrium potentials (V_{Na}). Because the permeability to K^+ is typically much greater than that to Na^+ or Cl^-, the resting potential of most neurons is slightly less negative than the K^+ equilibrium potential, but close to it.

●●● GRADED CHANGES IN MEMBRANE POTENTIAL

Neurons use localized changes in the probabilities of sets of ion channels being open or closed to cause membrane potential changes at specific sites. The potential changes are graded because the changes in probability are graded. All neurons have multiple sites like this, specialized for the production of depolarizing or hyperpolarizing graded potentials. Most are postsynaptic patches of membrane, abundant on neuronal dendrites but also found on the cell body and even on parts of the axon (see Fig. 3-4). Sensory receptor cells have analogous sites where physical stimuli are converted to graded electrical signals (see Chapter 4).

Increases or decreases in the permeability of a membrane to any ion with an electrochemical driving force causes the membrane potential to move toward or away from the equilibrium potential for that ion. For example, either decreasing the K^+ permeability or increasing the Na^+ permeability would cause the membrane potential to move closer to V_{Na} (i.e., depolarize). Opening relatively nonselective monovalent cation channels, which is common at excitatory synapses and in some sensory receptors, causes depolarization by moving the membrane potential toward some value roughly midway between V_{Na} and V_K.

Spread of Membrane Potential Changes

Because graded potentials are initiated at restricted sites, they spread along the membrane in a way determined by the electrical properties of both the cytoplasm and the membrane itself. Ions moving through an open channel constitute a current, which moves into and through the cytoplasm by interacting with other ions, repelling those with the same charge and attracting those with the opposite charge (Fig. 2-9). Current always flows in complete loops, so the ionic current must somehow cross the membrane to return to its starting point. It does so in two ways: partly by changing the charge on the membrane capacitance and partly by flowing through other open channels (Fig. 2-10), which are the electrical equivalent of a resistance. Electrical circuits with resistors and capacitors change the time course of signals, and in this case a step change in current flow causes an exponential change in membrane potential (see Fig. 2-10). The time required for the membrane potential to reach 63% (1 − 1/e) of its final value

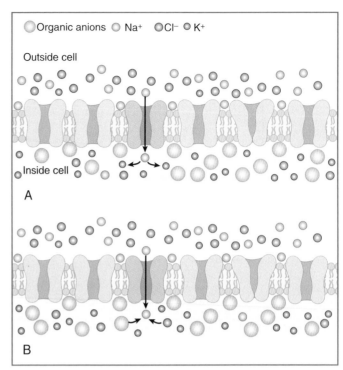

Figure 2-9. Current flow in ionic solutions. This is not the result of individual ions moving long distances through the solution but rather is caused by like charges repelling each other (**A**) and unlike charges attracting each other (**B**). (Cations moving in a given direction are electrically equivalent to anions moving in the opposite direction.)

is the time constant of the membrane. The time constant is directly proportional to both the resistance and the capacitance of the membrane, and is typically on the order of 10 ms or so.

Because some of the current entering through an open channel leaves across neighboring areas of membrane in this way, progressively less of it is available to cross subsequent areas of membrane. As a result, the membrane potential change becomes progressively smaller with increasing distance from a current source. The spatial profile of this decline is also exponential, and the distance required for a voltage change to decline to 37% (1/e) of its initial value is the length constant of a neuronal process (Fig. 2-11), typically a few hundred micrometers. The length constant is a function of both membrane properties and the diameter of a neuronal process. At any given point, current can either cross the membrane or continue through the cytoplasm. The more membrane channels are open, the easier it is for current to leave and the shorter the length constant. The larger the diameter of the process, the more cytoplasm is available for current to flow through, so larger diameter processes have longer length constants.

The result of all this is that graded potentials outlast the permeability changes that cause them (to an extent dictated by the time constant) and decline with distance from their origin (to an extent dictated by the length constant). This in turn affects the ways in which graded potentials interact (Fig. 2-12). Two successive permeability changes will cause

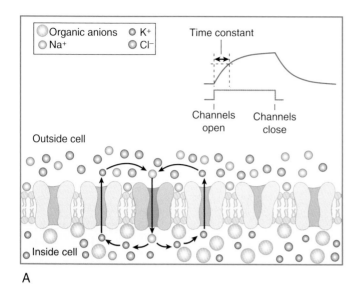

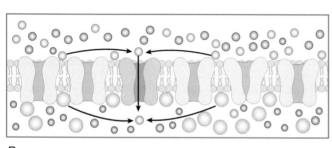

A

B

Figure 2-10. Passive current flow through neuronal processes and across their membranes. Current can flow across the membrane either by passing through ion channels (**A**) or by adding or removing charges on the membrane surface (**B**) (i.e., charging or discharging the membrane capacitance). Because of the parallel resistance and capacitance of the membrane, the voltage change caused by a step injection of current develops with an exponential time course (inset in **A**). During the early stages of this voltage change, current flows mainly through the membrane capacitance; during later stages it flows through ion channels.

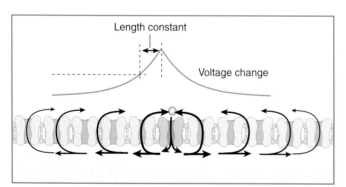

Figure 2-11. An injection of current at one point along a neuronal process causes a voltage change that declines exponentially with distance. (Not drawn to scale; real length constants are tens to hundreds of μm, whereas membranes and channels are orders of magnitude smaller.)

PHARMACOLOGY

Toxins That Block Voltage-gated Channels

Plants and animals have evolved a number of toxins that block the activity of different voltage-gated channels in a variety of ways. Probably the best known is tetrodotoxin, the puffer fish poison, which occludes the pore in voltage-gated Na^+ channels. This in turn blocks the production of action potentials in peripheral nerve fibers, causing numbness and weakness.

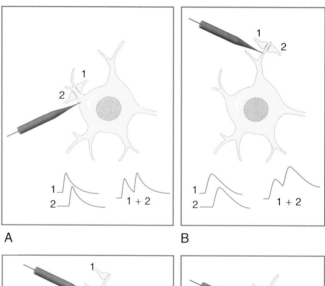

A   B

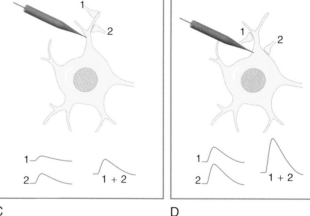

C   D

Figure 2-12. Temporal and spatial summation. Sequential activation of two synapses (1 and 2) in a neuronal process with a short time constant (**A**) results in little temporal summation. In a neuronal process with a long time constant (**B**), the response at the first synapse has decayed little when the response at the second synapse begins, allowing substantial temporal summation of the two responses. In a neuronal process with a short length constant (**C**), postsynaptic potentials decay substantially on their way to a recording site. In a neuronal process with a long length constant (**D**), postsynaptic potentials spread with less decrement to a recording site, allowing more significant spatial summation.

graded potentials that add to each other with a degree of temporal summation determined by the time constant. Two simultaneous permeability changes at neighboring sites will cause graded potentials that add to each other with a degree of spatial summation determined by the length constant.

●●● ACTION POTENTIALS

Neurons that are not much longer than their length constants can use graded potentials effectively to move signals from one part of the cell to another. Rods and cones of the retina and some small interneurons, for example, rely entirely on graded potentials. The vast majority of neurons, however, are distinguished by their ability to generate action potentials in response to sufficient depolarization (Fig. 2-13). These brief, depolarizing, all-or-none signals, different from graded potentials in almost every way (Table 2-3), are propagated actively from one end of an axon to the other without losing amplitude.

Voltage-gated Channels

Action potentials (or nerve impulses) are based on the activity of voltage-gated channels, usually voltage-gated Na^+ and K^+ channels (Fig. 2-14).

Depolarization causes both types of channel to open but with different time courses. The Na^+ channels open quickly and are responsible for the rising phase of the action potential: as each opens, the Na^+ permeability increases, causing more depolarization, which causes more Na^+ channels to open, and so on. In less than 1 ms, the normal balance of ionic permeabilities is reversed and the membrane potential at that site approaches V_{Na}. Once open, however, the Na^+ channels spontaneously move into a closed, inactivated state in which they cannot be made to open again until the membrane potential returns to something approaching its resting level; repolarization of the membrane "resets" (deinactivates) the Na^+ channels. As the Na^+ channels inactivate, the K^+ permeability returns to dominance and the membrane potential moves back toward V_K. This is abetted by voltage-gated K^+ channels, which open more slowly and help speed the falling phase of the action potential. Because these channels also close slowly, action potentials are usually followed by an afterhyperpolarization during which the added K^+ permeability moves the membrane potential even closer to V_K than usual.

Threshold and Trigger Zones

The all-or-none property of action potentials means that a stimulus producing less than a critical level of depolarization results in only a graded potential (see Fig. 2-13); i.e., there is a threshold voltage for triggering action potentials. The threshold is not the same in all parts of a neuron. Zones in which graded potentials are produced, for example, usually have too few voltage-gated Na^+ channels to produce action potentials at all. In contrast, neurons also have low-threshold trigger zones (Fig. 2-15) with relatively high densities of voltage-gated Na^+ channels; less depolarization is required at these

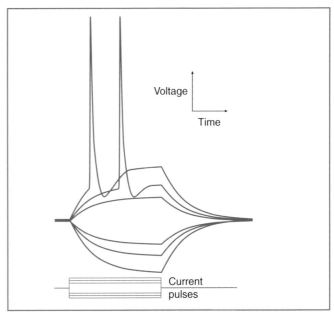

Figure 2-13. Successively larger hyperpolarizing current pulses cause successively larger voltage changes, each with an exponential rise and fall dictated by the time constant. Successively larger depolarizing current pulses, in contrast, cause successively larger voltage changes until a critical threshold is reached, at which point a brief action potential is produced. Depolarizations larger than this reach threshold more rapidly, but the resulting action potential is no larger.

TABLE 2-3. Properties of Graded Potentials and Action Potentials

Property	Graded Potential	Action Potential
Amplitude	Variable, rarely more than 10 to 20 mV	≈ 100 mV
Duration	1 ms to ≥ 1 s	≈ 1 ms
Degree of interaction	Spatial and temporal summation	Unitary, all or none
Propagation	Fades with distance	Actively propagated with constant amplitude
Polarity	Depolarizing or hyperpolarizing	Always depolarizing

sites to open the number of Na^+ channels required to initiate an action potential. In most neurons, the axon's initial segment is thought to be the principal trigger zone. Here, the graded potentials produced throughout the dendritic tree and cell body are summed temporally and spatially, and action potentials are initiated. Pseudounipolar neurons, in contrast, have trigger zones far out in the periphery, close to where graded potentials (usually receptor potentials) are produced.

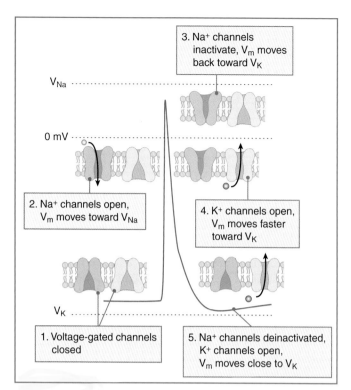

Figure 2-14. Na⁺ and K⁺ permeability changes underlying an action potential. V_K, potassium equilibrium potential; V_m, membrane potential; V_{Na}, sodium equilibrium potential.

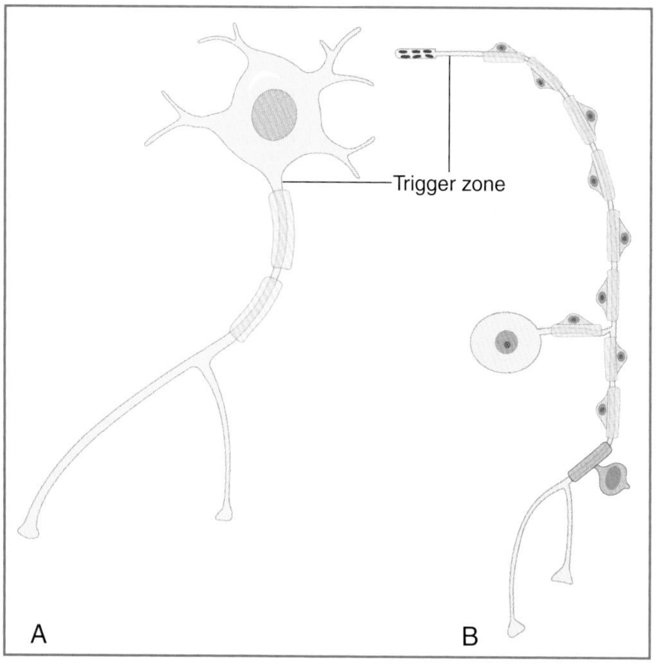

Figure 2-15. Trigger zones with a low threshold for action potential production in a typical neuron (**A**) and a pseudounipolar neuron (**B**). Pseudounipolar neurons are unusual in having the functional equivalent of a dendrite (receptive ending) continuing directly into an axon, almost as though the cell body had migrated along the axon.

Refractory Periods

Inactivation of voltage-gated Na⁺ channels helps terminate an action potential, but it has another important consequence. For a brief period following the peak of an action potential, most Na⁺ channels at that site are inactivated, and so few are available that the membrane is inexcitable. This absolute refractory period (Fig. 2-16) is the basis of the unitary nature of action potentials, their inability to sum (see Table 2-3). Its duration of about 1 ms also limits the maximum firing frequency of neurons to about 1000 Hz (although the maximum rate is considerably lower than this for most neurons).

Following the absolute refractory period, a patch of membrane is less excitable than normal for a few milliseconds,

Absolute refractory period: most Na⁺ channels inactivated

Relative refractory period: some Na⁺ channels inactivated, extra K⁺ channels open

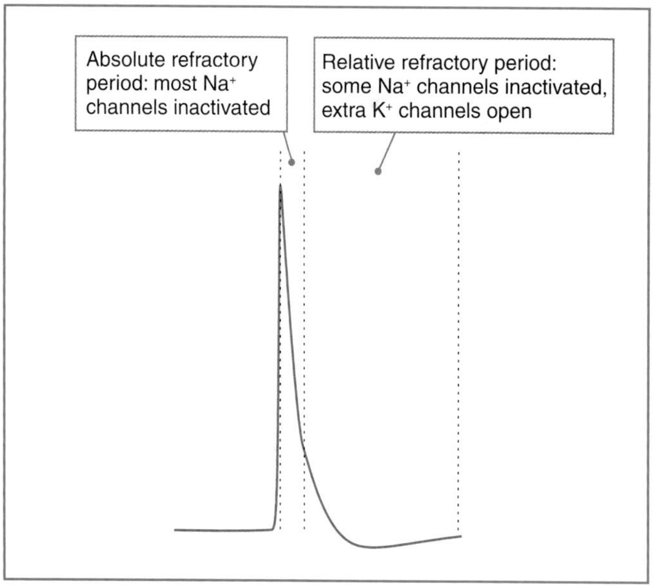

Figure 2-16. Absolute and relative refractory periods.

both because a full complement of voltage-gated Na⁺ channels is not yet available and because open voltage-gated K⁺ channels make it harder to depolarize. This relative refractory period is a period during which the threshold, infinite during the absolute refractory period, declines to its baseline level. As a result, the firing rate of a neuron is related to the magnitude

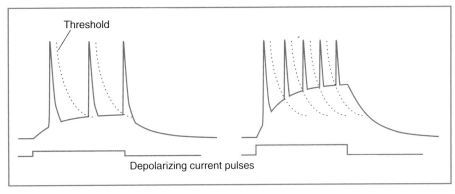

Figure 2-17. Effect of the relative refractory period on firing rate. The relative refractory period is a period of declining threshold, so the larger the level of background depolarization the more frequently threshold is reached.

of a depolarizing stimulus (Fig. 2-17), and the trigger zone is a site at which the amplitude code represented by graded potentials is converted into a rate code. Graded potentials can be thought of as analog signals like the ones that move loudspeaker cones in and out, and trains of action potentials as digital signals somewhat like the bit stream read to or from a CD. So neurons, like CD burners, need an analog-to-digital converter in which graded potentials are recoded as streams of action potentials, and this requirement is met at trigger zones. (The reverse process—converting a train of action potentials back to a graded potential—happens at synapses, as described in Chapter 3.)

Propagation of Action Potentials

As action potentials are initiated at trigger zones, they begin to spread to neighboring areas of membrane and depolarize them to threshold, in turn causing an action potential in the next neighboring area, and so on (Fig. 2-18). In an unmyelinated axon, the result is a smoothly continuous propagation of the action potential down the axon. Under ordinary circumstances, this propagation is unidirectional, away from the cell body and toward the axon's terminals, because the area just traversed by an action potential is refractory and inexcitable (Fig. 2-19). The rate at which the action potential moves (the conduction velocity) is a function of an axon's length constant. In essence, the longer the length constant, the farther an action potential can "reach" down an axon before declining to a subthreshold value (see Fig. 2-18). The most straightforward way to increase the length constant is to increase the diameter of the axon, a strategy used by invertebrates. The most extravagant example is the giant axons of squid, which attain diameters of hundreds of micrometers. These axons conduct impulses relatively rapidly to a squid's mantle muscle and help it escape from potential predators.

Such large-diameter axons are too costly (in terms of space requirement) to be widely used in complex nervous systems. Vertebrates have evolved the alternative strategy of myelination, which allows relatively thin axons to conduct rapidly.

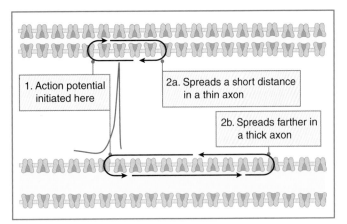

Figure 2-18. Propagation of action potentials along unmyelinated axons. The thicker the axon, the longer its length constant and the greater the conduction velocity. (This action potential is reversed relative to most others illustrated in this chapter because, in essence, time goes from right to left here as the action potential propagates from left to right.)

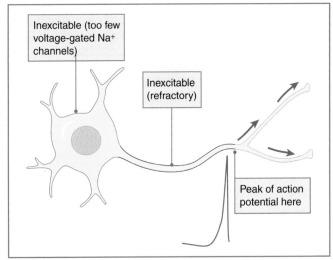

Figure 2-19. Action potentials initiated at a trigger zone (usually the beginning of the axon) begin propagating down the axon; in most neurons, they spread only passively into the cell body and dendrites because of a relative paucity of voltage-gated Na$^+$ channels there. Propagation continues unidirectionally down the axon because an area of membrane just traversed by an action potential is refractory.

CLINICAL MEDICINE

Testing Conduction Velocity

Nerve conduction studies involve stimulating a peripheral nerve at a point where it passes close to the skin, causing action potentials to be propagated both orthodromically (the normal, physiologic direction—toward the CNS in sensory axons and away from it in motor axons) and antidromically (the opposite direction). Stimulating the same nerve at two different sites and measuring the difference in the time required for some effect to be observed (e.g., muscle activity or the antidromic arrival of action potentials in sensory axons) provides a measure of the nerve's conduction velocity and some hints about pathologic processes. For example, processes involving loss of axons result in a smaller than normal effect but often a normal conduction velocity, whereas loss of myelin causes slowed conduction velocity.

CLINICAL MEDICINE

Demyelination

Demyelinating diseases cause the propagation of action potentials to be abnormally slow. The assortments of membrane proteins in the myelin made by Schwann cells and oligodendrocytes are overlapping but not identical, and there are even antigenic differences between the myelin of PNS sensory and motor fibers. As a result, any of these can be targeted selectively by certain disease processes. For example, multiple sclerosis is an autoimmune process that affects CNS myelin, whereas in the Guillain-Barré syndrome, PNS myelin is affected, primarily that on the axons of motor neurons.

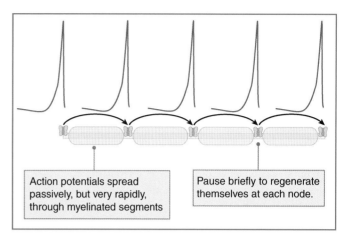

Figure 2-20. Saltatory conduction along a myelinated axon.

Action potentials spread passively, but very rapidly, through myelinated segments

Pause briefly to regenerate themselves at each node.

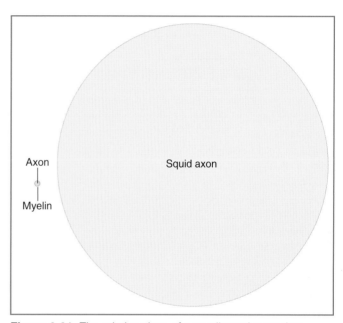

Figure 2-21. The relative sizes of a myelinated axon that conducts at about 25 m/s (*left*) and an unmyelinated squid giant axon with the same conduction velocity (*right*).

Axon

Myelin

Squid axon

Myelin acts as a low-capacitance insulating sheath, allowing an action potential to spread almost instantaneously along the axon until it reaches a node of Ranvier, where voltage-gated Na^+ channels are concentrated. As a result, action potentials skip from one node to the next and are generated anew at each, in a process called saltatory (Latin, *saltare*, "to leap" or "to dance") conduction (Fig. 2-20). The only part that takes much time is the regeneration at each node, and so a myelinated axon 10 µm in diameter (including the myelin) conducts as rapidly as a 500-µm unmyelinated axon (Fig. 2-21).

Categories of Peripheral Nervous System Axons

PNS axons come in a range of sizes and speeds, from unmyelinated axons less than 1 µm in diameter that conduct at less than 1 m/s to heavily myelinated 20-µm axons that conduct at 100 m/s. The size and conduction velocity of the axons in spinal nerves (and some cranial nerves) are correlated with function (Fig. 2-22 and Table 2-4). The smallest diameter axons (including both unmyelinated and thinly myelinated fibers) are mostly visceral afferents and efferents and afferents carrying pain and temperature information. Larger, more heavily myelinated axons deal with skin, skeletal muscles, and joints. These differences have anatomic correlates as well. Subsequent chapters will contrast the courses of large and small afferents once they enter the CNS, and the locations and connections of different types of motor neuron.

Diameter and conduction velocity have both been used to categorize PNS axons, and bits of arcane jargon from both systems are still in use (see Table 2-4). A Roman numeral system divides axons by diameter into groups I to IV, with group I the largest myelinated fibers and group IV the unmyelinated fibers. A letter-based system divides axons by conduction velocity into groups A to C, with groups A and B the myelinated and group C the unmyelinated fibers. Group A includes diverse fiber types and is subdivided into Aα (fastest) through Aδ (slowest myelinated).

TABLE 2-4. Diameters, Conduction Velocities, and Functions of PNS Axons*

Diameter (μm)	Group	Conduction Velocity (m/s)	Group	Function	Commonly Used Terminology
Myelinated					
12–20	I	70–120	Aα	Largest muscle afferents	Ia, Ib
				Lower motor neurons	α
6–12	II	30–70	Aβ	Touch, position	Aβ (or II)
2–10	II	10–50	Aγ	Efferent to muscle spindles†	γ
1–6	III	5–30	Aδ	Some pain and visceral receptors, cold receptors, preganglionic autonomic	δ
Unmyelinated					
<1.5	IV	0.5–2	C	Most pain receptors, warmth receptors, some visceral receptors, postganglionic autonomic	C

*The segregation of fiber types is not so absolute as this table seems to indicate. For example, some touch receptors have unmyelinated axons. Some of these subtleties are discussed in later chapters.
†Small motor neurons that adjust the sensitivity of muscle stretch receptors (see Fig. 4-7).

●●● A SIMPLE NEURONAL CIRCUIT

All of the preceding can be combined to explain a simple but real-life example of neural processing—the stretch reflex that is tested as a standard part of the neurologic examination. An examiner taps on the patellar tendon, stretching the quadriceps, and in response the quadriceps contracts. This is the simplest possible CNS reflex because it involves only two neurons (Fig. 2-23): a sensory neuron and a motor neuron (all other reflex arcs passing through the CNS include at least one interneuron).

The sensory neuron is a pseudounipolar cell with its cell body in a sensory ganglion near the spinal cord (a dorsal root ganglion). The peripheral process ends in the quadriceps in a receptor organ called a muscle spindle (see Chapter 9), and the central process ends in the gray matter of the spinal cord. Stretching the quadriceps causes a depolarizing slow potential in the peripheral ending, which then spreads to the nearby trigger zone. If the depolarizing slow potential is large enough, action potentials are initiated and conducted all the way into the CNS. The axon branches centrally and makes

synapses on every motor neuron that innervates the quadriceps, in addition to feeding into ascending sensory pathways (divergence; Fig. 2-24). In addition, there are hundreds of muscle spindles in the quadriceps, and the sensory neurons

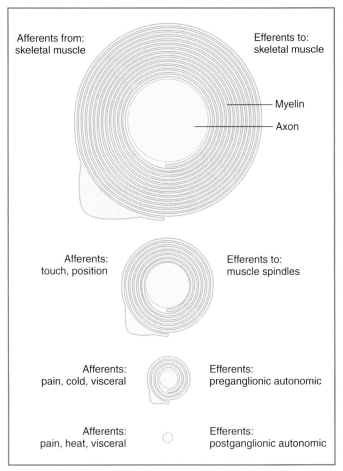

Figure 2-22. The spectrum of PNS axon diameters, with some functional correlates of each size group.

ANATOMY

Compression Blocks

Pressure on nerve fibers causes a progressive, size-dependent failure of action potential propagation, with larger axons affected first. Hence, peripheral nerves can be affected in places where they are close to the surface or where they pass through small, bony tunnels. In the upper extremity, pressure in the axilla can compress the radial nerve against the humerus ("Saturday night palsy"), the ulnar nerve can be compressed at the elbow as it passes between the olecranon and the median epicondyle, and the median nerve can be compressed by narrowing of the carpal tunnel.

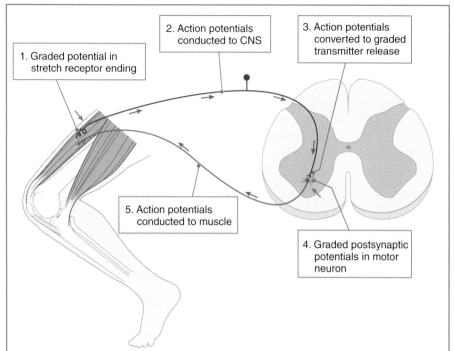

1. Graded potential in stretch receptor ending

2. Action potentials conducted to CNS

3. Action potentials converted to graded transmitter release

5. Action potentials conducted to muscle

4. Graded postsynaptic potentials in motor neuron

Figure 2-23. Sites of graded potentials and action potential propagation involved in the stretch reflex arc. Trigger zones, where graded potentials are converted to trains of action potentials, are indicated by red arrows.

from all of them project to any given quadriceps motor neuron (convergence; Fig. 2-25). Thus, in response to a vigorous tendon tap, hundreds of axon terminals will release neurotransmitters onto every quadriceps motor neuron. This causes hundreds of graded, excitatory potentials in each motor neuron. If the summed graded potentials depolarize a motor neuron's trigger zone to threshold, action potentials are initiated and conducted back out to the neuromuscular junction,

causing release of transmitter and depolarization of the muscle. The muscle then initiates its own action potentials, causing contraction.

However, there is more to the story. There is only one set of quadriceps motor neurons, and they are needed to contract (or not contract) the quadriceps during more than just stretch reflexes. The quadriceps are used to stand upright, to walk, to run after a handball, and to withdraw from some painful

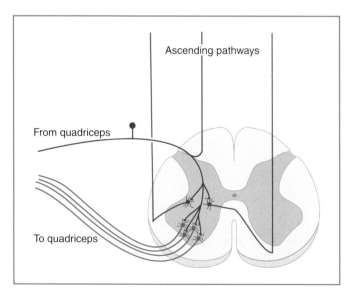

Ascending pathways

From quadriceps

To quadriceps

Figure 2-24. Divergence in the stretch reflex arc. Each afferent from a muscle stretch receptor diverges to contact not only every motor neuron for the muscle that it came from but also numerous other neurons that feed into ascending pathways to the thalamus, cerebellum, and other sites.

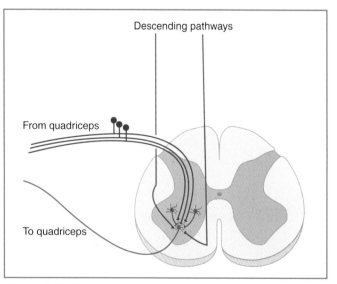

Descending pathways

From quadriceps

To quadriceps

Figure 2-25. Convergence onto motor neurons. Each motor neuron receives synaptic inputs not only from every stretch receptor in the muscle it innervates, but also from axons descending from the cerebral cortex, the brainstem, and other spinal levels.

stimuli. The quadriceps need to relax as part of sitting down and they, like other muscles, relax during sleep. Correspondingly, each quadriceps motor neuron receives thousands of synaptic inputs, possibly as many as 10,000, and only a few hundred come from stretch receptors. The rest come from a wide array of places (see Fig. 2-25): interneurons conveying other sensory information (e.g., from other muscle receptors or from pain receptors), other spinal neurons (coordinating different muscle actions), the brainstem (vestibular nuclei, many other places), and the cerebral cortex (voluntary contraction). Some of these synaptic inputs are excitatory, others inhibitory. The moment-to-moment temporal and spatial summation of all these inputs determines the firing rate of a quadriceps motor neuron, and the firing rate of the whole population determines the level of contraction of the quadriceps. This is part of the reason that damage at various sites in the CNS can cause either an increase or a decrease in muscle tone. If the net effect of the damage is to remove inhibitory inputs, for example, then motor neurons will be abnormally depolarized and muscle tone will increase.

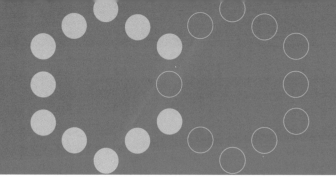

Synaptic Transmission   3

Chapters 1 and 2 described the ways in which neurons have adapted the organelles and electrical processes used by other cells to support neuronal structure and function. This chapter continues in the same vein, exploring the ways in which neurons transfer information between each other at localized sites of apposition called synapses (Greek, "fasten together"). Most synapses use adaptations of the secretory processes used by other cells as the basis of chemically mediated signal transfer.

⬤⬤⬤ ELECTRICAL SYNAPSES

The most straightforward way for information to pass between neurons is not by secreting chemicals but rather by having current (and voltage changes) simply spread passively from one to another (Fig. 3-1). Such electrical synapses do exist and, in fact, have a speed advantage over the chemical synapses described below. However, chemical synapses have so many other advantages that they are the dominant means of signal transfer between neurons.

Gap Junctions

Electrical synapses are based on gap junctions (Fig. 3-2). These are sites at which the separation between two adjoining neurons narrows to only a few nanometers and the gap is spanned by pairs of channels that provide a route for current to flow from one to the other. Each channel, called a connexon, is composed of six connexin molecules that surround a central pore larger than that of typical ion channels, large enough to allow not just ions but also a variety of small molecules to pass through it. Current generally can pass equally well in either direction, so depolarization and hyperpolarization can

spread from one neuron to another nearly instantaneously through gap junctions.

Because the basic properties of an electrical signal do not change much at these synapses, they cannot play a large role in the computational functions of the nervous system. However, because gap junctions are good at spreading electrical signals through networks of interconnected neurons, they can be effective in helping synchronize the activity of groups of neurons (in the minority of situations where this is functionally desirable). In addition, some networks of neurons are specialized to simply spread signals laterally over substantial distances, adding to them here and there; coupling by gap junctions allows them to function as an electrical syncytium. For example, retinal horizontal cells (see Chapter 12) are electrically coupled, allowing information about illumination in one part of the retina to spread to other parts. Finally, because the pores in connexons are large enough to let a variety of small molecules through, gap junctions provide a route for metabolic coupling between cells. This may be an important signaling mechanism for neurons during development, and it plays a role in the normal function of some cell populations (e.g., gap junctions between astrocytes allow metabolic substrates to move around within the CNS). Gap junctions can even be formed between different parts of an individual cell, allowing substances to take a short cut from

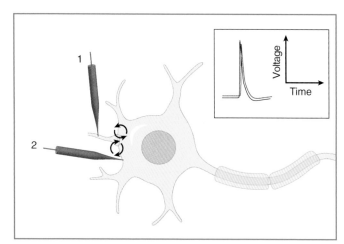

Figure 3-1. Passive, decremental spread of current (and voltage) from one neuron (1) to another (2) through an electrical synapse. There is little delay, and the direction of the voltage swing is unchanged.

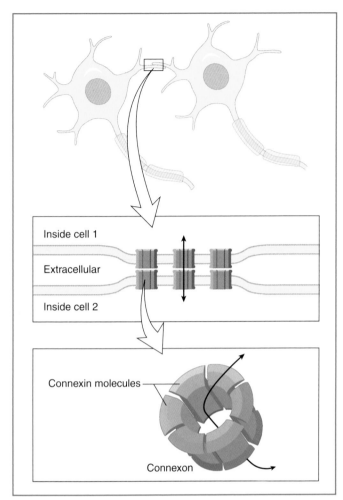

Figure 3-2. A gap junction, made up of a patch of channels (connexons).

one part of the cell to another. The utility of this is especially apparent in myelinating glial cells, where gap junctions between different parts of their small remaining fingers of cytoplasm (see Figs. 1-13 and 1-14) allow substances to move around without having to spiral through multiple turns of myelin.

Control of Transmission at Electrical Synapses

Connexons, like other channels, can switch between open and closed states. A variety of different intracellular parameters, such as pH, Ca^{++} concentration, and the voltage across a gap

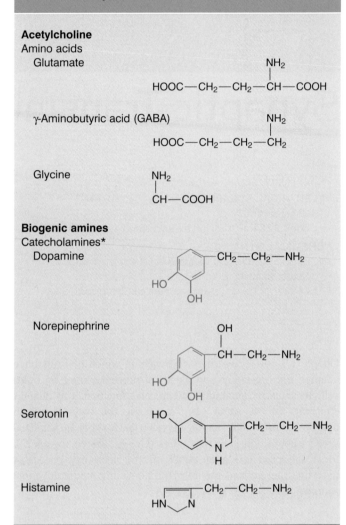

TABLE 3-1. Major Small-Molecule Neurotransmitters

Acetylcholine
Amino acids
  Glutamate

  γ-Aminobutyric acid (GABA)

  Glycine

Biogenic amines
Catecholamines*
  Dopamine

  Norepinephrine

  Serotonin

  Histamine

*Named for the catechol group (shown in color).

junction, can affect the probability of their being in one or the other state. In some networks of neurons, the degree of intercellular coupling is managed systematically. For example, the neurotransmitter dopamine (Table 3-1), released in the retina in response to light, sets in motion a multistep process that culminates in phosphorylation of connexin and an increased probability of connexons being closed. As a result, the extent to which information spreads laterally in the retina is different under light-adapted and dark-adapted conditions.

●●● CHEMICAL SYNAPSES

Chemical synapses allow much more signaling flexibility, and presumably because of this they are much more numerous than electrical synapses. The basic elements of a stereotypical chemical synapse are a presynaptic and a postsynaptic element, separated from one another by a synaptic cleft 10 nm or more across. Depolarization of the presynaptic element causes the release of the contents of synaptic vesicles containing one or more neurotransmitters. Transmitter molecules diffuse across

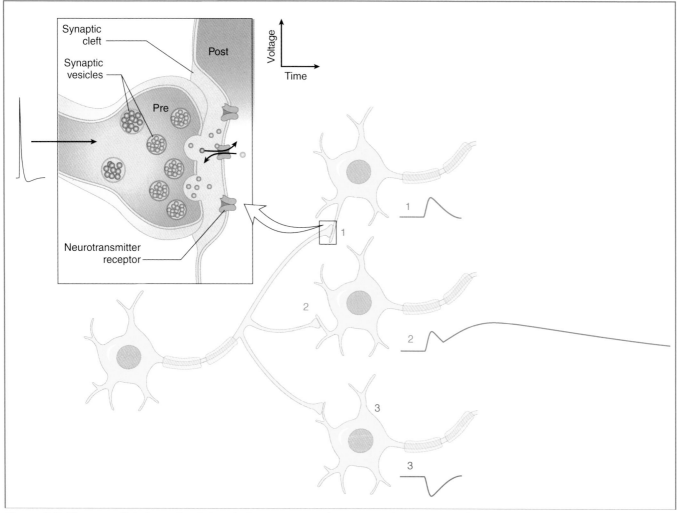

Figure 3-3. The essential elements of chemical synapses, and representative postsynaptic responses.

the synaptic cleft, bind to neurotransmitter receptor mole-cules in the postsynaptic membrane, and directly or indirectly cause a change in the ionic permeability of the postsynaptic membrane. The nature and duration of the permeability change depend on the properties of the receptor, so the resulting potential change can be depolarizing (excitatory postsynaptic potential, or EPSP) or hyperpolarizing (inhibitory postsynaptic potential, or IPSP), fast or slow (Fig. 3-3). Depolarization of a presynaptic element is typically the result of action potentials spreading into it, so this process is the reverse of that seen at neuronal trigger zones; at chemical synapses, the rate code embodied in a train of action potentials is converted into graded potentials.

Basic Structure and Function

Most presynaptic endings are parts of axons, synapsing[1] on dendrites of other neurons either as axon terminals or as

[1]Originally a noun, synapse is now commonly used as a verb referring to a presynaptic element making a synaptic contact with a postsynaptic element.

preterminal swellings as the axon passes by part of a dendrite. However, in various parts of the nervous system any part of a neuron can be presynaptic to any other part (Fig. 3-4). This gives rise to two-part names for synapses (much like the two-part names for tracts discussed in Chapter 1): axon terminals make axodendritic synapses with dendrites and axoaxonic synapses with other axon terminals, dendrites make dendro-dendritic synapses with each other, and so on.

Transmission at chemical synapses involves five essential steps:

1. Synthesis of the neurotransmitter, either in presynaptic terminals or in neuronal cell bodies.
2. Concentration and packaging of neurotransmitter molecules in preparation for release.
3. Release of neurotransmitter into the synaptic cleft.
4. Binding of neurotransmitter by postsynaptic receptor molecules, triggering some effect in the postsynaptic ending.
5. Termination of neurotransmitter action, preparing the synapse for subsequent release of transmitter.

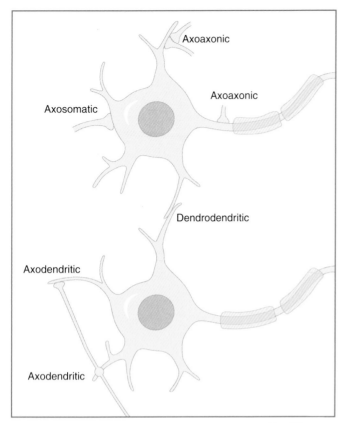

Figure 3-4. Terminology for chemical synapses with different presynaptic and postsynaptic components. Presynaptic parts of axons can be either terminal boutons ("buttons") or en passant ("in passing") endings.

Packaging of Neurotransmitters

More than 100 different chemicals are used as neurotransmitters, but almost all of them, as discussed later in this chapter, fall into two broad categories. Some are small-molecule neurotransmitters such as amino acids and small amines,

PHARMACOLOGY

Blocking the Filling of Synaptic Vesicles

There are specific vesicular transporters for different neurotransmitters or groups of transmitters, and drugs that block their activity diminish the amount of transmitter available for release. Through this mechanism, vesamicol and reserpine interfere with transmission at synapses that use acetylcholine and amine transmitters, respectively.

and others are neuropeptides up to a few dozen amino acids long. Both types are concentrated in membrane-bound synaptic vesicles, ready for release in response to presynaptic depolarization. Small-molecule neurotransmitters (e.g., glutamate, acetylcholine) are synthesized from locally available ingredients by cytoplasmic enzymes that arrive by slow axoplasmic transport. The transmitters are then loaded into small vesicles by specific transporters (Fig. 3-5), forming highly concentrated packets of neurotransmitter available for release. In contrast, neuropeptides are fragments of larger proteins that are synthesized in the cell body. The precursor proteins are packaged into somewhat larger vesicles that reach the synapse by fast axonal transport (see Fig. 3-5); the precursors are processed into neuropeptide transmitters during the journey. Individual presynaptic endings commonly contain both small and large vesicles.

Release of Neurotransmitters

Changes in intracellular Ca^{++} concentration initiate or modulate many cellular processes. At synapses, a rise in presynaptic Ca^{++} concentration is the key signal that initiates transmitter release. Presynaptic membranes contain voltage-gated Ca^{++} channels that open in response to depolarization; Ca^{++} influx results, because of both a voltage and a concentration gradient (see Tables 2-1 and 2-2). The resulting rise in presynaptic Ca^{++} concentration triggers an interaction between synaptic vesicle

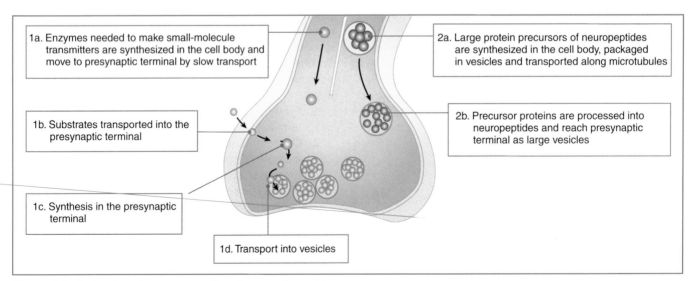

1a. Enzymes needed to make small-molecule transmitters are synthesized in the cell body and move to presynaptic terminal by slow transport

2a. Large protein precursors of neuropeptides are synthesized in the cell body, packaged in vesicles and transported along microtubules

1b. Substrates transported into the presynaptic terminal

2b. Precursor proteins are processed into neuropeptides and reach presynaptic terminal as large vesicles

1c. Synthesis in the presynaptic terminal

1d. Transport into vesicles

Figure 3-5. Packaging of neurotransmitters in synaptic vesicles.

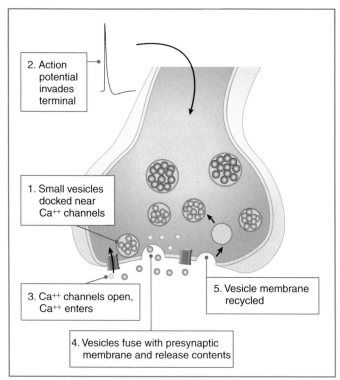

Figure 3-6. Release of small-molecule neurotransmitters.

MICROBIOLOGY & IMMUNOLOGY

Antibodies That Block Transmitter Release

Some patients with small-cell carcinoma of the lung or some other types of cancer develop Lambert-Eaton syndrome, in which antibodies to presynaptic voltage-gated Ca^{++} channels are produced. Packaging of transmitter remains normal, but fewer vesicles than normal are released in response to presynaptic depolarization, resulting in weakness and some autonomic disturbances.

PHARMACOLOGY

Blocking Acetylcholine Release

Botulinum toxin, ingested accidentally or injected on purpose into selected muscles, is taken up by the presynaptic terminals of motor neurons and cleaves proteins essential for fusing vesicles of acetylcholine with the presynaptic membrane. As a result, neuromuscular transmission is blocked.

membrane proteins and presynaptic membrane proteins, resulting in fusion of nearby synaptic vesicles with the surface membrane and discharge of their contents. A subset of the small synaptic vesicles form clusters in active zones near the presynaptic membrane, close to the voltage-gated Ca^{++} channels, so one or more vesicles of small-molecule transmitter are likely to release their contents in response to small depolarizations or single action potentials (Fig. 3-6). Large synaptic vesicles, in contrast, are located farther away from active zones. As a result, the Ca^{++} concentration required to trigger fusion of these vesicles with the presynaptic membrane is achieved only in response to large depolarizations or trains of action potentials (Fig. 3-7). In both cases, because transmitter is stored in and released from vesicles of relatively uniform size, neurotransmitters are released as discrete packets, or quanta.

Following fusion, synaptic vesicle membranes are retrieved by the synaptic terminal for reuse or degradation. Small vesicles are re-formed and refilled with transmitter multiple times (see Fig. 3-6), whereas the membranes of large vesicles are shipped back to the cell body for recycling or degradation (see Fig. 3-7).

Figure 3-7. Release of neuropeptides.

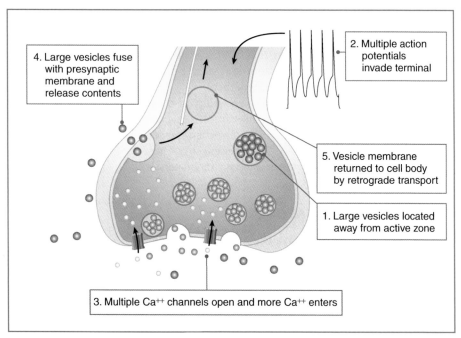

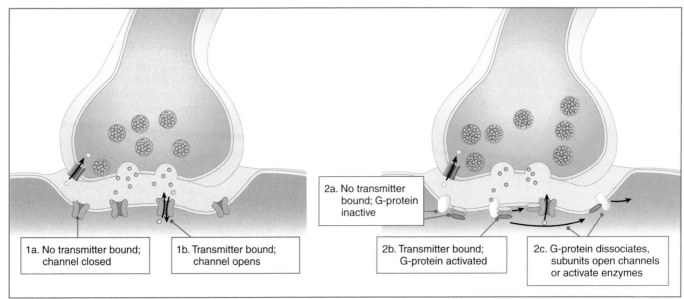

Figure 3-8. Ionotropic (*left*) and metabotropic (*right*) neurotransmitter receptors.

Postsynaptic Receptors

Neurotransmitter receptors fall into two categories (Fig. 3-8). Ionotropic receptors are themselves ligand-gated ion channels, with a specific neurotransmitter being the ligand. Binding of one or more molecules of that transmitter to the receptor increases the probability of the channel being open. Because of the direct coupling between transmitter binding and permeability changes, the postsynaptic potential mediated by an ionotropic receptor is usually relatively rapid (and brief). Its polarity depends on the ionic selectivity of the channel, in a straightforward way predicted by the Goldman equation (see Eq. 2-3). For example, either closing K^+ channels or opening Na^+ channels would cause an EPSP, moving the membrane potential closer to V_{Na} and making it more likely to reach threshold. Similarly, opening relatively nonselective monovalent cation channels (which is common at excitatory synapses) also causes depolarization, in this case by moving the membrane potential toward some value midway between V_{Na} and V_K. Opening K^+ channels or Cl^- channels would cause an IPSP, moving the membrane potential toward some value below threshold.

Ionotropic receptors are assemblies of four to five membrane-spanning subunits surrounding a central channel. Each such assembly includes subunits of two or more types, so numerous closely related receptors can be formed from different combinations of subunits. This has allowed both nature and pharmacologists to develop more or less selective agonists and antagonists that bind to receptors in particular parts of the nervous system and mimic or block the effects of specific neurotransmitters there.

Metabotropic receptors also cause EPSPs and IPSPs, but they do so indirectly, affecting the state of postsynaptic ion channels by way of second messengers (the neurotransmitter being the "first messenger"). These receptors are transmembrane proteins, usually monomers, with an extracellular binding

PHARMACOLOGY

Selective Cholinergic Antagonists

The ionotropic acetylcholine receptors (nicotinic receptors) of skeletal muscle are slightly different from those of autonomic ganglion cells, so *d*-tubocurarine (curare) blocks neuromuscular transmission, and hexamethonium blocks ganglionic transmission.

Figure 3-9. Mechanisms for removal of neurotransmitter after release. Different transmitters favor different mechanisms: enzymatic degradation of acetylcholine and neuropeptides, reuptake of other small-molecule neurotransmitters, internalization of neuropeptides bound to receptors.

site for a neurotransmitter and an intracellular binding site for a three-subunit GTP-binding protein, or G protein; hence they are also called G protein–coupled receptors. In the absence of neurotransmitter, G proteins bind GDP and are inactive. Binding of the appropriate neurotransmitter enables G proteins to bind transiently to the receptor, exchange GDP for GTP, and dissociate into subunits. Depending on the specifics of a given G protein, the subunits then participate in a variety of processes leading to postsynaptic voltage changes (see Fig. 3-8). Some bind directly to ion channels, causing them to open or close. Others stimulate or inhibit enzymes such as adenylate cyclase, whose products may affect either ion channels or other enzymes. The extra steps in postsynaptic processes mediated by metabotropic receptors provide opportunities for amplification and modulation but also result in postsynaptic potentials that develop more slowly and may be very long lasting.

Even though metabotropic receptors are monomeric proteins, almost all of them, like ionotropic receptors, come in several closely related forms. Hence, there are agonists and antagonists selective for subsets of these receptors as well.

Postsynaptic Effects of Neurotransmitters

Although some transmitters are usually excitatory (e.g., glutamate) and others are usually inhibitory (e.g., GABA), the effect of a transmitter at a given synapse is ultimately determined by the receptor to which it binds. For example, there are metabotropic receptors at which glutamate causes closing of nonselective cation channels (and consequently IPSPs). Many transmitters cause EPSPs at some synapses and IPSPs at others.

Termination of Neurotransmitter Action

At the same time neurotransmitters are binding to their receptors, other processes are in competition, trying to remove

PHARMACOLOGY

Prolonging Neurotransmitter Action

Agents that block the reuptake of a transmitter allow that transmitter to remain in the synaptic cleft longer than usual, thereby enhancing its effect. For example, the popular antidepressant fluoxetine works by inhibiting the reuptake of serotonin, and cocaine enhances the effects of dopamine and other amines by blocking their reuptake.

PHARMACOLOGY

Too Much Acetylcholine

Organophosphates, such as the nerve gas sarin and some insecticides, work by blocking acetylcholinesterase. This results in an extended presence of acetylcholine at muscle membranes, keeping them depolarized and their voltage-gated Na^+ channels in an inactivated state. This depolarization block makes the muscle fibers inexcitable and unable to contract.

transmitter molecules and "clear the decks" for subsequent releases (Fig. 3-9). At all synapses, some neurotransmitter simply diffuses out of the synaptic cleft and is taken up by nearby cells or degraded enzymatically; this is the principal route of removal for neuropeptides. The most common mechanism, however, is reuptake by specific transporters, either back into the presynaptic terminal or into glial processes surrounding the synapse. (The glial processes subsequently ship the neurotransmitter or its metabolites back into the presynaptic terminal for reuse.) The major exception is acetylcholine, which is hydrolyzed to acetate and choline by acetylcholinesterase located adjacent to the synaptic cleft. The choline is then transported back into the presynaptic terminal and used to make more acetylcholine.

Neurotransmitters

About ten neurotransmitters are small, soluble molecules (see Table 3-1), many of which interact with both ionotropic and metabotropic receptors. The rest are neuropeptides, all of which interact with metabotropic receptors.

Small-Molecule Transmitters

The principal small-molecule transmitters (see Table 3-1) are acetylcholine, a few amino acids (glutamate, γ-aminobutyric acid [GABA], and glycine), and a diverse group of biogenic amines. The latter include serotonin, histamine, and the catecholamines dopamine and norepinephrine.

Acetylcholine

Acetylcholine (Table 3-2) is the major transmitter mediating fast excitatory transmission in the PNS, acting at nicotinic receptors (called this because nicotine is a potent agonist at these sites). Nicotinic receptors are most prominent on skeletal muscle fibers, where they mediate neuromuscular transmission (there are no inhibitory synapses on vertebrate skeletal muscles), but they are also found on autonomic ganglion cells (see Chapter 18). Acetylcholine also works through

TABLE 3-2. Locations of Cholinergic Neurons and Their Synapses

Location/Type of Neuron	Location of Terminal
Motor neurons	Skeletal muscle
Preganglionic autonomic neurons	Autonomic ganglia
Postganglionic parasympathetic neurons	Smooth and cardiac muscle, glands
Reticular formation*	Thalamus
Basal nucleus (nucleus basalis of Meynert)*	Cerebral cortex, amygdala
Septal nuclei*	Hippocampus
Caudate nucleus, putamen	Local connections

*See Chapter 5.

MICROBIOLOGY & IMMUNOLOGY

Antibodies to Neurotransmitter Receptors

Myasthenia gravis is an autoimmune disorder caused by the production of antibodies to skeletal muscle nicotinic receptors. Because an abnormally small number of functional nicotinic receptors are available, acetylcholinesterase wins the competition for acetylcholine and weakness results. Anticholinesterases usually provide effective therapy.

PATHOLOGY

Excitotoxicity

Although an increase in Ca^{++} concentration is an important signal for a variety of intracellular processes, excessive increases initiate destructive and even fatal events for the neurons in which they occur. For this reason, prolonged exposure to glutamate can be excitotoxic, allowing harmful levels of Ca^{++} influx through NMDA channels.

TABLE 3-3. Major Locations of Neurons Using Amino Acids as Transmitters

Transmitter	Location/Type of Neuron	Location of Terminal
Glutamate	Interneurons, many CNS sites	Local connections
	Primary afferent neurons	Secondary neurons in CNS
	Cortical pyramidal cells*	Other cortical areas, many subcortical sites
GABA	Interneurons, many CNS sites	Local connections
	Cerebellar Purkinje cells†	Deep cerebellar nuclei†
	Caudate nucleus, putamen	Globus pallidus, substantia nigra
	Globus pallidus, substantia nigra‡	Thalamus, subthalamic nucleus‡
	Thalamic reticular nucleus*	Thalamus
Glycine	Interneurons, spinal cord and brainstem	Local connections

*See Chapter 5.
†See Chapter 16.
‡See Chapter 15.

TABLE 3-4. Major Locations of Neurons Using Biogenic Amines as Transmitters

Transmitter	Location/Type of Neuron	Location of Terminal
Dopamine	Substantia nigra*	Caudate nucleus, putamen
	Ventral tegmental area*	Frontal lobe, limbic structures
Norepinephrine	Postganglionic sympathetic neurons	Smooth and cardiac muscle, glands
	Locus ceruleus†	Widespread CNS areas
Serotonin	Raphe nuclei†	Widespread CNS areas
Histamine	Hypothalamus	Widespread CNS areas

*See Chapter 15.
†See Chapter 5.

metabotropic muscarinic receptors (called this because muscarine, produced by *Amanita muscaria*, a poisonous mushroom, is a potent agonist at these sites). In the PNS, muscarinic receptors are found in the smooth muscles and glands targeted by some autonomic axons, and they coexist with nicotinic receptors on autonomic ganglion cells. The role of acetylcholine in the CNS is important but more limited, usually involving muscarinic receptors. Some interneurons in certain CNS nuclei are cholinergic, and there are a few collections of cholinergic neurons that provide modulatory inputs to widespread areas of the CNS (see Chapter 5).

Amino Acids

Glutamate (Table 3-3) is the major neurotransmitter mediating fast excitatory transmission throughout the CNS. There are multiple types of ionotropic glutamate receptors, the two most widespread being AMPA and NMDA receptors (acronyms for the agonists α-amino-3-hydroxyl-5-methyl-4-isoxazolepropionate and N-methyl-D-aspartate). AMPA receptors, like nicotinic acetylcholine receptors, are nonselective monovalent cation channels. NMDA receptors, in contrast, have two special properties (Fig. 3-10)—voltage dependency and Ca^{++} permeability—that allow them to play unique roles in the CNS. The central pore of these receptors contains a Mg^{++} binding site that is occupied at normal resting potentials, occluding the pore even if it changes shape in response to the binding of glutamate. Depolarization of the postsynaptic membrane (e.g., by activation of nearby AMPA receptors) is required to expel the Mg^{++} ion and allow current to flow through the pore. Once open, NMDA receptors allow the passage of not just Na^+ and K^+ but also Ca^{++} ions. The resulting Ca^{++} influx not only contributes to the EPSP but also provides a second messenger that sets in motion a series of intracellular processes that can lead to long-term changes in the structure and function of that synapse. For this reason, NMDA receptors are thought to play a central role in learning and memory and in other processes involving synaptic plasticity (see Chapter 20). Like acetylcholine, glutamate also acts at a variety of metabotropic receptors, producing slow EPSPs and IPSPs in CNS neurons.

GABA and glycine (Table 3-4) are the major neurotransmitters mediating fast inhibitory transmission throughout the

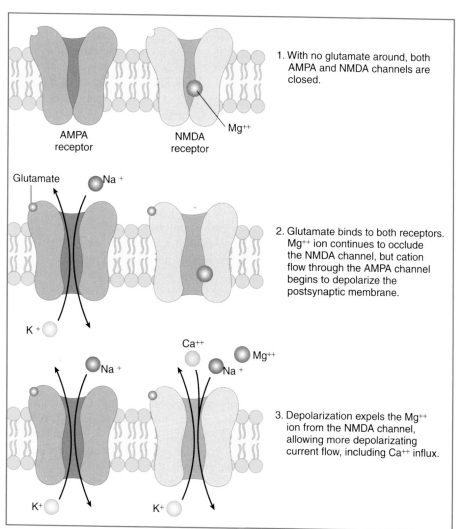

Figure 3-10. Opening of NMDA channels requires both binding of glutamate and concurrent postsynaptic depolarization.

1. With no glutamate around, both AMPA and NMDA channels are closed.

AMPA receptor

NMDA receptor

Mg++

Glutamate

Na +

2. Glutamate binds to both receptors. Mg++ ion continues to occlude the NMDA channel, but cation flow through the AMPA channel begins to depolarize the postsynaptic membrane.

K +

Ca++

Na +

Mg++

Na +

3. Depolarization expels the Mg++ ion from the NMDA channel, allowing more depolarizing current flow, including Ca++ influx.

K+

K+

CNS. Both have substantial roles in the spinal cord, but GABA is dominant everyplace else. Both work through closely related ionotropic receptors that are Cl⁻ channels; GABA acts at metabotropic receptors as well. Activation of the ionotropic receptors causes brief IPSPs. These may be very small because the Cl⁻ equilibrium potential is often close to the resting membrane potential. Nevertheless, they can have a potent inhibitory effect by increasing the weight of the Cl⁻ term in the Goldman equation (see Eq. 2-3) and making it harder to move the membrane potential toward threshold. Activation of metabotropic GABA receptors also causes IPSPs,

in this case slower ones often mediated by the opening of K^+ channels.

Biogenic Amines

Amine neurotransmitters (see Table 3-4), such as norepinephrine, are important in many PNS autonomic synapses (see Chapter 18). In the CNS, most aminergic neurons have cell bodies clustered in discrete locations but axons with many branches spread over wide areas of the brain and spinal cord (see Figs. 5-22 and 5-23). This diffusely projecting pattern of

---

PHARMACOLOGY

Excitation from Blocking Inhibition

Strychnine, a selective antagonist of glycine, reduces the level of inhibition in the spinal cord and brainstem. At relatively low doses, motor neurons become hyperexcitable, and excessive muscle contraction ensues. Higher doses lead to convulsions and death.

PHARMACOLOGY

Drugs That Enhance Inhibition

GABA_A receptors are the most common inhibitory ionotropic receptors in the brain, and drugs that enhance their effects can be effective tranquilizers. Benzodiazepines accomplish this by increasing the frequency of opening of channels that have bound GABA, and barbiturates do so by increasing the duration of each open period.

Targeting Biogenic Amines to Affect Mental Status

Because of the widespread distribution of biogenic amines, drugs or clinical conditions that affect their function can have broad effects on mood, mental state, and cognition. A few examples: amphetamine and cocaine have stimulant effects, amphetamine by increasing the release of norepinephrine and dopamine, and cocaine by blocking their reuptake; blockers of serotonin reuptake, such as fluoxetine, are antidepressants; the antipsychotic drug haloperidol is an antagonist at some dopaminergic synapses.

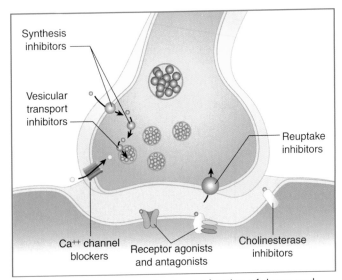

Figure 3-11. Common mechanisms of action of drugs and toxins that affect the nervous system by modifying synaptic transmission. Other changes in synaptic transmission (not shown) occur physiologically and involve changes in channel permeability (through phosphorylation and other mechanisms), and longer lasting changes such as up- or down-regulation of receptors and transporters.

connections makes these neurons poorly suited for transmitting discrete bits of information but well suited for modulating the activity of large CNS areas, as required for things such as changes in attention and alertness. For example, fluctuations in the activity of different populations of aminergic neurons are key features of the sleep-wake cycle (see Chapter 19). With a single exception, the biogenic amines act entirely through families of G protein–coupled receptors (although most serotonin receptors are metabotropic, one type is a ligand-gated cation channel).

Neuropeptides

More than 50 different peptides, from a few to a few dozen amino acids in length, have been implicated as neurotransmitters. Most or all of them are also used as signaling molecules elsewhere in the body or the brain, such as in the GI tract (e.g., enkephalin, substance P), as pituitary hormones

(e.g., ACTH, vasopressin), or as pituitary-regulating factors released by the hypothalamus (e.g., somatostatin, thyrotropin-releasing hormone). Neuropeptides produce slow postsynaptic potentials, and sometimes longer-lasting metabolic and even structural changes, through G protein–coupled receptors. Few if any presynaptic endings use only neuropeptides, to the exclusion of small-molecule transmitters; instead, neuropeptide release provides an additional phase of synaptic signaling in response to prolonged presynaptic depolarization.

Control of Transmission at Chemical Synapses

Transmission at an individual chemical synapse need not be an all-or-nothing event. The multiple steps involved—synthesizing and packaging neurotransmitter, Ca^{++} influx, transmitter release, receptor binding, opening or closing of ion channels—provide numerous opportunities for short- and long-term changes in the effect of a presynaptic action potential on postsynaptic electrical activity (Fig. 3-11). Some of these changes are a straightforward consequence of synaptic physiology. For example, repeated presynaptic action potentials can cause a buildup of Ca^{++} ions in the presynaptic terminal, leading not only to release of neuropeptides but also to enhanced release of small-molecule transmitters; on the other hand, a really prolonged or rapid burst of action potentials can partially deplete the population of vesicles available for fusion with the presynaptic membrane, leading to temporarily reduced postsynaptic potentials.

Other changes in synaptic efficacy involve chemical messengers that, unlike conventional neurotransmitters, are not released as vesicular contents. One example is the long-term changes set in motion by Ca^{++} ions entering postsynaptic cells through NMDA channels; these are thought to play a major role in the synaptic changes underlying learning and memory (see Chapter 20) and in some other forms of synaptic plasticity. Another example is the growth factors exchanged between neurons and their targets as part of the processes involved in the establishment and maintenance of connections (see Chapter 20). In addition, some small molecules modulate synaptic function on a moment-to-moment basis. Prominent examples are adenosine, endocannabinoids, and the gases nitric oxide (NO) and carbon monoxide (CO).

ATP, adenosine, and some other purines affect widespread areas of the nervous system. Surprisingly, ATP is packaged

Adenosine Receptors and Alertness

Xanthine derivatives such as theophylline and caffeine are purinergic receptor antagonists. Theophylline relaxes airway smooth muscle and is used as a bronchodilator. The stimulant effects of caffeine, probably the most widely used pharmacologically active substance in the world, are based in large part on blocking CNS adenosine receptors.

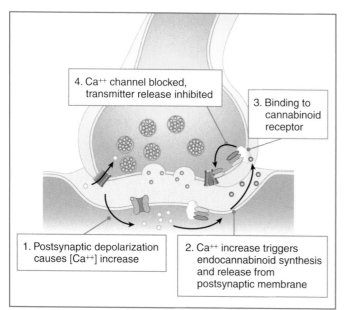

Figure 3-12. Retrograde synaptic signaling by endocannabinoids. Postsynaptic depolarization results in Ca^{++} influx through voltage-gated Ca^{++} channels, or Ca^{++} release from intracellular stores. This in turn causes synthesis and release of endocannabinoids from membrane lipids. Activation of presynaptic cannabinoid receptors inhibits transmitter release in part by blocking voltage-gated Ca^{++} channels, but other mechanisms are also involved.

PHARMACOLOGY

Vasodilatory Effects of Nitrous Oxide

The signaling function of NO was first appreciated when it was found to be an agent that is released from endothelial cells and causes relaxation of nearby vascular smooth muscle cells by increasing their cyclic GMP concentration. This vasodilatory effect is exploited pharmacologically by using nitroglycerin (which releases NO) to increase cardiac blood flow, and sildenafil, which inhibits phosphodiesterase V (an enzyme that breaks down cyclic GMP), to relax the smooth muscle of the corpus cavernosum.

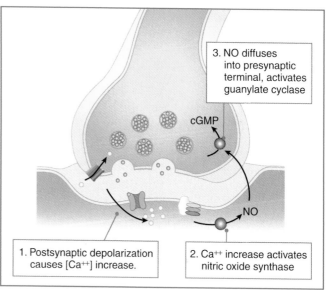

Figure 3-13. Retrograde synaptic signaling by NO (CO acts similarly). The most common effect of NO is to activate guanylate cyclase; the resulting increase in cyclic GMP concentration then affects channels or other enzymes. Although NO and CO most commonly function as retrograde signals, at some synapses they are produced in the presynaptic ending and diffuse in an anterograde direction.

with better known neurotransmitters in synaptic vesicles and released along with them. At some synapses, especially neuromuscular junctions, peripheral autonomic synapses, and synapses of somatosensory receptors, ATP binds to ionotropic and metabotropic receptors and behaves much like other small-molecule neurotransmitters. However, adenosine, a breakdown product of ATP, is not packaged in vesicles and has a different mode of action. It diffuses from areas of ATP hydrolysis, freely crosses cell membranes, and binds to widely distributed metabotropic receptors. Its generally inhibitory effect promotes sleepiness and decreased activity.

Marijuana (*Cannabis sativa*) has been used medicinally and recreationally by humans for thousands of years. Its active ingredient, Δ^9-tetrahydrocannabinol (Δ^9-THC) acts in the brain by binding to G protein–coupled receptors in presynaptic terminals and suppressing the release of neurotransmitter (Fig. 3-12). These same receptors are normally acted upon by endocannabinoids (endogenous cannabinoids) that are quickly synthesized from postsynaptic membrane lipids in response to depolarization, diffuse across the membrane, and reach cannabinoid receptors in nearby terminals. Hence, these substances are retrograde messengers, conveying signals in a postsynaptic to presynaptic direction. Cannabinoid receptors are widely distributed, but concentrated in the cerebral cortex, hippocampus, hypothalamus,

cerebellum, and basal ganglia. This is presumably related to the effects of marijuana use on subjective experience, memory, appetite, and movement.

Similarly, NO and CO are synthesized in processes of some neurons in response to depolarization, diffuse across the membrane, and reach nearby neurons (Fig. 3-13). In this case, however, no membrane receptors are involved: these small, soluble gases simply diffuse into other cells, where they activate guanylate cyclase and thereby increase the concentration of cyclic GMP, which in turn affects the activity of ion channels or other enzymes. Although these gaseous messengers often convey retrograde signals, in some parts of the nervous system they move in the same direction as conventional neurotransmitters.

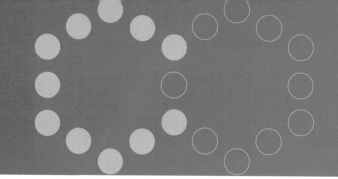

Sensory Receptors

4

CONTENTS

TABLE 4-1. Adequate Stimulus of Different Receptor Types

Adequate Stimulus	Types of Receptor
Chemicals	Olfactory receptors
	Taste receptors
	Some nociceptors
	Hypothalamic chemoreceptors
	Visceral chemoreceptors
Mechanical stimuli	Mechanoreceptors of skin, muscles, and joints
	Some nociceptors
	Auditory and vestibular receptors
	Visceral mechanoreceptors
	Hypothalamic osmoreceptors
Photons	Retinal photoreceptors
Temperature change	Cool receptors
	Warm receptors
	Some nociceptors
	Hypothalamic thermoreceptors

Whatever we "know" about our own bodies and the world around us has its origins in sensory receptors that convert some kind of physical stimulus into an electrical signal and pass this electrical signal along toward the central nervous system. The brain takes this information, factors in past experience, current mood, and other factors, and makes its best guess about what is really going on out (or in) there. Although it feels as if perceptions are accurate reflections of physical reality, this best guess is sometimes wrong—this is the basis of such things as visual illusions.

●●● FUNCTIONAL ANATOMY OF SENSORY RECEPTORS

Sensory receptors are specialized cells, usually neurons but sometimes specialized epithelial cells, that are able to transduce (Latin, "lead across") some kind of stimulus energy into graded electrical signals called receptor potentials. Receptor potentials are much like postsynaptic potentials: they are relatively slow (at least compared with action potentials) and, depending on the receptor, can be either depolarizing or hyperpolarizing. A given kind of receptor responds best to a particular kind of stimulus, termed the adequate stimulus for that receptor type (much as a postsynaptic receptor molecule selectively binds a particular neurotransmitter). This gives rise to a fairly straightforward classification system for receptors, based on their adequate stimulus (Table 4-1)—chemoreceptors,

mechanoreceptors, photoreceptors, and thermoreceptors.[1] Many pain receptors can respond to more than one kind of tissue-damaging stimulus, and so pain receptors are usually referred to as a separate category of nociceptors. That is, the sensory ending of a single nociceptor may contain the machinery needed to detect intense mechanical stimuli, damaging heat or cold, and chemicals released in injured tissues.

Anatomic/Functional Zones

All receptors have a cell body and three general functional areas, each of which makes sense in view of the role of sensory receptors. There is a zone specialized for receiving and transducing stimuli, a nearby zone rich in mitochondria that support the energy requirements of the transduction

---

[1]There are, of course, other forms of energy in the environment, and various animals have evolved receptors for them. Some aquatic animals have electroreceptors that allow them to communicate or to detect objects by sensing changes in electric fields. Other animals have magnetoreceptors that are used as navigational aids.

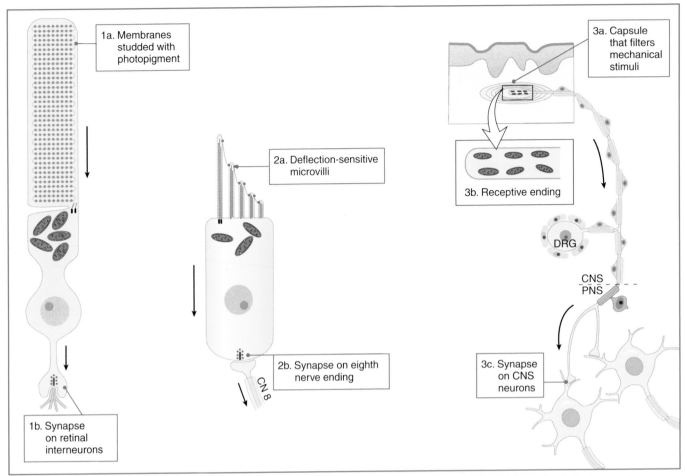

Figure 4-1. Functional anatomic zones of a few representative sensory receptors; from left to right, a retinal photoreceptor, an auditory/vestibular receptor (hair cell), and a pacinian corpuscle (a touch/vibration receptor).

process, and a zone where information is passed on toward or into the CNS.

Some receptors have transduction zones with anatomic features more or less obviously suited to the function of those receptors (Fig. 4-1). For example, photoreceptors contain stacks of membranes loaded with photopigment (see Fig. 12-7); cochlear and vestibular receptors have arrays of rigid, actin-filled microvilli that enable them to respond to physical deflection (see Fig. 10-6); and many somatosensory receptors have peripheral terminals with capsules or accessory structures that filter mechanical stimuli (see Fig. 9-1). Others, particularly some somatosensory and visceral receptors, have transduction zones that are simply free nerve endings that bear the molecules required for transduction but lack any obvious anatomic specializations. For example, although all unmyelinated sensory fibers (C fibers) have free nerve endings, various individual C fibers are selectively sensitive to touch, warmth, painful stimuli, or distention of hollow organs.

Short Versus Long Receptors

Receptor potentials are not propagated actively; rather, they decay over a short distance, like postsynaptic potentials. This is easy for receptors that signal over short distances (a couple of hundred micrometers or less), and they do not need to produce action potentials. Instead, they synapse on the peripheral processes of primary afferent neurons whose cell bodies lie in peripheral ganglia (or on interneurons, in the case of the retina). The receptor potential changes the rate at which the receptor releases transmitter, and this in turn

---

HISTOLOGY

Multiple Uses for Microvilli and Cilia

The microvilli and cilia used for various purposes by other cells have been adapted as transduction zones by some sensory receptors. Almost all the sensory "hairs" for which auditory and vestibular receptors (hair cells) are named are actin-filled microvilli. The photosensitive part of a retinal rod or cone is actually an elaborately modified cilium, with a longitudinally running microtubule array and a surface membrane greatly expanded to accommodate its content of photopigment. Each olfactory receptor cell has a dendrite from which a series of chemosensitive cilia emerge.

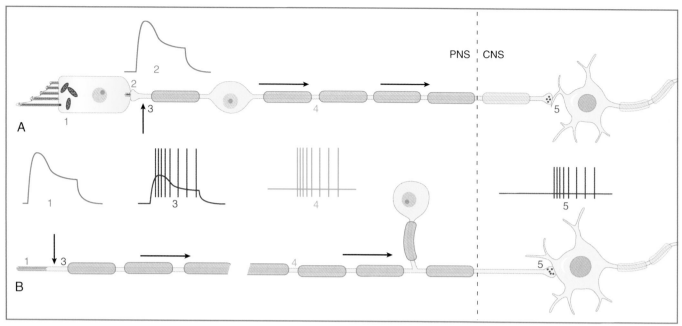

PNS | CNS

A

B

Figure 4-2. Electrical signaling associated with short receptors and long receptors. Delivery of an adequate stimulus to either a short receptor (**A**, here an auditory/vestibular receptor) or a long receptor (**B**) elicits a receptor potential (1). In the long receptor, the receptor potential spreads passively to the nearby trigger zone (*arrow*) and initiates a train of action potentials (3) that propagate (4) toward the CNS and spread into presynaptic terminals in the CNS (5). In the short receptor, the receptor potential modulates the rate of transmitter release onto a primary afferent (here a terminal of an eighth nerve fiber), causing a postsynaptic potential (2) that spreads passively to the nearby trigger zone (*arrow*) and initiates a train of action potentials (3) that propagate (4) toward the CNS and spread into presynaptic terminals in the CNS (5).

changes the rate at which the primary afferent neuron sends action potentials into the CNS (Fig. 4-2). Thus, for these kinds of receptors, the generation of receptor potentials and the modulation of action potential frequency happen in different cells; i.e., the sensory receptor and the primary afferent are two separate cells. Many of these short receptors depolarize and increase their rate of transmitter release in response to a stimulus. Others hyperpolarize and decrease their rate of transmitter release, and some can do either depending on the properties of the stimulus. Examples of short receptors are taste receptor cells, retinal rods and cones, and hair cells of the inner ear (Table 4-2).

On the other hand, consider the problem faced by receptors that signal over long distances. A receptor potential in such a cell would die out long before reaching a synaptic ending, and so it must generate action potentials as well as receptor potentials. An example is a receptor that signals something touching your big toe. A long receptor like this produces a receptor potential in response to touch, and the receptor potential in turn spreads to a nearby trigger zone and causes action potentials that are conducted all the way into the CNS (see Fig. 4-2). The receptor potential itself dies out near the receptive ending. So in this case, the generation of receptor potentials and the modulation of action potential frequency happen in adjacent parts of a single cell; i.e., the same cell serves as both sensory receptor and primary afferent. (The trigger zone in long receptors is in an unusual but necessary place, often far from the cell body. The recep-

tive ending in such a cell corresponds to the dendrites of a typical neuron, and the nearby trigger zone corresponds to the axon initial segment.) The receptors that convey information about somatic sensation (touch, pain, etc.), olfactory receptors, and most visceral receptors are receptors with long axons (see Table 4-2). Although there is no reason from first principles why a long receptor could not signal a stimulus by firing less frequently (and some invertebrate receptors do just that), all vertebrate long receptors depolarize and fire faster in response to an adequate stimulus.

TABLE 4-2. Short Receptors and Long Receptors

Short Receptors
Taste receptors
Hypothalamic receptors
Some visceral chemoreceptors
Auditory and vestibular receptors
Photoreceptors

Long Receptors
Olfactory receptors
Most visceral receptors
Mechanoreceptors of skin, muscles, and joints*
Nociceptors
Cool and warm receptors

*Merkel receptors are a possible exception; see Chapter 9.

●●● SENSORY TRANSDUCTION

The transducing membranes of sensory receptors are a lot like postsynaptic membranes, differing mainly by being sensitive to some physical stimulus rather than to a transmitter released by another neuron. Just as at synapses, there are two broad categories of sensory transduction mechanisms: ionotropic (stimulus-gated ion channels) and metabotropic (G protein–coupled) mechanisms (Table 4-3). In some cases, the molecules in sensory receptors that interact directly with the physical stimulus are actually closely related to postsynaptic receptor molecules.

Like their synaptic counterparts, ionotropic transduction mechanisms are fast, so they are found in receptors where speed is important (although not exclusively in such receptors). These include auditory and vestibular receptors and mechanoreceptors in skin, muscles, and joints. Despite the lack of enzymatic cascades, accessory structures that couple the stimulus to the transduction channel often make these receptors exquisitely sensitive as well (see Chapters 9–11). In contrast, the amplification provided by metabotropic transduction mechanisms provides enhanced sensitivity in receptors where speed is less important. Olfactory receptors and photoreceptors, for example, can respond to single odorant molecules or single photons (see Chapters 12 and 13), but they are significantly slower than auditory and vestibular receptors.

Ionotropic Mechanisms

Some taste receptor cells have the ultimately simple ionotropic transduction mechanism, not even requiring a receptor (Fig. 4-3): increases in extracellular Na^+ concentration resulting from salty foods cause a depolarizing current flow through open Na^+ channels, moving the membrane potential toward a level predicted by the Goldman equation

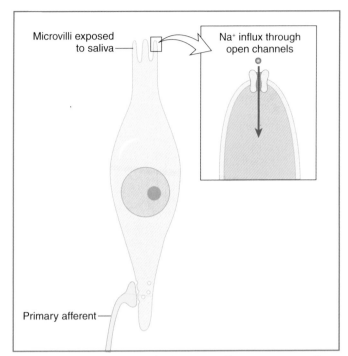

Figure 4-3. Transduction of salty tastes. Taste receptor cells (see Chapter 13) are short receptors that make synapses on peripheral processes of cranial nerve fibers. They also have microvillous processes that are exposed to saliva and contain transduction machinery. Some contain normally open Na^+ channels, so an increased Na^+ concentration resulting from chewing salty foods causes a depolarizing influx of Na^+ ions.

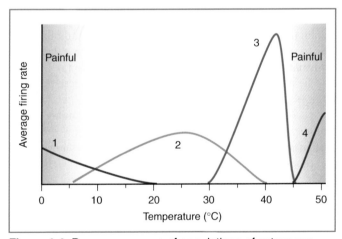

Figure 4-4. Response ranges of populations of cutaneous temperature receptors. Different receptors are selective for warming (3, 4) or cooling (1, 2) in either innocuous (2, 3) or painful (1, 4) ranges.

(see Eq. 2-3). Similarly, at least part of the basis for transducing sour tastes is a depolarizing influx of protons through cation channels. Other receptors have cation channels gated by temperature increases (warm receptors) or decreases (cool receptors) in particular ranges, some innocuous and others painful (Fig. 4-4).

TABLE 4-3. Transduction Mechanisms of Different Receptor Types	
Transduction Mechanism	**Receptor Type**
Ionotropic (stimulus-gated channels)	Mechanoreceptors of skin, muscles, and joints Auditory and vestibular receptors Nociceptors Temperature receptors Some visceral receptors Some taste receptors Hypothalamic receptors?
Metabotropic (mediated by G proteins)	Retinal photoreceptors Olfactory receptors Some taste receptors Some visceral receptors

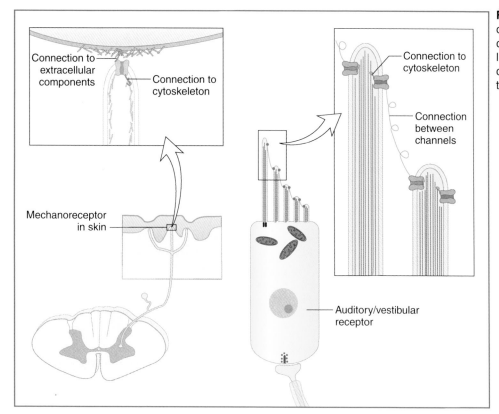

Figure 4-5. Transduction channels of many mechanoreceptors are coupled to stimuli by proteins that link the channels to the cytoskeleton and to connective tissue elements or to each other.

Mechanoreceptors have the most diverse kinds of specializations, suiting them to detect stimuli as varied as touch, position, sound, painful prodding, and osmolality changes (see Chapters 9–11). Most, however, use channels that are linked to both the cytoskeleton and to some extracellular structure, allowing them to be directly gated by mechanical deformation (Fig. 4-5).

Metabotropic Mechanisms

Many receptors tap into second-messenger machinery similar to that of postsynaptic neurons, using G protein–coupled receptors related to those in postsynaptic membranes (Fig. 4-6). Photoreceptors and olfactory receptors, for example, have cyclic nucleotide–gated ion channels. Stimulation by a photon or an odorant causes changes in cyclic nucleotide concentration through activation of an enzyme by a G protein.

PHARMACOLOGY

Spicy Foods

Some temperature-sensitive channels have binding sites for chemicals as well, accounting for the cool sensation engendered by menthol and the burning sensation produced by capsaicin, the compound responsible for the spiciness of chili peppers.

Control of Signaling by Sensory Receptors

Just as synapses are adjustable, the multiple steps involved in sensory reception—delivering a stimulus to a receptor, transduction, and transmission of a signal to the CNS—provide multiple opportunities for controlling and adjusting this process. This shows up partly as the adaptation shown by almost all receptors in the face of maintained stimulation (described later in this chapter). Longer term changes in receptor sensitivity can be initiated by events such as Ca^{++} entry through transduction channels. In addition, projections from the CNS can adjust the sensitivity of some receptors on a moment-to-moment basis. Two prominent examples (Fig. 4-7) are the stretch receptors of skeletal muscle and auditory receptors.

●●● CODING BY SENSORY RECEPTORS

The signals provided by sensory receptors are used by the CNS to judge not just the nature of stimuli but also their timing, intensity, and often their location. These could most simply be coded by, respectively, the type of receptor responding, the duration and size of its receptor potentials, and its location, but there is more to it than that.

Nature of a Stimulus

The classical sensory modalities correspond to the "five senses"—touch, vision, hearing, taste and smell. However, it

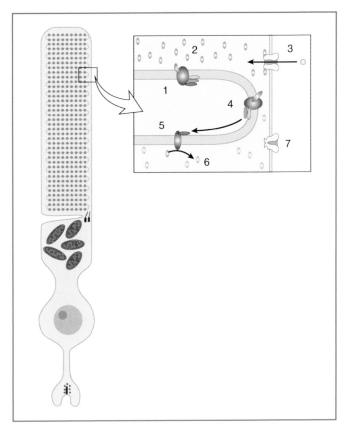

Figure 4-6. Phototransduction in rods as an example of a metabotropic transduction mechanism. In the dark, G proteins are not activated by rhodopsin (1), the cyclic GMP concentration is relatively high (2), and cyclic GMP–gated cation channels are open (3). Absorption of a photon changes the conformation of rhodopsin, activating G proteins (4). This in turn activates phosphodiesterase (5), the enzyme that hydrolyzes cyclic GMP. Cyclic GMP levels decline (6), and cyclic GMP-gated cation channels close (7).

is clear that there are additional modalities (e.g., balance, pain, temperature) and that there are submodalities or qualities associated with stimuli (e.g., color). In some cases, there is a straightforward one-to-one mapping between receptor type and sensory modality. For example, anything that deflects the sensory microvilli of vestibular receptors—either a natural movement of the head or some pathologic process—causes a sensation of movement; this is the basis of the vertigo experienced in some diseases or after overindulgence in ethanol. However, some kinds of receptors cause no conscious sensation when stimulated. Most commonly these are visceral receptors working behind the scenes to keep track of things such as blood chemistry. In addition, individual receptors are rarely stimulated in isolation except under laboratory conditions, and the CNS normally compares and combines information from multiple receptors to decide what is going on. For example, something touching the skin will stimulate several different kinds of receptors (see Fig. 9-1), whose combined outputs may lead to a sensation of not just touch but also the texture of the object.

Timing of a Stimulus

The duration of a stimulus is often encoded simply by the duration of a receptor potential. However, a little twist is added to duration coding by the fact that receptors usually do not respond in a constant way throughout a maintained stimulus. Although a few receptors interested in critical physiologic variables such as blood pH may provide a constant output reflecting the absolute value of a stimulus, sensory receptors typically adapt to some degree during a maintained stimulus. This shows up in common experiences, such as being dazzled only temporarily when stepping out of a dimly lit room into a more brightly lit space, adapting to the temperature of water that at first feels shockingly cold, and losing track of the constant touch of clothing. Adaptation phenomena such as these partly occur in the CNS, but partly reflect changes at the level of receptors themselves. In response to a constant stimulus, some receptors are slowly adapting and others are rapidly adapting (Fig. 4-8); some even adapt to such an extent that they completely shut down. Many rapidly adapting receptors encode the duration of a stimulus by signaling its beginning and its end. Receptor-level adaptation can be based on almost any conceivable aspect of receptor function (Fig. 4-9), from filtering stimuli before they even reach the receptor to effects on ion channels in the receptor. These mechanisms usually decrease the response of a receptor, but tissue damage can make nociceptors *more* sensitive (Fig. 4-10) to maintained or successive stimulation (again corresponding to common experience).

Amplitude of a Stimulus

Increasing intensity of a stimulus could theoretically be encoded either by having a homogeneous population of receptors produce larger and larger receptor potentials, or by having progressively less sensitive receptors become active (Fig. 4-11). In fact, both strategies are used. Grading the size of the receptor potential is typically the more important mechanism, but multiple receptor populations are also used; the most obvious example of the latter is the retina, where rods detect dim light and cones detect brighter light (see Chapter 12). The lowest stimulus intensity a subject can detect is termed the sensory threshold, which is determined partly by the sensitivity of receptors and partly by CNS mechanisms. Sensory thresholds are not invariant: they can be influenced by experience, fatigue, or the context in which the stimulus is presented. The threshold for pain, for example, is often raised in hazardous situations and lowered in situations where more pain is anticipated, by mechanisms described in Chapter 9.

Location of a Stimulus

Orderly mapping is a common wiring principle of the nervous system (see Figs. 9-5 and 12-13), so it is easy to imagine that the location of a stimulus is coded by the location of the

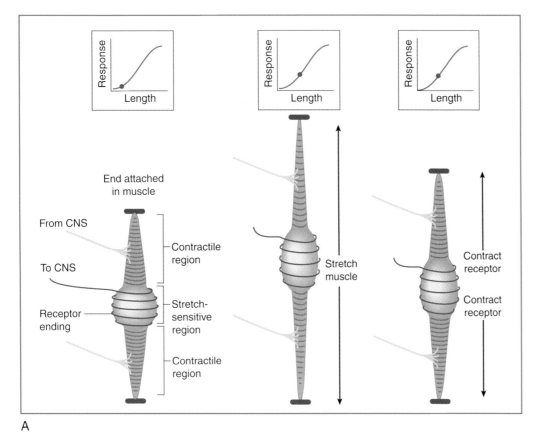

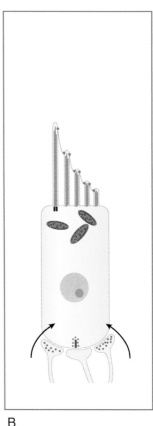

A

B

Figure 4-7. Control of the sensitivity of stretch receptors (**A**) and auditory receptors (**B**) by projections from the CNS. Skeletal muscle stretch receptors are based on small, special muscle fibers contained in muscle spindles (see Chapter 9). Each of these muscle fibers contains a central, stretch-sensitive, noncontractile region flanked by contractile zones (A1). The sensory part of the fiber can be stretched and thereby moved into a more sensitive part of its response range, either by stretch of the muscle (A2) or by stimulation of efferents to its contractile zones (A3). **B**, The sensitivity of many auditory receptors can be adjusted by inhibitory synapses made directly onto the receptors by efferents from the CNS (see Chapter 10).

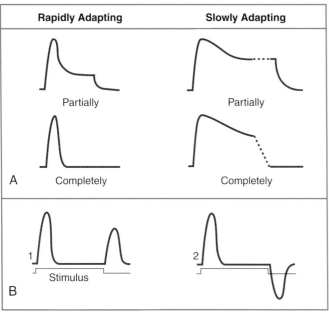

Figure 4-8. Adaptation in receptors. **A**, Although almost all receptors adapt to some degree, some are slowly adapting and may produce a substantial response throughout a maintained stimulus; others adapt rapidly and produce little or no sustained response. **B**, Receptors often produce a transiently enhanced response at the beginning and end of a stimulus. Sometimes (B1), as in pacinian corpuscles (see Chapter 9), the transient responses are in the same direction. In others (B2), such as many temperature receptors, the transient responses are in opposite directions.

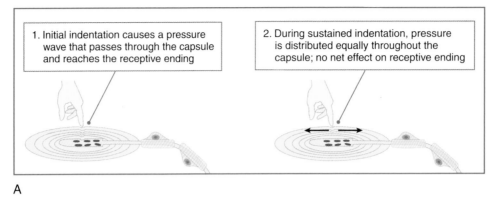

1. Initial indentation causes a pressure wave that passes through the capsule and reaches the receptive ending

2. During sustained indentation, pressure is distributed equally throughout the capsule; no net effect on receptive ending

A

1. Some channels open, some channels closed

2. All channels open

3. Channels move along cell membrane, decreasing effect of stimulation

B

1. Odorant binds to G-protein coupled receptor, cAMP synthesized, cation channels open, allowing Na$^+$ and Ca^{++} influx

Na$^+$
Ca^{++}

2. Increased [Ca^{++}] affects channels and enzymes

C

Figure 4-9. Three examples of receptor-level adaptation mechanisms. **A,** The capsule of pacinian corpuscles acts as a mechanical filter: the pressure change caused by an indenting mechanical stimulus initially is transmitted to the receptive ending but quickly becomes uniformly distributed throughout the fluids and cell layers of the capsule. **B,** Transduction channels of hair cells are connected to the cytoskeleton and to filamentous extracellular proteins. Increased tension on these filamentous proteins increases the probability of channel opening (B2). The tension is quickly relieved by movement of the transduction channels, ratcheted along by their cytoskeletal attachments (B3). **C,** Calcium entering through the transduction channels of olfactory (and other) receptors decreases the opening of channels and decreases the activity of enzymes activated by G proteins.

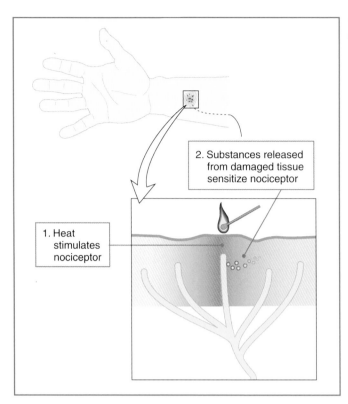

Figure 4-10. Substances released in response to tissue damage—histamine, serotonin, prostaglandins, and others—make nociceptive endings more sensitive to sustained or repeated stimuli.

2. Substances released from damaged tissue sensitize nociceptor

1. Heat stimulates nociceptor

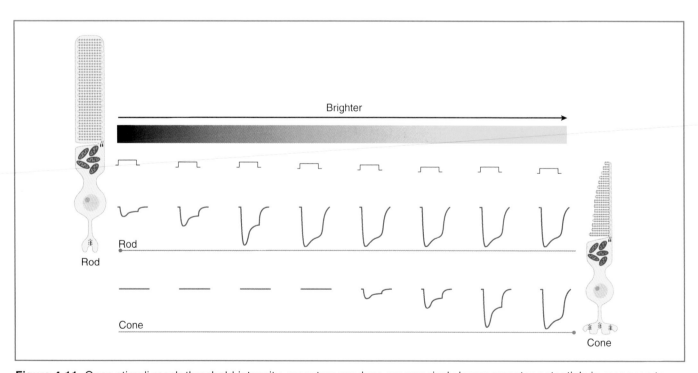

Brighter

Rod

Cone

Rod

Cone

Figure 4-11. Once stimuli reach threshold intensity, receptors produce progressively larger receptor potentials in response to stimuli of progressively greater magnitude, until saturation is reached. The threshold of retinal cones is near the level of light intensity at which rods saturate, allowing the retina to respond over a greater range of intensities than would be possible with rods or cones alone.

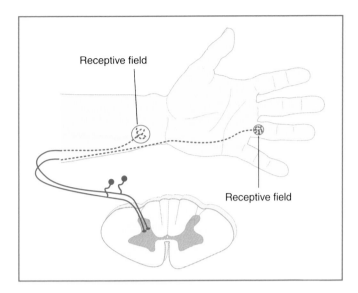

Figure 4-12. Cutaneous receptive fields of two touch receptors.

stimulated receptor. The location of a visual object is reflected in the locations of the photoreceptors that catch photons coming from it; each photoreceptor has a receptive field corresponding to some small area of the visual world. A similar strategy can yield the location of a tactile stimulus (i.e., tactile receptors have cutaneous receptive fields; Fig. 4-12), but localizing something like a sound, smell, or taste is trickier and requires some central processing. The notion of localization does not even make much sense for things like balance.

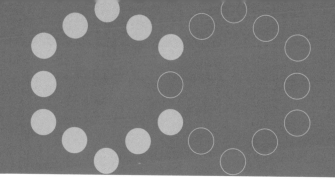

General Organization of the Nervous System

5

CONTENTS

The major parts of the CNS introduced in Chapter 1 have functions based on systematic patterns of connections. This chapter provides a preliminary look at these functions and patterns of connections and is largely the basis for the more detailed considerations of functional systems in Chapters 9–19.

●●● PLANES AND DIRECTIONS IN THE CENTRAL NERVOUS SYSTEM

Nervous systems are often studied, both experimentally and clinically, by slicing them up (either literally or virtually) in various planes. Most commonly used, and easiest to understand, are three sets of planes, each at right angles to the other two (Fig. 5-1). Coronal (or frontal) planes are parallel to the front of your face. Axial (or transverse, or horizontal) planes are more or less perpendicular to the long axis of your body. Several different variations of axial planes are used in clinical studies, based on anatomic landmarks, but for the purposes of this book they are all lumped together. Finally, sagittal planes are parallel to the one that divides your body into two symmetric halves.

Most vertebrates move through the world horizontally, with a CNS that is also laid out mostly horizontally. As a result, various directional terms have the same meaning for all parts of the body and CNS of a typical vertebrate (Fig. 5-2A). Dorsal ("toward the back") is the same direction as superior ("toward the sky"), and the dorsoventral axis is perpendicular to the anteroposterior axis. Rostral ("toward the beak") and caudal ("toward the tail") have roughly the same meaning as anterior and posterior. The upright posture of humans complicates this terminology a bit, because our heads move through the world horizontally like those of other vertebrates, but our bodies are vertical (see Fig. 5-2B). Superior continues to mean toward the sky, and anterior continues to be the direction in which we are heading. However, the bend between the long axis of the cerebrum and the long axis of the brainstem and spinal cord, the result of a flexure that forms during the development of the CNS (see Chapter 6), corresponds to a bend in the dorsoventral axis: dorsal is equivalent to posterior in the brainstem and spinal cord, but its meaning changes in the cerebrum, where it is equivalent to *superior*. In addition, the tremendously expanded growth of our cerebral hemispheres adds an element of confusion to the meaning of rostral and caudal. For the spinal cord and brainstem, it's easy: caudal means toward the sacral spinal cord and rostral means toward the midbrain. In the cerebrum, rostral should technically mean toward the nose. This would mean, for example, that the

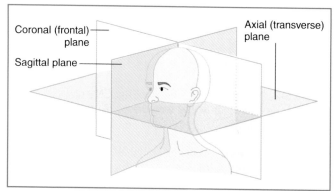

Figure 5-1. Planes commonly used to study the CNS (and other parts of the body).

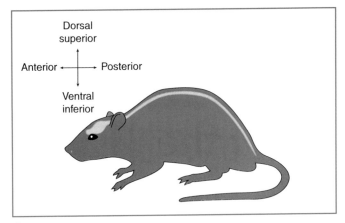

A

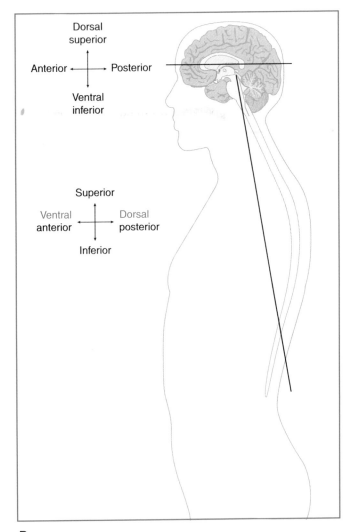

B

Figure 5-2. Directional terms used for the CNS of quadrupeds and other typical vertebrates (**A**) and for the CNS of humans (**B**).

diencephalon is rostral to the occipital lobes. However, rostral and caudal are often used in a more functional sense, referring to the way in which parts of the CNS develop as a linear sequence of structures (see Figs. 6-5 and 6-6). In this sense, all parts of the cerebral cortex are rostral to the diencephalon.

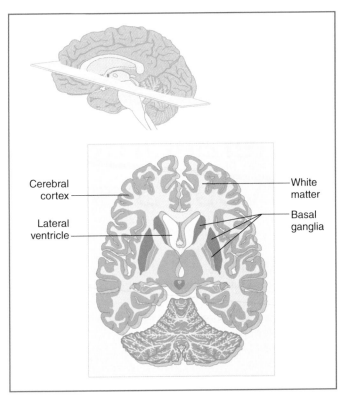

Figure 5-3. Arrangement of gray and white matter in the interior of the cerebral hemispheres.

●●● MAJOR STRUCTURES OF THE CEREBRAL HEMISPHERES

Each cerebral hemisphere includes a covering of cerebral cortex a few millimeters thick, a core of white matter interconnecting cortical areas with each other and with various subcortical structures, and areas of gray matter that are major components of the basal ganglia and limbic system (Fig. 5-3). In addition, as described further in Chapters 6 and 7, the CNS develops from a hollow epithelial tube, and fluid-filled remnants of the cavity of the tube extend through most parts of the adult CNS. The portion in each cerebral hemisphere is a lateral ventricle (see Fig. 7-9).

Cerebral Cortex

Cerebral cortex covers nearly the entire surface of each cerebral hemisphere. Almost all of this is neocortex, so named because it has a six-layered structure found only in mammals. (The hippocampus and some small olfactory areas have a different, simpler structure that merges with neocortex through transitional areas of cortex.) Humans have much more neocortex than most other mammals do, and the human brain is prominently corrugated into a series of gyri and sulci to accommodate this increased area. Three prominent sulci—the central, lateral, and parieto-occipital sulci—are used as landmarks to divide each hemisphere into frontal, parietal, occipital, and temporal lobes (Fig. 5-4). In addition, the corpus callosum, a thick fiber bundle interconnecting the two hemispheres, is

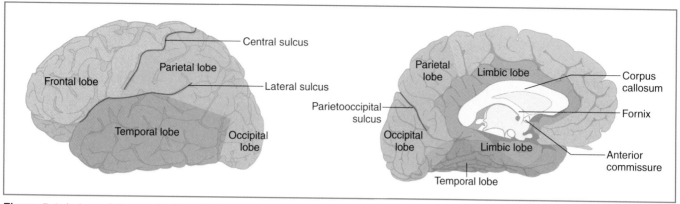

Figure 5-4. Lobes of the cerebral hemisphere as seen on the lateral and medial surfaces.

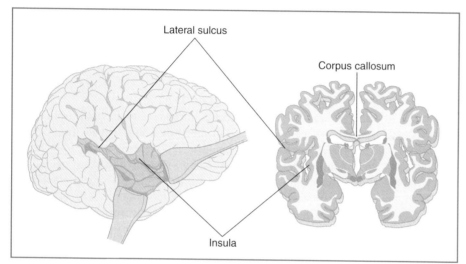

Figure 5-5. The insula, as seen by prying open the lateral sulcus and in a coronal section.

nearly encircled by a ring of cortex often recognized as a distinct limbic lobe (see Fig. 5-4). Finally, the insula is a separate area of cortex, not part of any of these lobes, buried in the lateral sulcus (Fig. 5-5).

The configuration of gyri and sulci is similar from one brain to another, and many of those in the frontal, parietal, temporal, and limbic lobes have commonly used names (Fig. 5-6).

Neocortical Structure

There are two main classes of cortical neurons (Fig. 5-7)—pyramidal cells and a diverse class of nonpyramidal cells. Pyramidal cells are more numerous and often fairly large, many with cell bodies in the 30- to 40-μm range (the largest are 100 μm or so). As the name implies, pyramidal cells are somewhat conical; the apex points toward the cortical surface, and emits a long apical dendrite that extends to the most superficial cortical layer. Additional basal dendrites emerge from the base of the pyramid and extend horizontally in the cortex. Pyramidal cells are the principal output neurons of the cortex; they all make excitatory (glutamate) synapses on their targets. The neurons whose axons cross in the corpus callosum, for example, are pyramidal cells. Many nonpyramidal cells are small, multipolar neurons with relatively short

axons. Others have a variety of distinctive shapes, but few have axons that leave the cortex. Collectively, nonpyramidal cells are the principal interneurons of the cortex, helping to process information in small cortical areas; most of them make inhibitory (GABA) synapses on their targets.

The basal and apical dendrites of pyramidal cells reflect two perpendicular directions of cortical organization: pyramidal and nonpyramidal cells are arranged anatomically in layers parallel to the cortical surface, but they are also organized functionally into columns about 50 to 500 μm wide. The most superficial cortical layer contains few neurons and is primarily a place where synaptic interactions occur, e.g., as certain incoming fibers end on the apical dendrites of pyramidal

---

PHARMACOLOGY

Uses of Barbiturates

Barbiturates are agonists at ionotropic GABA receptors, so they suppress cortical activity, making them useful as antianxiety and antiseizure drugs.

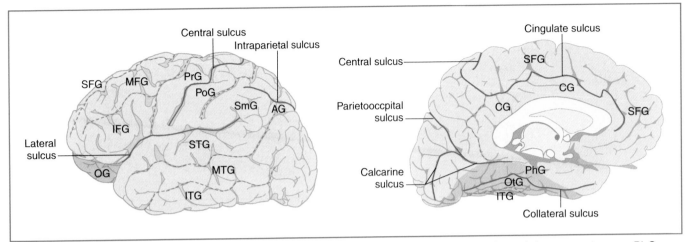

Figure 5-6. Major sulci and gyri. AG, angular gyrus; CG, cingulate gyrus; OG, orbital gyri; OtG, occipitotemporal gyrus; PhG, parahippocampal gyrus; PoG, postcentral gyrus; PrG, precentral gyrus; SFG, MFG, IFG, superior, middle, and inferior frontal gyri; SmG, supramarginal gyrus; STG, MTG, ITG, superior, middle, and inferior temporal gyri.

cells. Beneath this layer are four alternating layers with different proportions of cell types (layers III and V are mostly pyramidal cells, layer IV mostly nonpyramidal cells, and layer II a mix of nonpyramidal cells and small pyramidal cells). Finally, layer VI is a mix of pyramidal cells and other cell types. The layering is a mechanism for sorting inputs and outputs, and each layer has a distinctive pattern of connections. For example, many incoming fibers from subcortical sites end in layer IV; the pyramidal cells in layer III send their axons to other cortical areas; and the pyramidal cells in layer V send their axons to the basal ganglia, brainstem, and spinal cord.

Cortical columns, in contrast, run perpendicular to the surface of the brain. The columns in visual cortex (see Chapter 12), in which most of the neurons in any vertical array have similar functional properties, are the most obvious and best understood, but the same sort of arrangement is found in other sensory areas of cortex. This kind of columnar organization is probably a general feature of neocortex. Even in areas where the functional properties of the neurons are difficult to define, columns can be demonstrated anatomically: tracers injected into such areas are transported down the axons of pyramidal cells and wind up in terminals arranged in 50- to 500-μm wide columns in other cortical areas.

Columns are one manifestation of a modular organization of neocortex. Beneath each square millimeter of almost all parts of the cerebral surface of any mammal lie nearly the same number of neurons, about 75% of them pyramidal cells. The size and complexity of the cells and the numbers of synapses vary from area to area and from species to species, but the basic construction and patterns of connections are constant; the details of the inputs and outputs of a given module determine its functional role. Presumably, the processing power of human cerebral hemispheres is based largely on an increased number of modules contained in an expanded cortical surface.

Neocortical Connections

Each area of neocortex receives inputs both from other cortical areas and from subcortical sites. Inputs from cortical areas in the same hemisphere (Fig. 5-8) arrive from neighboring areas via short U-fibers that dip under just one or two sulci, and from faraway areas through longer association bundles. The arcuate fasciculus, for example, is an association bundle that arcs above the insula and interconnects anterior and posterior parts of a hemisphere. Inputs from cortical areas in the contralateral hemisphere arrive through two commissures. (A commissure is a set of crossing axons that interconnect similar areas of the CNS. In contrast, a decussation is a site where axons cross the midline on their way from one part of the CNS to a different part.) The corpus callosum (see Figs. 5-4 and 5-8) is the largest commissure in the human CNS, interconnecting most areas of each hemisphere's cortex with mirror-image and related sites in the contralateral hemisphere. The major exception is the temporal lobe, which sends many of its interconnecting fibers through the anterior commissure (see Fig. 5-4) instead.

Subcortical inputs, described later in this chapter, arise primarily in the thalamus and in a series of small nuclei, most of them in the brainstem, that provide widespread modulatory inputs.

Cortical pyramidal cells project to other cortical areas but also influence many other areas of the CNS by projecting to a wide variety of subcortical sites—parts of the basal ganglia and limbic system, the thalamus, numerous brainstem nuclei, and the spinal cord—as detailed in subsequent chapters.

Cortical Maps

Despite the modular structure of neocortex, different areas have somewhat different appearances, often in ways consistent with what they do. For example, areas that give rise to particularly long axons have populations of large pyramidal cells and as a result are thicker than other areas. Various

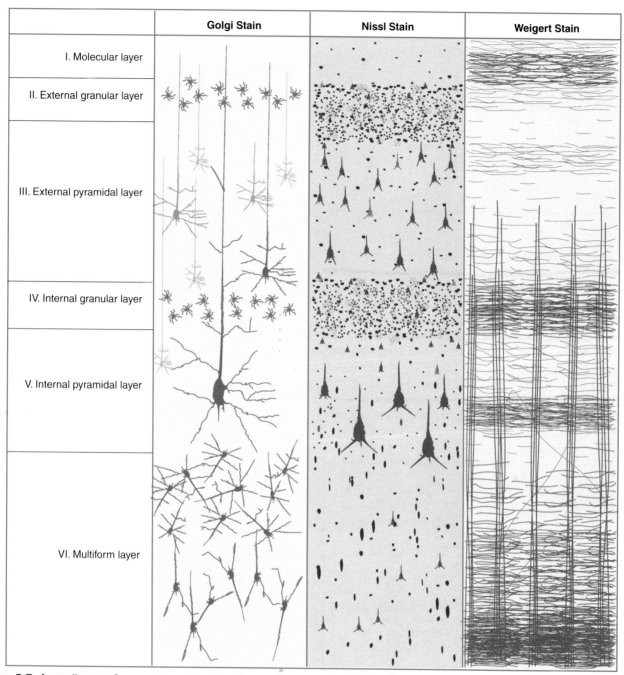

	Golgi Stain	Nissl Stain	Weigert Stain
I. Molecular layer			
II. External granular layer			
III. External pyramidal layer			
IV. Internal granular layer			
V. Internal pyramidal layer			
VI. Multiform layer			

Figure 5-7. A small area of neocortex, stained by three different methods. The Golgi stain reveals details of the shapes of a few neurons and leaves the others unstained. The Nissl stain shows the cell bodies of all neurons, revealing how different types are distributed among the six layers. The Weigert stain for myelin (see Fig. 1-4) demonstrates vertically oriented bundles of axons entering and leaving the cortex, and horizontally coursing fibers that interconnect neurons within a layer. (Based on Brodmann K. Vergleichende Lokalisation lehre der Grosshirnrinde in ihren Prinzipien dargestellt auf Grund des Zellenbaues, Leipzig, JA Barth, 1909.)

people over the years have utilized such variations to construct anatomic maps of the cerebral cortex, using criteria such as the sizes of different cell types and the thickness of different layers to divide it up into areas. Many of the differences are subtle, but some of these anatomically defined areas correspond to areas with a particular functional significance. The mapping system in most common usage parcels the neocortex into a series of Brodmann's areas, based on a numerical system devised by Brodmann early in the 20th century.

Functional Localization

Neocortex can be carved up in a functional sense into primary areas, unimodal association areas, multimodal association areas, and limbic areas. Primary areas (Fig. 5-9) account for a rela-

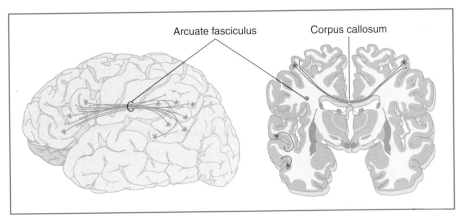

Figure 5-8. Fibers interconnecting cortical areas. The arcuate fasciculus is shown as an example of a long association bundle. In addition, many fibers interconnecting the temporal lobes travel through the anterior commissure rather than the corpus callosum.

tively small proportion of human neocortex, but they deal most directly with elemental functions like somatic sensation, vision, and voluntary movement. Adjacent to or near each primary area are unimodal association areas (see Fig. 5-9) that receive major inputs from the primary area and work on more complex or refined aspects of the same function. For example, different areas of visual association cortex specialize in analyzing the shape, color, or movement of objects (see Fig. 12-16).

Multimodal association areas (Fig. 5-10) receive major inputs from unimodal areas of multiple types, and they are critically involved in the higher cognitive functions described in Chapter 19. The two major expanses of multimodal association cortex are the parts of the frontal lobe anterior to motor association areas (prefrontal cortex) and the parts of the parietal and temporal lobes bordered by somatosensory, visual, and auditory association cortex. Finally, limbic areas of cortex (see Fig. 5-10), including the cingulate and parahippocampal gyri, orbital and anterior temporal cortex, and much of the insula, receive converging inputs from multimodal areas and from other parts of the limbic system. These connections, together with projections back to multimodal areas, allow limbic cortex

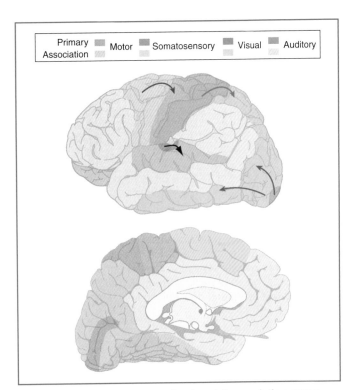

Figure 5-9. Primary areas and unimodal association areas. Unimodal areas receive major inputs (*arrows*) from primary areas (or, in the case of motor association areas, provide major inputs *to* primary motor cortex). Additional primary and unimodal areas are touched on in subsequent chapters, e.g., taste cortex in the insula.

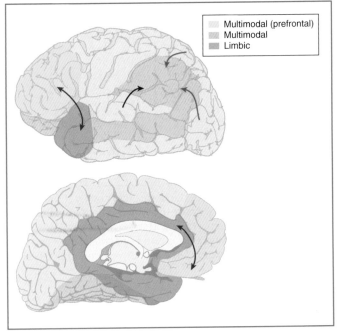

Figure 5-10. Multimodal association areas and limbic areas. To keep things simple, converging projections (*single-headed arrows*) from unimodal areas are shown only for the parietotemporal multimodal area, although the same is true of prefrontal cortex. Similarly, both multimodal areas are interconnected with limbic cortex, but this is shown only for prefrontal cortex (*double-headed arrows*).

to play an important role in directing behavior by helping determine emotional and motivational states.

Basal Ganglia

The basal ganglia (also, and more appropriately, called the basal nuclei), a group of nuclei and their interconnections located partially in the cerebrum and partially in the brainstem, are prominently involved in the initiation and control of movement but actually play a much broader role in cerebral functions. The major elements of the basal ganglia situated in each cerebral hemisphere are the caudate nucleus (named for its long, curving tail), putamen, and globus pallidus (Fig. 5-11). Although they have different patterns of connections, the putamen and globus pallidus together are referred to as the lenticular nucleus because of their physical adjacency. As described further in Chapter 15, the basal ganglia function by affecting the output of the cerebral cortex (see Fig. 5-11). The caudate nucleus and putamen are the major input structures, receiving projections from the cerebral cortex; the globus pallidus is the major output structure, projecting back to the cortex by way of the thalamus. Since this circuit of basal ganglia connections does not cross the midline, it winds up affecting cortex on the ipsilateral side. Because each cerebral hemisphere controls muscles on the contralateral side of the body, unilateral damage to the basal ganglia affects movements on the contralateral side.

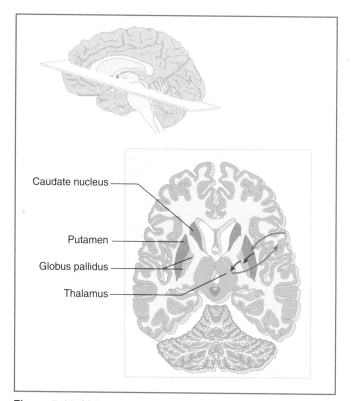

Figure 5-11. Major components of the basal ganglia in each cerebral hemisphere, and some of their principal connections. Only projections from cortex to putamen are indicated, but the caudate nucleus is part of a similar cortex/caudate/globus pallidus/thalamus/cortex loop involving different cortical areas.

Limbic System

The limbic system (see Chapter 18), a collective term for limbic areas of cortex, together with the hippocampus, the amygdala, and some diencephalic structures, is centrally involved in drives, emotions, and some forms of memory. The hippocampus (Fig. 5-12), named for its fancied resemblance to a seahorse, is a strip of three-layered cortex rolled into the medial part of the temporal (or limbic) lobe but still continuous with the parahippocampal gyrus. The amygdala (see Fig. 5-12), in contrast, is a collection of nuclei at the anterior end of the hippocampus.

●●● DIENCEPHALON

The diencephalon (Fig. 5-13), interposed between the cerebral hemispheres and the brainstem, includes the pineal

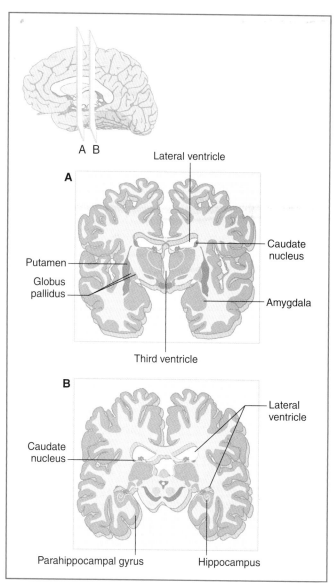

Figure 5-12. The amygdala and hippocampus, major components of the limbic system in each cerebral hemisphere, as seen in coronal sections.

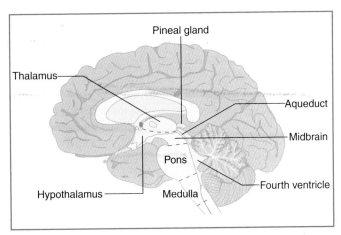

Figure 5-13. Major components of the diencephalon and brainstem.

gland, thalamus, hypothalamus, and a few other nuclei not visible except in sections; its portion of the ventricular system is the third ventricle, a midline slit (see Fig. 5-12). The pineal is a neuroendocrine gland involved in circadian rhythms and seasonal cycles. The thalamus and hypothalamus are groups of nuclei, each group having a distinctive function.

Thalamus

Although there are a variety of diffuse modulatory projections (introduced later in this chapter) to the cerebral cortex, almost all specific functional pathways reach the cortex only after passing through the thalamus. The job of the thalamus is not to do much processing of information but rather to act as a bank of switches that regulate the access of these functional pathways to their cortical targets.

Physiology of the Thalamus

With the exception of a meshwork of neurons and white matter (the reticular nucleus) that covers the lateral and anterior surfaces of the thalamus, all thalamic nuclei are constructed and behave similarly (Fig. 5-14). Most of the neurons are thalamocortical neurons whose axons synapse directly in the cerebral cortex. Their switch function is based on the two stable physiologic states in which these neurons can exist. Much of the time they are in a tonic mode that is well suited for the accurate transmission of incoming data. In this state, thalamocortical neurons behave like the prototypical neurons described in Chapter 2, producing a steady stream of action potentials in response to maintained depolarization. However, slight hyperpolarization deinactivates a population of voltage-gated Ca^{++} channels and moves thalamocortical neurons into a burst mode that is less well suited for accurate data transmission. The voltage-gated Ca^{++} channels behave like the voltage-gated Na^+ channels that underlie typical action potentials, but on a slower time scale. Depolarizing a neuron in burst mode causes the voltage-gated Ca^{++} channels to open, then inactivate and close, resulting in a depolarizing, Ca^{++}-based wave that carries the membrane potential through threshold and causes a brief burst of Na^+-based action potentials (see Fig. 5-14). The slow time course of the opening/inactivation/deinactivation cycle of the voltage-gated Ca^{++} channels results in a refractory period of about 100 ms, so Ca^{++}-based waves and bursts of action potentials can recur only about 10 times per second. The functional significance of the burst mode is still uncertain, but the probability of a neuron being in this state increases in states of sleep or diminished attention.

Connections of the Thalamus

Corresponding to these two physiologic states, each thalamocortical neuron receives two kinds of inputs—specific

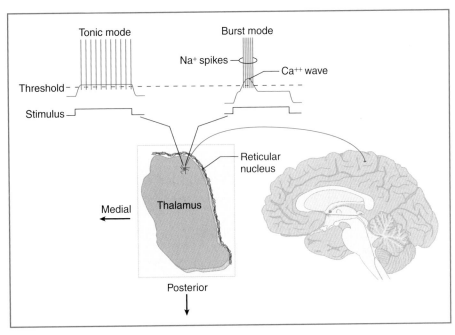

Figure 5-14. An axial section through the thalamus, showing the location of the reticular nucleus and the physiologic states of thalamocortical neurons.

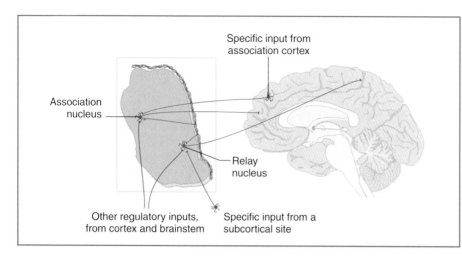

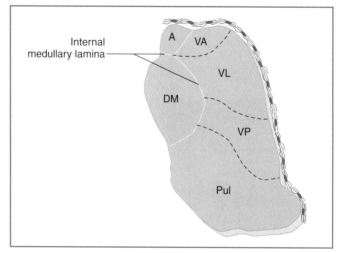

Figure 5-15. Thalamocortical neurons in relay and association nuclei. Both types of nucleus receive some regulatory inputs from the reticular nucleus and others, some excitatory and some inhibitory, from the cerebral cortex and the brainstem. The balance of these regulatory inputs determines the physiologic state of a given neuron. The major difference is the source of specific inputs, which come from a variety of subcortical sites in the case of relay nuclei, but from association cortex for association nuclei.

inputs conveying the information that *can* be passed along accurately to the cortex, and regulatory inputs that collectively determine the physiologic state of the neuron (i.e., *whether* the information gets passed along faithfully). Most thalamic nuclei (other than the reticular nucleus) fall into one of two categories, based on the source of their specific inputs (Fig. 5-15). Relay nuclei receive specific inputs from subcortical structures and project to primary and unimodal association areas; this is how information from sensory systems, the basal ganglia, cerebellum, and some limbic structures reaches the cortex. Association nuclei, in contrast, receive specific inputs primarily from association cortex and project back to association cortex; they provide a mechanism for controlling connections between cortical areas. Regulatory inputs are provided to both kinds of thalamic nuclei by the thalamic reticular nucleus (see Fig. 5-15), by diffuse modulatory projections from the brainstem, and by the cerebral cortex itself.

Thalamic Nuclei

A thin layer of white matter (the internal medullary lamina) partitions the thalamus into anterior, medial, and lateral divisions (Fig. 5-16). The anterior and medial divisions contain one large nucleus apiece, the anterior and dorsomedial nuclei, respectively. The larger lateral division includes three nuclei arranged in an anteroposterior sequence—the ventral anterior (VA), ventral lateral (VL), and ventral posterior (VP) nuclei, followed by the pulvinar, the largest nucleus in the thalamus. Appended to the bottom of the pulvinar is a little curved extension containing the medial geniculate nucleus (MGN) and lateral geniculate nucleus (LGN).

Each of these nuclei has a specific pattern of connections (Fig. 5-17 and Table 5-1). The dorsomedial nucleus and pulvinar are the association nuclei for prefrontal cortex and for parietal-occipital-temporal association areas, respectively. All the rest are relay nuclei: VP, MGN, and LGN for the somatosensory, auditory, and visual systems; VA and VL for the basal ganglia and cerebellum; and the anterior nucleus for the hippocampus.

Internal Capsule

Thalamocortical axons, together with the axons of cortical pyramidal cells on their way to subcortical sites, funnel into a

small cleft bordered laterally by the lenticular nucleus and medially by the thalamus and caudate nucleus. Here they form the internal capsule (Fig. 5-18), a sheet of fibers that partially encapsulates the lenticular nucleus. The internal capsule is divided into parts based on their relationship to the lenticular nucleus and its neighbors: an anterior limb between the lenticular and caudate nuclei, a posterior limb between the lenticular nucleus and the thalamus, a genu at the junction between the anterior and posterior limbs, a retrolenticular part just behind the lenticular nucleus, and a sublenticular part that dips underneath the most posterior part of the lenticular nucleus. In general, the content of each of these parts is predictable, based on its relationship to the thalamus and various cortical areas (Table 5-2).

Hypothalamus

The hypothalamus is the major control center for the autonomic nervous system (ANS) and for drive-related behavior

Figure 5-16. Topographic arrangement of major thalamic nuclei (the lateral and medial geniculate nuclei are inferior to this plane of section). A, anterior nucleus; DM, dorsomedial nucleus; Pul, pulvinar; VA, ventral anterior nucleus; VL, ventral lateral nucleus; VP, ventral posterior nucleus (commonly subdivided into a lateral and medial part, VPL and VPM, as discussed in Chapter 9).

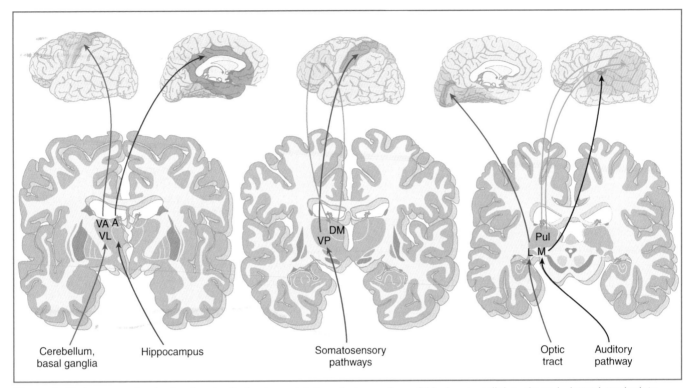

Figure 5-17. Inputs and outputs of major thalamic nuclei. A, anterior nucleus; DM, dorsomedial nucleus; L, lateral geniculate nucleus; M, medial geniculate nucleus; Pul, pulvinar; VA, ventral anterior nucleus; VL, ventral lateral nucleus; VP, ventral posterior nucleus.

TABLE 5-1. Connections of Major Thalamic Nuclei

Name	Type	Input from	Output to
Anterior	Relay	Mammillothalamic tract	Cingulate gyrus
Dorsomedial	Association	Prefrontal cortex	Prefrontal cortex
Lateral geniculate	Relay	Optic tract	Visual cortex
Medial geniculate	Relay	Inferior brachium	Auditory cortex
Pulvinar	Association	Parietal/occipital/temporal association cortex	Parietal/occipital/temporal association cortex
Ventral anterior, ventral lateral	Relay	Cerebellum, basal ganglia	Motor cortex, motor association cortex
Ventral posterior	Relay	Somatosensory pathways	Postcentral gyrus
Reticular		Cerebral cortex, other thalamic nuclei	Other thalamic nuclei

TABLE 5-2. Principal Contents of Parts of the Internal Capsule*

Part of Internal Capsule	To and from Thalamic Nuclei	To Other Subcortical Sites
Anterior limb	Anterior nucleus Dorsomedial nucleus	Prefrontal to pons[†]
Posterior limb	Ventral anterior nucleus Ventral lateral nucleus Ventral posterior nucleus Pulvinar	Motor neurons in the spinal cord and brainstem Frontal, parietal to pons[†]
Retrolenticular part	Lateral geniculate nucleus Pulvinar	Parietal, occipital to pons[†]
Sublenticular part	Lateral geniculate nucleus Medial geniculate nucleus Pulvinar	Temporal to pons[†]

*The genu is not indicated, because it is essentially a transition zone between the anterior and posterior limbs.
[†]And from there to the cerebellum (see Chapter 16).

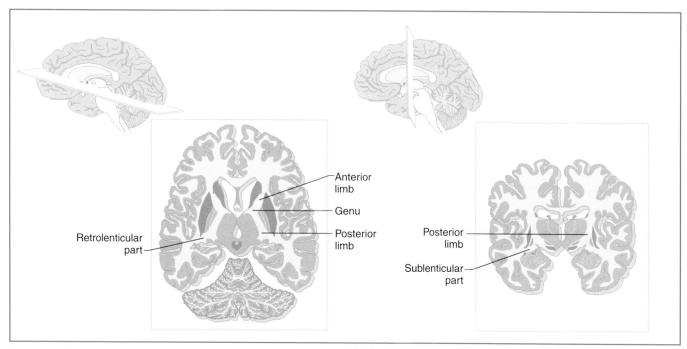

Figure 5-18. Internal capsule, as seen in axial (*left*) and coronal (*right*) sections.

in general (hunger, thirst, sex, temperature regulation, etc.). As described in more detail in Chapter 18, it accomplishes this by monitoring the status of the body through visceral and other inputs, then affecting behavior and physiology in three different ways: neuroendocrine control via the pituitary gland, projections to autonomic motor neurons, and interactions with the limbic system that influence motivation and behavior (Fig. 5-19).

●●● BRAINSTEM

Many structures are packed together in the brainstem: long tracts on their way to the thalamus, long tracts on their way downstream from the cerebral cortex and other places, and

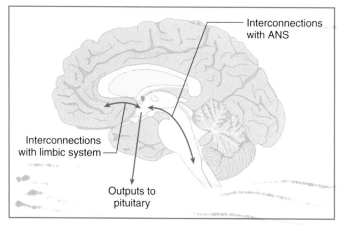

Figure 5-19. General pattern of connections of the hypothalamus. ANS, autonomic nervous system.

tracts and nuclei related to cranial nerves, all embedded in a neural matrix called the reticular formation (which has some distinctive functions of its own). Some general aspects of brainstem anatomy are presented here, to be revisited in subsequent chapters as parts of functional systems.

External Anatomy of the Brainstem

The brainstem (see Fig. 5-13) is subdivided into the midbrain (continuous with the diencephalon), pons, and medulla (continuous with the spinal cord). Each subdivision is characterized by a set of surface landmarks and cranial nerve (CN) attachment points (Fig. 5-20).

Midbrain

Dorsally are two pairs of bumps, the superior and inferior colliculi (Latin *colliculus*, "little hill"). On the ventral surface are two massive fiber bundles, the cerebral peduncles, separated by a cleft into which the oculomotor nerve (CN III) emerges. The trochlear nerve (CN IV) leaves dorsally (the only one to do so) at the junction between the midbrain and pons. The third ventricle funnels down into a small canal, the cerebral aqueduct, which traverses the midbrain.

Pons

The pons (Latin for "bridge") was named after the basal pons, a large bulge on its anterior surface that looks as if it interconnects the two halves of the cerebellum. (In fact, the interconnection is between one side of the pons and the other side of the cerebellum; see Fig. 5-24.) Posteriorly, three cerebellar peduncles tether the cerebellum to the brainstem, conveying cerebellar inputs and outputs. The trigeminal nerve

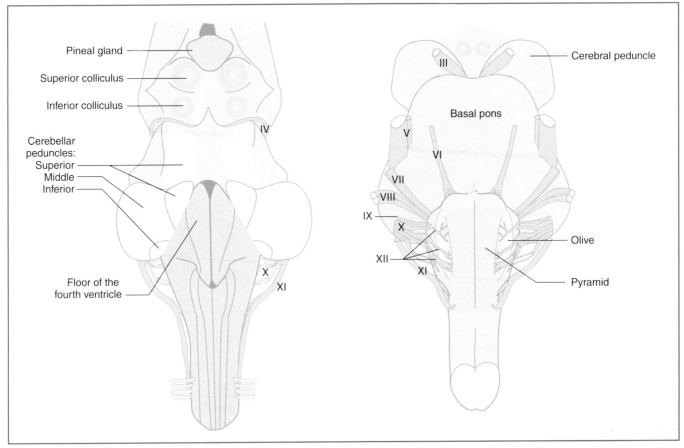

Figure 5-20. Surface features of the brainstem, as seen in a posterior view (*left*) and an anterior view (*right*).

(CN V) is attached to the side of the pons at a midpontine level, and the abducens, facial, and vestibulocochlear nerves (CNs VI, VII, and VIII) emerge at the junction between the pons and medulla. The aqueduct opens up into the fourth ventricle, which extends through the entire length of the pons and into the medulla.

Medulla

The pyramids form two longitudinal elevations on the anterior surface of the medulla, in line with the cerebral peduncles but smaller. Just lateral and posterior to each pyramid in the rostral half of the medulla is an ovoid bump called the olive. The glossopharyngeal and vagus nerves (CNs IX and X) emerge as a series of filaments just dorsal to the olive; the hypoglossal nerve (CN XII) emerges as another series of filaments in the groove between the pyramid and the olive. The accessory nerve (CN XI) arises from upper levels of the spinal cord but then moves up alongside the medulla. The fourth ventricle continues into the rostral half of the medulla, then narrows into a microscopically small central canal that continues into the spinal cord.

Internal Anatomy of the Brainstem

The interior of the brainstem is a combination of the neural structures underlying the surface features just described, long

tracts, and sensory and motor nuclei dealing with CNs III to XII, all surrounding or embedded in the reticular formation (Fig. 5-21).

Cranial Nerves

Cranial nerves fall into three different categories (Table 5-3). Some (I, II, and VIII) are special sensory nerves, dealing with the senses of olfaction, vision, and hearing/balance. Others (III, IV, VI, and XII) are somatic motor nerves, primarily or exclusively conveying axons of motor neurons for skeletal muscles. The remaining nerves (V, VII, IX, X, and XI) also innervate skeletal muscle, but in this case muscles derived embryologically from branchial arches, so they are often referred to as branchiomeric nerves; all but one of them contain additional components. All are discussed in more detail in subsequent chapters, but a brief account of their major functions is included here.

Cranial nerve I (olfactory). CN I is the special sensory nerve containing the axons of olfactory receptor neurons in the olfactory mucosa; they penetrate the base of the skull and terminate in the olfactory bulb. CN I is the only cranial nerve that projects directly to a cerebral hemisphere, so it breaks some rules—its information reaches the ipsilateral cerebral cortex, and it does so without passing through the thalamus.

Cranial nerve II (optic). CN II consists of the axons of ganglion cells, the output cells of the retina. Half of them

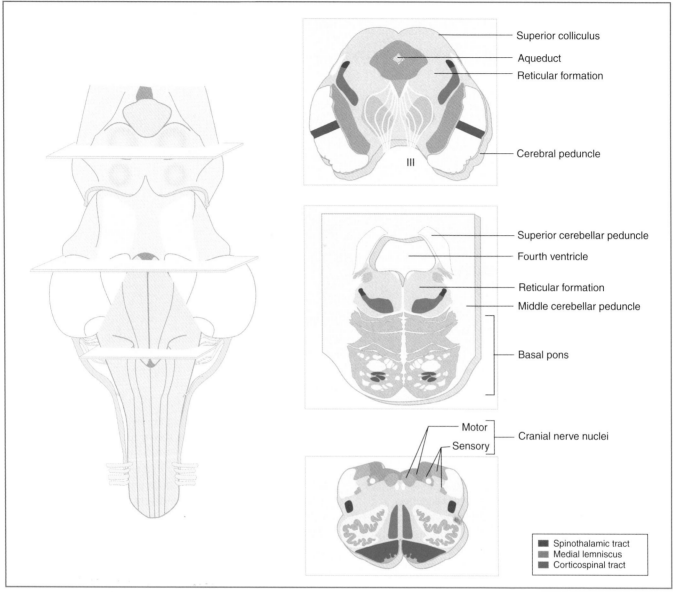

Figure 5-21. Internal anatomy of the brainstem, showing the locations of the reticular formation and some long tracts, and the way in which surface features are reflected in the internal anatomy. The corticospinal tract, the major descending pathway carrying instructions for voluntary movements to spinal cord motor neurons, is discussed in Chapter 14. The medial lemniscus and spinothalamic tract convey touch/position and pain/temperature information, respectively, to the thalamus. Both are discussed in Chapter 9.

cross in the optic chiasm, and then the crossed and uncrossed fibers regroup as the optic tract and project to the lateral geniculate nucleus (and to a few other sites in the CNS). Anatomically, it's a tract of the CNS.

Cranial nerve III (oculomotor). CN III is the motor nerve for four of the six extraocular muscles and the principal muscle that raises the eyelid. CN III is unlike the other somatic motor nerves in that it also contains a contingent of preganglionic autonomic fibers, those responsible for constricting the pupil and for adjusting the focus of the lens.

Cranial nerve IV (trochlear). CN IV is the motor nerve for the superior oblique, one of the extraocular muscles. It got its name because the tendon of the superior oblique

passes through the trochlea, a connective tissue pulley (Greek, *trochlea*, "pulley"), before inserting in the wall of the eye.

Cranial nerve V (trigeminal). CN V is the principal somatosensory nerve for the face and the motor nerve for the muscles used for chewing.

Cranial nerve VI (abducens). CN VI is the motor nerve for the lateral rectus, which moves the eye laterally. (Latin, *abducens*, "leading away.")

Cranial nerve VII (facial). CN VII is the motor nerve for facial muscles and the sensory nerve for taste buds on the anterior two thirds of the tongue.

Cranial nerve VIII (vestibulocochlear). CN VIII is the sensory nerve for hearing and balance. Unlike CNs I and II, it includes a contingent of efferent fibers that synapse on

TABLE 5-3. Major Contents of Cranial Nerves*

Cranial Nerve	Preganglionic Parasympathetics for	Motor Axons to	Primary Afferents from
I (olfactory)			Olfactory receptors
II (optic)			Retina
III (oculomotor)	Pupillary sphincter, ciliary muscle	All extraocular muscles except lateral rectus and superior oblique	
IV (trochlear)		Superior oblique	
V (trigeminal)		Muscles of mastication	Face, dura mater of the head
VI (abducens)		Lateral rectus	
VII (facial)		Muscles of facial expression	Taste buds
VIII (vestibulocochlear)			Inner ear
IX (glossopharyngeal)			Taste buds, heart
X (vagus)	Thoracic and abdominal viscera	Larynx and pharynx	Thoracic and abdominal viscera
XI (accessory)		Trapezius, sternocleidomastoid	
XII (hypoglossal)		Tongue	

*Relatively minor, although often functionally important, components are not included in the table but are discussed in subsequent chapters. For example, the facial and glossopharyngeal nerves contain preganglionic parasympathetics for salivary and lacrimal glands, and the vestibulocochlear nerve contains efferent fibers that regulate the sensitivity of receptor cells in the inner ear.

cochlear and vestibular receptor cells and regulate their sensitivity.

Cranial nerve IX (glossopharyngeal). CN IX innervates the taste buds on the posterior third of the tongue and is the most important nerve for taste. It also contains some visceral sensory fibers important for cardiovascular function.

Cranial nerve X (vagus). Vagus means "wanderer," and CN X was so named because its preganglionic autonomic and visceral afferent fibers wander throughout the thoracic and abdominal cavities. It also contains the motor axons for striated muscles of the larynx and pharynx.

Cranial nerve XI (accessory). CN XI originates from the spinal cord but is nevertheless considered a cranial nerve, in part because it ascends into the skull and leaves with the vagus nerve. CN XI is the motor nerve for muscles that shrug the shoulder and turn the head. (Some accounts of cranial nerves include a portion of the motor axons for pharyngeal and laryngeal muscles as the cranial part of the accessory nerve; in this book, all such fibers are considered part of the vagus.)

Cranial nerve XII (hypoglossal). CN XII is the motor nerve for most tongue muscles.

Cranial Nerve Nuclei

The sensory and motor neurons that receive or give rise to the axons in cranial nerves III to XII reside in a fairly systematically arranged set of nuclei in the brainstem (and, in the case of CN XI, the upper cervical spinal cord). All are located relatively close to the aqueduct, fourth ventricle, or central canal. At least to a first approximation, each is located at a longitudinal brainstem level close to the attachment point of its cranial nerve; e.g., the hypoglossal, trochlear, and oculomotor nuclei are in the rostral medulla, caudal midbrain, and rostral midbrain, respectively. (However, some sets of cranial nerve nuclei are more extensive than this, extending rostrally or caudally beyond the cranial nerve's level of attachment; the trigeminal and vestibular nuclei, considered in more detail in Chapters 9 and 11, are two prominent examples.) Finally, because of the way sensory and motor neurons in the CNS develop (see Fig. 6-12), cranial nerve sensory nuclei are typically located lateral to motor nuclei.

Reticular Formation

Reticular means "like a fine network," and the reticular formation was named for its appearance as a seemingly diffuse network of neurons and connections occupying much of the core of the brainstem (see Fig. 5-21). Although it contains dozens of nuclei and their interconnections, neither the nuclei nor the tracts of the reticular formation are as compact as most of those related to cranial nerves or long tracts. Despite the diffuse appearance, however, different regions of the reticular formation are specialized for particular functions. Some of its nuclei give rise to widespread modulatory projections that regulate levels of consciousness and alertness and play a critical role in sleep-wake cycles (see Chapter 19). Prominent among these are the locus ceruleus (Latin, "blue place," named for its pigmented neurons) of the rostral pons and the midline raphe nuclei, which distribute norepinephrine and serotonin, respectively, to large expanses of the cerebrum (Figs. 5-22 and 5-23). Other regions of the reticular formation, discussed in later chapters, are important in the control of movement and of visceral functions. Finally,

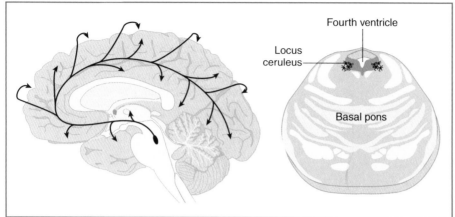

Figure 5-22. Location (*right*) and projections (arrows, *left*) of the locus ceruleus, the major collection of norepinephrine-containing (noradrenergic) neurons in the brainstem. Additional noradrenergic neurons (not shown), mostly in more caudal levels of the reticular formation, provide similarly widespread projections to the cerebellum and spinal cord.

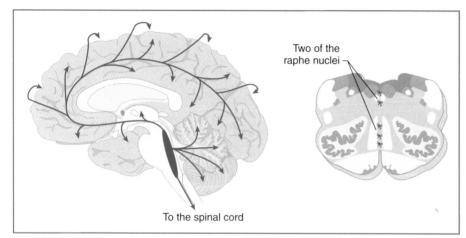

Figure 5-23. The raphe nuclei have serotonin-containing neurons with widespread projections throughout the CNS. Although only the rostral medulla is shown, these are a series of plate-like nuclei near the midline at most levels of the brainstem.

parts of the reticular formation control the flow of information through some sensory and reflex pathways; a prominent example is the modulation of transmission of pain and temperature information (see Fig. 9-9).

CEREBELLUM

Humans have not only a great deal of neocortex but also a very large cerebellum that roofs the fourth ventricle and spreads superiorly over part of the midbrain and inferiorly over the medulla (see Fig. 5-13). A distinctive cerebellar cortex covers its surface and receives most of the input, and a series of deep nuclei embedded beneath the cortex provide the output (Fig. 5-24). Like the basal ganglia, the cerebellum is primarily involved in the regulation of movement and does so largely by affecting the output of the cerebral cortex, but also like the basal ganglia it is now known to have a broader role in other cerebral functions as well. A major difference between the cerebellum and the basal ganglia (and most other parts of the CNS) is that one side of the cerebellum affects the ipsilateral side of the body. Part of the anatomic basis

for this is a crossing of the midline by neural traffic between the cerebrum and the cerebellum (see Fig. 5-24).

SPINAL CORD

The spinal cord is in some ways a simplified version of the brainstem: spinal nerves contain no special sensory fibers and innervate no branchial muscles, and the reticular formation does not extend into the spinal cord. Although there are some level-to-level variations, the basic cross-sectional anatomy of the spinal cord is similar everywhere (Fig. 5-25), with a central H-shaped core of gray matter surrounded by white matter. The posterior extension of the gray matter is the posterior (or dorsal) horn, the anterior extension is the anterior (or ventral) horn, and the two meet in the intermediate gray matter. The substantia gelatinosa, a layer of densely packed interneurons important in the processing of pain and temperature information, forms the most superficial part of the posterior horn at all levels. The horns of gray matter subdivide the white matter into poste-

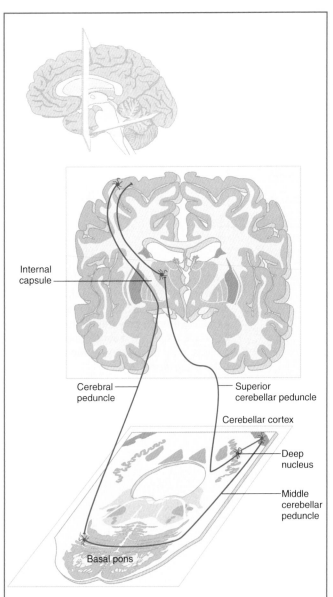

Figure 5-24. Arrangement of cerebellar cortex and deep nuclei, and the general pattern of cerebellar connections. Cerebellar cortex and connections are described in more detail in Chapter 16, but a major circuit is the loop from cerebral cortex to cerebellum and from there back to cerebral cortex. Because there is a crossing of the midline on the way into and out of the cerebellum, one side of the cerebellum affects the ipsilateral side of the body.

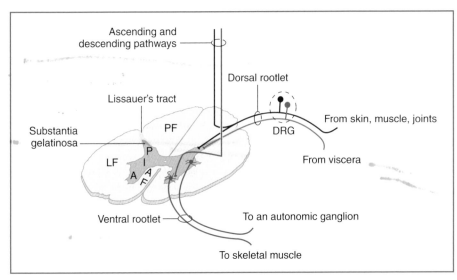

Figure 5-25. Internal anatomy of the spinal cord, using the thoracic cord as an example. Primary afferents mostly terminate in the posterior horn, motor neurons live in the anterior horn, and preganglionic autonomic neurons (at levels where they occur) live in the intermediate gray matter. A, anterior horn; AF, anterior funiculus; DRG, dorsal root ganglion; I, intermediate gray matter; LF, lateral funiculus; P, posterior horn; PF, posterior funiculus.

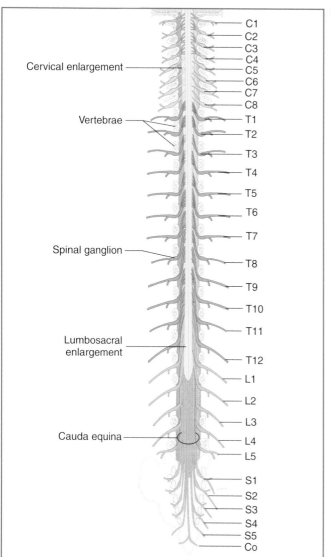

Figure 5-26. Segmentation of the spinal cord.

Labels on figure: Cervical enlargement, Vertebrae, Spinal ganglion, Lumbosacral enlargement, Cauda equina; C1, C2, C3, C4, C5, C6, C7, C8, T1, T2, T3, T4, T5, T6, T7, T8, T9, T10, T11, T12, L1, L2, L3, L4, L5, S1, S2, S3, S4, S5, Co

rior, lateral, and anterior funiculi (Latin, *funiculus*, "little cord") full of ascending and descending pathways. The white matter adjacent to the substantia gelatinosa is Lissauer's tract, a collection of thinly myelinated and unmyelinated afferents conveying pain and temperature information.

A series of dorsal and ventral rootlets join the spinal cord along its entire length. The central processes of somatic and visceral primary afferents, their cell bodies in nearby dorsal root ganglia, enter the cord through dorsal rootlets; most of their branches terminate in the posterior horn. Ventral rootlets, in contrast, contain axons on their way to skeletal muscle from motor neurons in the anterior horn. At some cord levels, ventral rootlets also contain the axons of preganglionic autonomic neurons, originating from cell bodies in the intermediate gray matter. Groups of dorsal and ventral rootlets coalesce into dorsal and ventral roots, which in turn join to form spinal nerves. Spinal nerves define a segmentation of the spinal cord, in which the length of cord that gives rise to a single nerve is a segment (Fig. 5-26). Human spinal cords have 31 segments: 8 cervical (C1–C8), 12 thoracic (T1–T12), 5 lumbar (L1–L5), 5 sacral (S1–S5), and 1 coccygeal (Co). Particular spinal cord segments are related to predictable parts of the body. Each dorsal root, for example, conveys information from a restricted area of skin (a dermatome; Fig. 5-27), and each ventral root innervates muscles in a restricted part of the body.

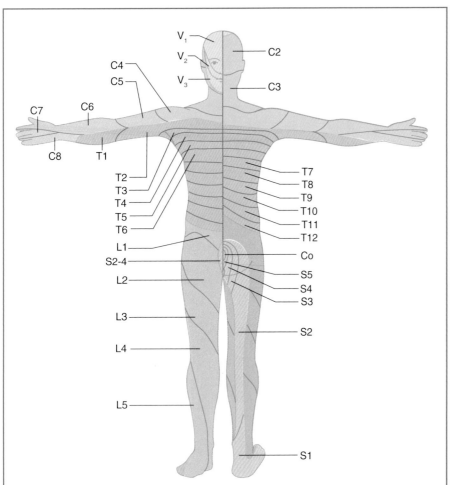

Figure 5-27. Each spinal cord segment receives cutaneous sensory information from a predictable region of the body surface, resulting in a series of dermatomes. The mapping continues into trigeminal territory.

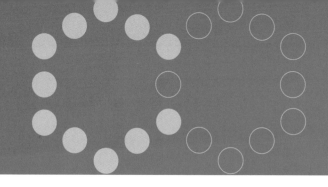

Development of the Nervous System

6

CONTENTS

Somehow humans wind up with something like 10^{11} neurons, wired up in a fairly predictable fashion, and arranged in brains that are reasonably similar to one another in shape. This requires an elaborate process in which chemical signals released in a carefully orchestrated temporal and spatial pattern induce various groups of stem cells to differentiate into distinct parts of the nervous system. The whole CNS develops from a simple tube with a few bulges and bends, so understanding a little about the process helps make sense of how things are arranged in adult brains and helps make sense of some malformations.

●●● NOTOCHORD AND NEURAL PLATE

At the end of the first week of development, the cells that will give rise to all the tissues and organs of the body live in a small epithelial disk (the epiblast) one cell layer thick. The process of gastrulation during the second week establishes the three tissue layers of the embryo (ectoderm, mesoderm, and endoderm), as well as the midline and the rostral-caudal axis of the future body. Starting at about day 8 a band of rapidly dividing cells forms the primitive streak, arranged like a radius extending halfway across the epiblast, with a

primitive node at the end of the streak near the center of the epiblast (Fig. 6-1). At the primitive streak and node, newborn cells dive through the epiblast and spread out to form mesodermal and endodermal layers; epiblast cells that stay behind form the ectoderm, which will develop into skin and the nervous system.

Some of the cells that move through the primitive node form a mesodermal rod, the notochord, which extends away from the primitive streak but in line with it. The primitive streak and notochord define the midline of the embryo (remnants of

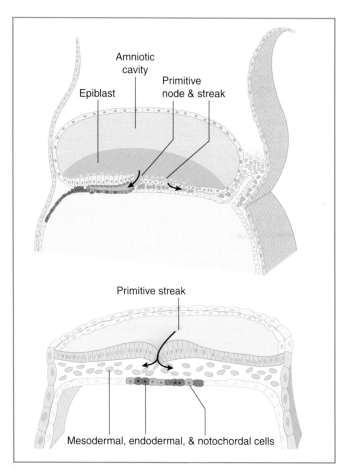

Figure 6-1. Gastrulation during the second week of development.

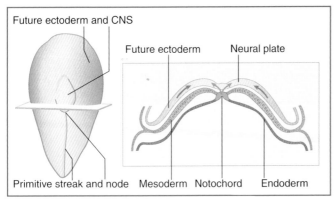

Future ectoderm and CNS

Future ectoderm   Neural plate

Primitive streak and node   Mesoderm   Notochord   Endoderm

Figure 6-2. Induction of the neural plate. Even before the neural tube forms, opposing gradients of signaling molecules begin to determine the future development of stem cells.

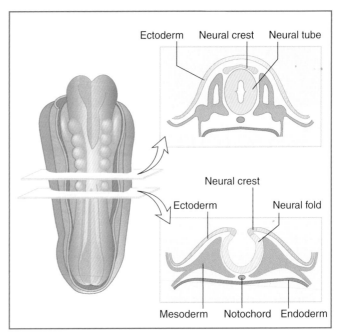

Ectoderm   Neural crest   Neural tube

Neural crest

Ectoderm   Neural fold

Mesoderm   Notochord   Endoderm

Figure 6-3. Formation of the neural tube. Closure begins at about the end of the third week.

the notochord persist after birth as the nucleus pulposus of each intervertebral disk). The notochord defines the rostral-caudal axis of the CNS: its origin near the primitive node underlies the future lumbar spinal cord, and the notochord ends near the future diencephalon. The importance of the notochord extends far beyond this, however, because it secretes signaling molecules (sonic hedgehog and others) that induce the overlying midline ectoderm to thicken into a pseudostratified columnar epithelium, the neural plate.

At the same time the notochord is inducing the neural plate, the ectoderm and nearby tissues are secreting their own set of signaling molecules. The opposing gradients of these molecules (Fig. 6-2) cause graded changes in patterns of differentiation and growth: cells near the midline begin to develop into motor neurons, those in more lateral parts of the neural plate into sensory neurons, and those at the junction between the neural plate and the rest of the ectoderm into a special population of neural crest cells.

NEURAL TUBE FORMATION

During the third week of development, a longitudinal groove (the neural groove) appears in the neural plate, flanked on either side by a neural fold. Cells of the neural crest grow at the apex of each neural fold. The neural folds get bigger and bigger, finally meeting in the midline at about the level of the future cervical spinal cord to form the beginning of the neural tube (Fig. 6-3). Additional sites of closure soon appear, and all of them proceed to zip up in rostral and caudal directions. As this closure progresses, the neural crest cells separate from the neural folds and form a layer draped over the neural tube, between it and the surface ectoderm. The entire neural tube is closed up and detached from the surface ectoderm by about the end of the fourth week. This process of neurulation—formation of the neural tube—is a major developmental event, because the neural tube will go on to become the entire CNS (Fig. 6-4); its cavity becomes the ventricular system of the brain. (The sacral spinal cord forms after neural tube closure by a process of secondary neurulation, in which the cavity of

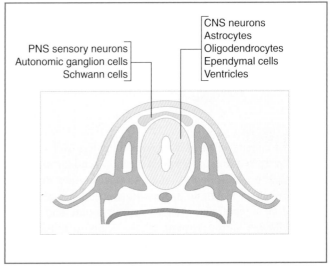

PNS sensory neurons
Autonomic ganglion cells
Schwann cells

CNS neurons
Astrocytes
Oligodendrocytes
Ependymal cells
Ventricles

Figure 6-4. Derivatives of the neural tube and neural crest. (Most consider microglial cells to be blood-borne invaders and not neural tube derivatives, but this is not certain.)

the neural tube extends into a mass of stem cells at the caudal end of the spinal cord.) Neural crest cells, in contrast, begin to migrate and go on to form the neurons and glial cells of the peripheral nervous system (as well as cutaneous melanocytes, the adrenal medulla, and an assortment of nonneural tissues in the head). These include the primary sensory neurons of spinal and most cranial nerve ganglia, postganglionic autonomic neurons, and the Schwann cells and satellite cells of peripheral nerves and ganglia. Placodes of neural crest–like cells that initially remain in the surface ectoderm detach later and form the balance of the PNS in the head.

Defective Neurulation

Problems with neurulation are surprisingly common, affecting approximately 0.1% of infants and even higher percentages of fetuses that do not survive to term. Neural tube defects result in a spectrum of abnormalities in the CNS, some of them profound. In addition, because the axial skeleton forms around the neural tube as it closes, neural tube defects are accompanied by abnormalities in posterior parts of the skull and vertebrae. At one extreme is a fatal condition (craniorachischisis) in which the neural tube does not close at all, and a furrowed mass of neural tissue is continuous with the skin of the back. If only the rostral end of the neural tube fails to close, anencephaly can result, in which dorsal and posterior parts of the skull are absent and most of the cerebrum is replaced by an open, exposed mass of neural tissue. The face and the rest of the skull develop under the influence of the notochord and ventral parts of the neural tube. As a result, the face of anencephalic fetuses, although not normal, is much more extensively developed than the cerebrum and the dorsal and posterior skull. If the caudal end of the neural tube fails to close, various types of spina bifida result, ranging from forms in which the caudal spinal cord is open and exposed, to less severe forms in which vertebral arches are deficient and parts of the spinal cord or meninges herniate into a membranecovered sac on the back. The mildest forms, usually resulting from aberrant secondary neurulation, may be asymptomatic and involve a single defective vertebra; in these cases the kinship between the CNS and surface ectoderm is often indicated by an overlying tuft of hair or a dimple.

Things can also go wrong with the proliferation or migration of neural crest cells. One of the best-known examples is Hirschsprung's disease, in which there is defective innervation of a segment of the colon by autonomic neurons involved in peristalsis. The affected segment is tonically constricted, restricting the passage of intestinal contents, and as a result more proximal portions of the colon dilate (hence the alternative term congenital megacolon).

CLINICAL MEDICINE

Detecting Neural Tube Defects

α-Fetoprotein (AFP) is synthesized in the fetal liver and is a major component of fetal serum. Some is normally excreted into amniotic fluid as part of fetal urine. In cases of open neural tube defects, much more than the normal amount of AFP leaks out into cerebrospinal fluid and reaches amniotic fluid and maternal serum. Hence, measuring levels of this protein at specified times during gestation is a useful screening test for neural tube defects.

BIOCHEMISTRY

Preventing Neural Tube Defects

Because of its role in DNA synthesis, an adequate supply of folic acid is essential for rapidly dividing cells. These include cells of the neural plate during neurulation, and folic acid supplementation can prevent more than 50% of neural tube defects. Neurulation occurs so early in development that the supplementation must be provided near the time of conception, and for this reason folate is added to parts of the food supply in some countries.

●●● BRAIN VESICLES

The neural tube is neither cylindrical nor straight. Even before it closes, the brain part of the tube develops a series of curves and creases that lay the groundwork for the arrangement of its future parts (Table 6-1).

Primary and Secondary Vesicles

First to appear (Fig. 6-5), during the fourth week, are three primary vesicles: the prosencephalon (or forebrain), mesencephalon (or midbrain), and rhombencephalon (or hindbrain). The prosencephalon is the forerunner of the cerebrum, and the mesencephalon, as its name implies, will form the midbrain. The rhombencephalon, named for its diamond-shaped cavity (the incipient fourth ventricle), will form the pons, medulla, and cerebellum.

Less than a week later, a bulge begins to grow on each side of the prosencephalon and differences in the rostral and caudal halves of the rhombencephalon become apparent. The result

TABLE 6-1. Major Derivatives of Neural Tube Vesicles

Primary Vesicle	Secondary Vesicle	Cavity	Major Derivative
Prosencephalon	Telencephalon	Lateral ventricles	Cerebral cortex, hippocampus, amygdala Caudate, putamen, globus pallidus
	Diencephalon	Third ventricle	Thalamus, hypothalamus, retina, pineal gland
Mesencephalon	Mesencephalon	Aqueduct	Midbrain
Rhombencephalon	Metencephalon	Rostral fourth ventricle	Pons, cerebellum
	Myelencephalon	Caudal fourth ventricle	Medulla

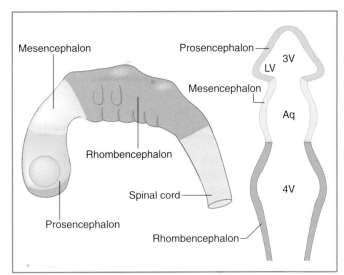

Figure 6-5. Primary brain vesicles at about the time of neural tube closure (about 4 weeks). 3V, 4V, third and fourth ventricles; Aq, aqueduct; LV, lateral ventricle.

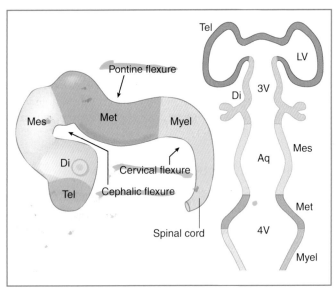

Figure 6-6. Secondary brain vesicles during the sixth week. Di, diencephalon; Mes, mesencephalon; Met, metencephalon; Myel, myelencephalon; Tel, telencephalon.

is five secondary vesicles (Fig. 6-6)—the prosencephalon gives rise to the telencephalon ("endbrain") and diencephalon ("in-between-brain"), the rhombencephalon to the metencephalon and myelencephalon, and the mesencephalon remains undivided. Each telencephalic vesicle will develop into a cerebral hemisphere; the diencephalon into the thalamus, hypothalamus, and a few other structures; the metencephalon into the pons and cerebellum; and the myelencephalon into the medulla. The cavity of the neural tube persists as a system of ventricles (see Chapter 7).

Flexures in the Neural Tube

Three prominent bends appear at the same time the embryonic vesicles are forming (see Fig. 6-6); two of them have major consequences for the later configuration of the CNS. In the first, the midbrain bends around the rostral end of the notochord, forming the cephalic (or mesencephalic) flexure. The cephalic flexure persists and accounts for the bend in the long axis of the CNS between the brainstem and cerebrum (see Fig. 5-2). Next, the cervical flexure appears between the spinal cord and brainstem; this one straightens out later in development. Finally, the brainstem bends anteriorly in the pontine flexure. The pontine flexure does not cause a long-term bend in the brainstem but, as explained below, it is important in determining the shape of the fourth ventricle and the position of the cerebellum.

"Rotation" of the Cerebral Hemispheres

Once the secondary embryonic vesicles form, the remaining development of the CNS is dominated by massive growth of the telencephalon. Initially a simple outpouching from the diencephalon, each telencephalic vesicle expands in all available directions. The medial and inferior part of the vesicle, where the basal ganglia will form, folds down alongside the diencephalon and fuses with it (Fig. 6-7). This area of fusion proceeds to develop a cortical covering (the insula) and establishes a fixed pivot point as the hemisphere continues to expand anteriorly, posteriorly, and inferiorly (Fig. 6-8). Eventually the insula is completely overgrown by parts of the frontal, parietal, and temporal lobes (see Fig. 6-7), and many telencephalic structures, such as the lateral ventricle and the caudate nucleus (see Fig. 6-8), are dragged around into a great C shape.

Malformation of the Prosencephalon

The prosencephalon subdivides early in development, not long after the neural tube closes. Problems with this subdivision can cause a spectrum of abnormalities called holoprosencephaly, indicating that they affect the entire cerebrum. In the most severe forms, the olfactory bulbs and tracts and the optic chiasm are missing, and the cerebral hemispheres are undivided, with an absent corpus callosum and a single ventricle that spans the midline. Effects on the skull and face are almost the opposite of those seen in anencephaly: dorsal and posterior parts of the skull are present but, because signaling molecules released by the notochord and nearby tissues influence the development of both the face and the cerebrum, holoprosencephaly is accompanied by marked facial abnormalities.

●●● PROLIFERATION, MIGRATION, AND DIFFERENTIATION OF NEURONS

Neural tube closure and the basic formation of the prosencephalon occur during the first month or so of development. This is followed, during the third and fourth months and later, by a period of massive proliferation of neurons and glial cells, followed by migration of these cells to their final locations and differentiation into specific cell types.

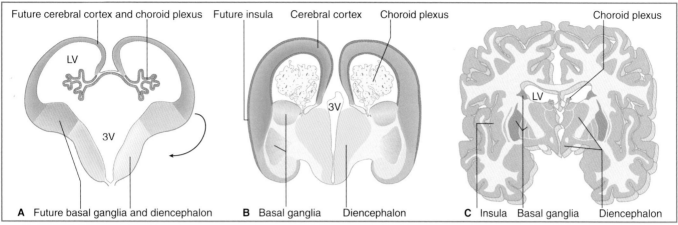

Figure 6-7. A, During the second month, the telencephalon starts to grow faster than most other parts of the CNS and balloons outward and downward as indicated. The continuity between the lateral ventricle (LV) and third ventricle (3V) is apparent, as is a thinned-out, nonneural area of the roof of the neural tube that will form the choroid plexus of these ventricles (see Chapter 7). **B,** By the end of the third month, the diencephalon and telencephalon have fused, establishing the basic locations of the insula and other parts of the cerebrum. **C,** By birth the telencephalon has expanded further and the insula is buried in the lateral sulcus.

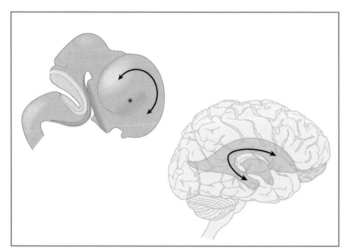

Figure 6-8. Growth of the telencephalon into a C-shaped cerebral hemisphere, with the future insula (*) as the pivot point.

Neurogenesis

The simple neural tube of early development has an equally simple wall, a pseudostratified columnar epithelium a single cell thick (Fig. 6-9). These are the stem cells that will give rise to the neurons and glial cells of the CNS. Early on, each cell spans the entire epithelium most of the time, with its nucleus shuttling back and forth between the ventricular surface and the external surface of the neural tube (see Fig. 6-9). As the nucleus moves outward, its DNA is replicated. As it moves back inward, the cell retracts its surface-directed process and then divides when it reaches the lumen of the neural tube. The two daughter cells then either repeat the process, or one or both leave the mitotic cycle, commit to being a neural or glial progenitor cell, and migrate to a final destination. The final round of mitosis happens before birth in almost all areas

of the CNS, and the last cells left near the lumen of the neural tube become the ependymal cells that line the ventricles.

The neural progenitors begin to accumulate outside the mitotic area, dividing the wall of the neural tube into three concentric zones (Fig. 6-10): a ventricular zone in which stem cell nuclei shuttle and divide, an intermediate zone of committed precursor cells, and a relatively cell-free marginal zone with surface-directed processes of stem cells.

The development of these three zones into parts of the adult CNS is most apparent in the spinal cord (see Fig. 6-10), where the ventricular zone winds up being the ependymal cells surrounding its tiny central canal, the intermediate zone becomes the spinal gray matter, and the marginal zone is soon invaded by ascending and descending tracts and becomes the white matter. The sequence in some other parts of the CNS is more complex. In the telencephalon, for example, some neurons follow the spinal cord pattern and stay close to the lateral ventricles, forming the basal ganglia and amygdala. Others migrate longer distances to form the cerebral cortex, with successive waves of newborn neurons migrating past those cortical neurons already present, so that the cortex is built from the inside out.

Abnormalities of Proliferation and Migration

Once the basic parts of the CNS have developed, the number of divisions undergone by neural stem cells, the timing of these divisions, and the subsequent migration of newborn neurons all need to be carefully controlled in order for the CNS to be wired up properly. If too few cycles of cell division occur, or if too few stem cells are formed in the first place, different types of microencephaly ("small brain") can result. In contrast, if the migration of neurons to the cerebral cortex is abnormal, gyri do not form properly. An extreme case is lissencephaly ("smooth brain"), in which a large percentage of neurons stop before reaching the cortex; as a result, the surface area of the cortex is reduced and gyri do not form. In less severe cases,

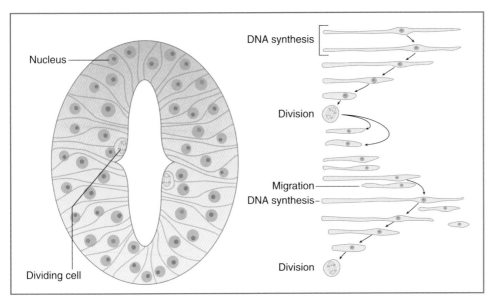

Figure 6-9. Multiplication of stem cells in the walls of the early neural tube. The pseudostratified columnar epithelium in the wall of the neural tube (*left*) is a population of stem cells with nuclei shuttling back and forth, replicating DNA and dividing (*right*).

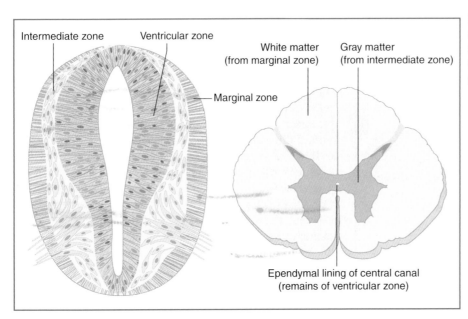

Figure 6-10. The three concentric zones of the walls of the neural tube. In the spinal cord, these develop into the ependymal lining of the central canal, the gray matter, and the white matter.

clusters of neurons get "stuck" in the white matter before reaching the cortex, forming heterotopic ("in a different place") clumps of gray matter.

Longitudinal Zones in the Central Nervous System

The signaling molecules released by the surface ectoderm and the notochord induce the parts of the neural tube closest to them to form the roof plate and the floor plate, secondary signaling centers that release the same molecules (Fig. 6-11). The roof and floor plates thin out, and most parts of the CNS develop from the lateral walls of the neural tube. This too is seen most clearly in the spinal cord (see Fig. 6-11), where the part of the tube near the roof plate thickens into an alar plate and the part near the notochord and floor plate thickens into

a basal plate, separated from the alar plate by a longitudinally running sulcus limitans. These then go on to form the posterior and anterior horns, containing sensory and motor neurons, respectively; preganglionic autonomic neurons (at levels where they occur) live in the intermediate gray matter, near where the sulcus limitans used to be. The cavity of the neural tube shrinks down into a tiny central canal, and very little neural tissue remains dorsal and ventral to this canal, where the roof plate and floor plate used to be.

The same basic organization continues into the rhombencephalon, but the pontine flexure spreads the walls of the neural tube apart and the roof plate stretches out into a thin, nonneural membrane that forms the roof of the fourth ventricle (Fig. 6-12). The alar and basal plates now form the floor of the fourth ventricle, so in the medulla and pons the alar plate ends up lateral to the basal plate. The same development into

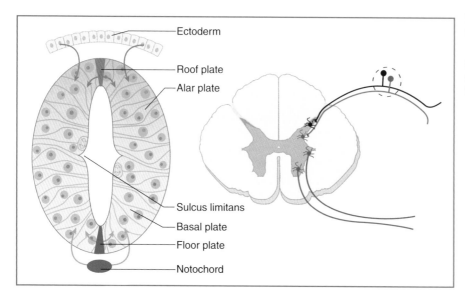

Figure 6-11. Longitudinal subdivision of the spinal cord part of the neural tube (*left*) into roof, alar, basal, and floor plates. This leads to the subsequent arrangement arrangement of cell types in the spinal cord (*right*).

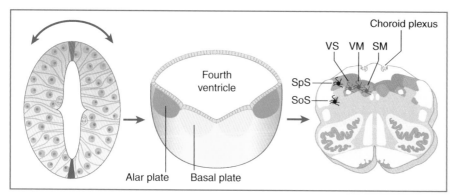

Figure 6-12. Opening up of the neural tube in the rhombencephalon, so that the walls of the neural tube become the floor of the fourth ventricle and sensory nuclei are generally lateral to motor nuclei. The roof plate stretches out into an ependymal membrane, and choroid plexus forms in the roof of the fourth ventricle. Not shown are motor neurons for skeletal muscles derived from branchial arches; many of these migrate away from the floor of the fourth ventricle (see Fig. 14-6).

sensory and motor structures occurs, however, and as a result cranial nerve sensory nuclei wind up lateral to cranial nerve motor nuclei. As in the spinal cord, visceral nuclei are near the sulcus limitans, in this case visceral sensory nuclei just lateral to it (see Fig. 13-4) and visceral motor nuclei just medial to it (see Fig. 18-3). In contrast to the spinal cord, however, the alar and basal plates in the brainstem do not form continuous columns of cells like the posterior and anterior horns. Instead, they form a series of discrete nuclei at levels roughly corresponding to the attachment points of related cranial nerves. Parts of the alar plate also form structures that are not sensory nuclei, at least not in any simple sense. Some of these migrate into anterior parts of the brainstem as cerebellum-related nuclei (e.g., the inferior olivary nucleus and pontine nuclei

described in Chapter 16), and the alar plate of the metencephalon grows dorsally and expands tremendously to form the cerebellum itself.

Whether the alar and basal plates and the sulcus limitans continue beyond the brainstem has been a subject of much debate, but sensory and motor nuclei of the kind found in the spinal cord and brainstem do not. The roof plate, however, continues as another thinned-out membrane that roofs over the third ventricle in the diencephalon and continues onto the surface of the telencephalon (see Fig. 6-7). Blood vessels outside the neural tube invaginate the roof plate–derived membranes of all four ventricles, forming the choroid plexus that produces the cerebrospinal fluid that fills the ventricles and bathes the outside of the CNS (see Chapter 7).

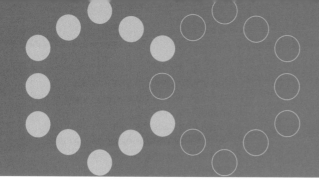

Tissues Supporting the Nervous System

7

Neurons are powerful information processors, but they need a lot of help to do their jobs. Their elaborate shapes make them even more delicate than most other cells, and the cytoskeleton by itself is inadequate to protect them from damage as we move through the world. For this, the CNS depends on collaboration with the ventricles and a series of external meninges (Greek, "membranes") that keep it safely suspended in a watery bath of cerebrospinal fluid. In addition, neurons use prodigious amounts of energy to run their ion pumps and synthetic machinery, so the CNS requires a copious, stable blood supply.

●●● MENINGES

A series of three meninges surround the brain—a relatively thick, collagenous dura mater attached to the inner surface of the skull; a thinner, more cellular arachnoid mater attached to the inner surface of the dura; and an even thinner pia mater attached to the surface of the brain (Fig. 7-1). (In common usage, "mater" is often dropped, and the three are referred to as the dura, arachnoid, and pia.) The intracranial dura has two parts—an outer, somewhat vascular part that serves as the periosteum for the inner table of the skull and an inner, less vascular part.

Although under some pathologic conditions (described later in this chapter) the dura can be separated from the skull and the arachnoid can be separated from the dura, the only space normally present within or around the meninges is the sub-arachnoid space between the arachnoid and pia. The extent of this space varies with the separation between the skull and the surface of the brain. It is narrow over the crests of cerebral gyri, extends into sulci, and is enlarged into subarachnoid cisterns in locations where there are larger depressions in the surface of the brain (Fig. 7-2).

Mechanical Suspension

There are three things in subarachnoid space: cerebrospinal fluid (CSF, produced in the ventricles, as described later in

PATHOLOGY

Tumors of the Meninges
Meningiomas, derived from arachnoid cells, are the most common benign intracranial tumors.

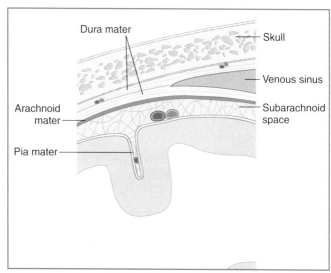

Figure 7-1. The basic arrangement of intracranial meninges.

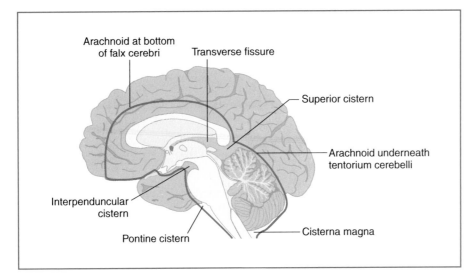

Figure 7-2. Locations where the arachnoid would be cut when a brain is hemisected, defining subarachnoid spaces and cisterns near the midline. The superior cistern extends into the transverse fissure, which leads off laterally into the choroid plexus of the body of the lateral ventricle (see Fig. 7-10). The median and lateral apertures of the fourth ventricle (see Fig. 7-11) open into the pontine cistern and cisterna magna, respectively. The interpeduncular cistern houses most of the circle of Willis (see Fig. 7-12).

this chapter), minute strands of connective tissue called arachnoid trabeculae that span the space and interconnect the arachnoid and pia, and a network of arteries and veins that provide the brain's blood supply. The CSF and arachnoid trabeculae are the basis of the mechanical suspension function of the meninges (Fig. 7-3). The brain has almost the same density as CSF, effectively making it nearly weightless inside the head. This near-weightlessness makes it possible for the arachnoid trabeculae to stabilize the position of the brain

within its CSF bath, so that the brain keeps up with the head when someone moves.

This mechanical suspension needs to be continued inward wherever there are especially deep clefts in the surface of the brain. This is accomplished by infoldings of the inner dural layer to form dural septa that carry along with them an arachnoid lining and a series of arachnoid trabeculae (Fig. 7-4). The major dural septa are the falx cerebri ("sickle of the cerebrum") between the cerebral hemispheres and the tentorium cerebelli ("tent over the cerebellum") between the cerebellum and the overlying occipital and temporal lobes (Fig. 7-5).

Dural Venous Sinuses

As the inner dural layer folds inward to form septa, an endothelium-lined triangular space is created between the two dural layers. The resulting longitudinal channels are dural venous sinuses, essentially veins running within the dura mater (see Figs. 7-4 and 7-5); they provide the major venous drainage paths for the brain. Hence, there is a superior sagittal sinus in the line of attachment between the falx cerebri and the top of

Figure 7-3. Schematic view of the suspension of the CNS within the meninges. CSF is made in the ventricles (see Fig. 7-10) but flows out to fill subarachnoid space (see Fig. 7-11), providing a partial flotation effect. Arachnoid trabeculae complete the suspension.

CLINICAL MEDICINE

Dural Septa as Hazards

Dural septa are effective in their mechanical suspension role because they are stretched tight, making them fairly rigid, but this rigidity can also cause problems. Because brain tissue is soft, an expanding intracranial mass can cause part of the brain to herniate from one side of a dural septum to another. For example, one cingulate gyrus can herniate under the falx cerebri and compress the contralateral cingulate gyrus. More seriously, the most medial part of one temporal lobe (the uncus) can herniate through the tentorial notch, compressing the midbrain against the free edge of the tentorium on the opposite side.

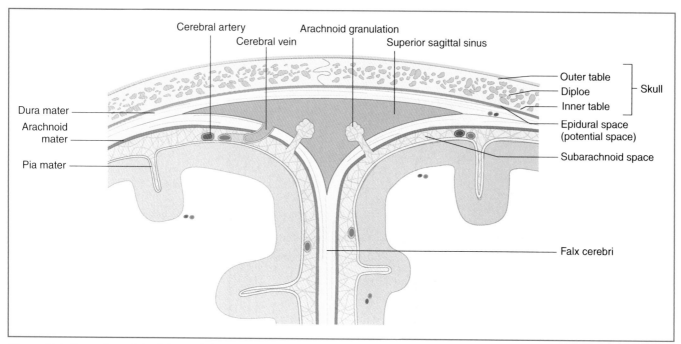

Figure 7-4. Formation of the falx cerebri, one of the dural septa, by an infolding of the inner dural layer. At sites like this, the two dural layers separate to enclose a venous sinus, in this case the superior sagittal sinus.

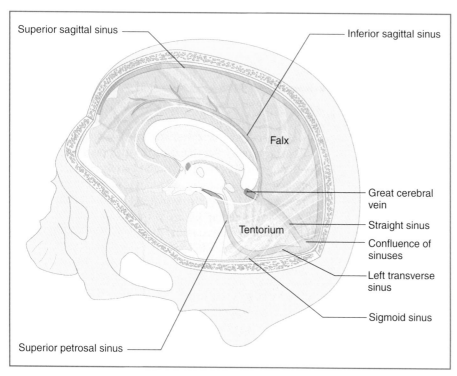

Figure 7-5. The falx cerebri and tentorium cerebelli, the two largest dural septa. The line of attachment between the two slopes anteriorly upward, so that the tentorium forms a "tent" (hence its name) over the top of the cerebellum.

the skull, and a transverse sinus on each side along the line of attachment between the tentorium cerebelli and the back of the skull. Blood flows posteriorly through the superior sagittal sinus and enters the transverse sinuses at the confluens of the sinuses. Each transverse sinus then curves downward into the sigmoid sinus, which in turn empties into the internal jugular vein, providing a major route for venous outflow from the CNS. Other venous sinuses form along edges of dural septa not attached to the skull, e.g., a small inferior sagittal sinus in the free edge of the falx cerebri. The major member of this category is the straight sinus, along the line of attachment between the falx cerebri and the tentorium cerebelli, through which blood also flows posteriorly to the confluens of the sinuses.

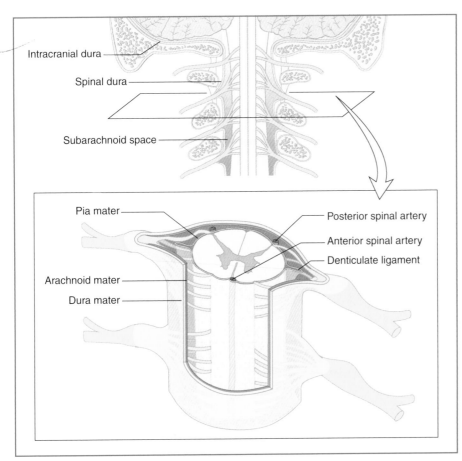

Figure 7-6. Transition from intracranial dura mater to the dural sheath of the spinal cord.

Potential Meningeal Spaces

The dura is normally tightly attached to the skull, and the arachnoid to the dura, so no epidural or subdural spaces exist. These are, however, potential spaces that can be opened up by different types of bleeding. Epidural bleeding is most commonly caused by tearing of a meningeal artery. Because these are in the outer part of the dura, near the skull, arterial pressure can pry the dura away from the inner table of the skull (see Fig. 8-6). Subdural bleeding is most commonly caused by tearing of a cerebral vein as it enters a dural venous sinus. The sinuses are rigidly fixed in place, so they do not move relative to the skull. In response to sudden acceleration or deceleration (e.g., from a blow to the head) the brain and its arteries and veins can move a little, tearing a vein just as it penetrates the arachnoid on its way into a sinus (see Fig. 7-4). The resulting venous bleeding can peel the arachnoid away from the dura[1] (see Fig. 8-7).

Spinal Meninges

The meningeal coverings of the spinal cord are fundamentally similar to those of the brain, except for a difference in the way the dura mater is configured (Fig. 7-6). As the intracranial dura passes through the foramen magnum, its two layers split and the periosteal part stays attached to the skull and continues onto its external surface. The inner layer continues as a dural sheath around the spinal cord. Vertebrae have their own individual periosteal coats, so in the vertebral canal there is a normally present epidural space that is located between dura and periosteum (as opposed to the potential epidural space between periosteum and bone in the skull).

Spinal dura, like intracranial dura, is lined with arachnoid, and the cord is suspended in subarachnoid space by strands of connective tissue that extend from arachnoid to pia. Those emerging from pia on the sides of the spinal cord are thickened to form a long, toothed denticulate ligament on each side. The dural sheath extends to about the level of the S2 vertebra, but the spinal cord itself ends, on average, between the L1 and L2 vertebrae. Between these two vertebral levels, the dural sac contains a subarachnoid cistern (the lumbar

CLINICAL MEDICINE

Sampling CSF from a Cistern

The lumbar cistern is the favored site for sampling CSF for diagnostic purposes because a needle can be inserted here with little risk of CNS damage.

---

[1]At a microscopic level, the splitting actually occurs in the innermost cellular layers of the dura mater, so the arachnoid and a bit of dura peel away from the rest of the dura mater.

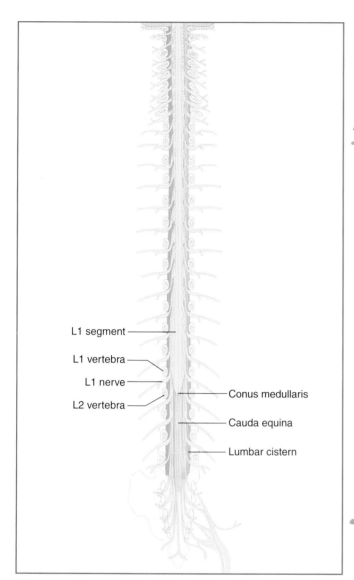

L1 segment

L1 vertebra

L1 nerve

L2 vertebra

Conus medullaris

Cauda equina

Lumbar cistern

Figure 7-7. Cauda equina and lumbar cistern.

cistern), through which dorsal and ventral roots from caudal levels of the spinal cord travel as the cauda equina ("horse's tail") on their way to their exit levels (Fig. 7-7).

Meningeal Extensions Around Peripheral Nerves

Axons of peripheral nerves have the same mechanical stability issues as CNS neurons. In some ways the problems in the PNS are even greater, because peripheral nerves need to extend over great distances, bending and twisting during body movements. This is addressed by a continuation of the meninges into peripheral nerves (Fig. 7-8). The dura mater continues as the epineurium, a relatively thick, collagenous sheath covering entire peripheral nerves, here too providing most of the mechanical strength. The arachnoid continues as the perineurium, a compact, more cellular sheath covering individual bundles of nerve fibers (fascicles) within a peripheral

nerve. Finally, wisps of connective tissue interspersed among the axons in nerve fascicles constitute the endoneurium.

●●● VENTRICLES

The cavity of the neural tube persists in the adult CNS as a continuous system of ventricles (Fig. 7-9). Each cerebral hemisphere contains a C-shaped lateral ventricle, with an anterior horn that protrudes into the frontal lobe, a body that extends through the parietal lobe and curves into an inferior horn in the temporal lobe, and a posterior horn that protrudes into the occipital lobe from the back of the curve. The body, posterior horn, and inferior horn meet in a roughly triangular area called the atrium, near the back of the corpus callosum. Each lateral ventricle is continuous through an interventricular foramen with the third ventricle, a slit-shaped cavity in the diencephalon walled by the thalamus and hypothalamus. The third ventricle ends anteriorly at the lamina terminalis (which started out as the rostral end of the neural tube). Posteriorly, it funnels down into the cerebral aqueduct, which traverses the midbrain. At the junction between the midbrain and pons, the aqueduct opens up into the diamond-shaped fourth ventricle, which reaches its greatest width at the pontomedullary junction. Halfway through the medulla, the fourth ventricle narrows into the microscopically small central canal, which continues through the length of the spinal cord.

The ventricles communicate with subarachnoid space through three apertures in the fourth ventricle, a single median aperture above the caudal end of the ventricle and a lateral aperture on each side at the pontomedullary junction. These are the routes through which CSF, made in the ventricles, reaches and fills subarachnoid space.

Cerebrospinal Fluid

CSF is a clear, colorless liquid, low in protein, with a precisely controlled ionic composition. It is produced in the lateral, third, and fourth ventricles by choroid plexus, a specialization of the thinned-out nonneural membranes derived from the roof plate of the neural tube (see Figs. 6-7 and 6-12). Although choroid plexus is multiply folded and convoluted, conceptually its organization is simple (Fig. 7-10). The roof plate contributes an ependymal layer, here specialized as a secretory epithelium (choroid epithelium), so on one side of any bit of choroid plexus is part of a ventricle. This is the only part contributed by the neural tube, and the pia mater that covers the CNS continues over the choroid epithelium; at these sites, the pia is sparse and discontinuous. Pia mater here and elsewhere faces subarachnoid space, where the CNS blood supply travels, and small arteries and veins that invaginate the pia/ependyma membrane complete the choroid plexus. The lateral ventricles contain most of the choroid plexus, in the form of a long strand in each that follows the C shape of the ventricle, from the inferior horn, through the atrium and body of the ventricle (there is none in the anterior or posterior horn). Both continue through the interventricular foramina and form two narrow, delicate strands in the roof of the third ventricle.

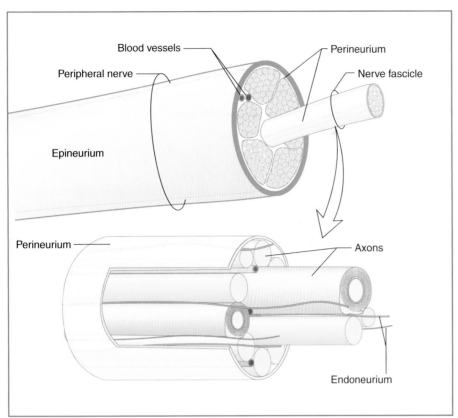

Figure 7-8. Connective tissue coverings of peripheral nerves.

A separate patch of choroid plexus is formed in the roof of the caudal half of the fourth ventricle.

Serum components leak out of choroidal capillaries, diffuse past the pial elements, and are transported across the choroid epithelium as newly formed CSF. The transport process is regulated in such a way that the overall composition of CSF remains constant. If something causes ventricular pH to increase, for example, more protons are secreted in new CSF to compensate.

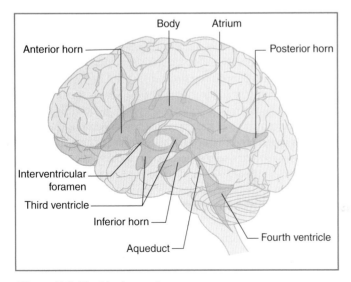

Figure 7-9. Ventricular system.

Circulation of Cerebrospinal Fluid

Enough CSF is produced to replace the entire volume of the ventricles and subarachnoid space several times a day, so it must constantly move away from its sites of production and be reabsorbed (Fig. 7-11). Newly formed CSF pushes that already present through the ventricles, out the apertures of the fourth ventricle, and into the subarachnoid cisterns of the posterior fossa. From there most of it moves upward through the tentorial notch, the hole in the tentorium cerebelli through which the brainstem passes, until it reaches arachnoid villi in one of the dural venous sinuses. Arachnoid villi (see Fig. 7-4), found in all the sinuses but mostly the superior sagittal sinus, are small herniations of arachnoid through the sinus wall. They are the principal sites of CSF reabsorption, acting as one-way flap valves that allow bulk CSF to be pushed from subarachnoid space into the venous circulation.

CLINICAL MEDICINE

CSF Alterations in Neurologic Disorders

The normally constant, cell-free, low-protein composition of CSF is what makes it so useful for diagnostic purposes. The presence of erythrocytes, for example, can indicate subarachnoid bleeding, and the presence of white blood cells can indicate an infection. In cases of meningitis, increased protein levels can indicate that the pathogen is bacterial rather than viral.

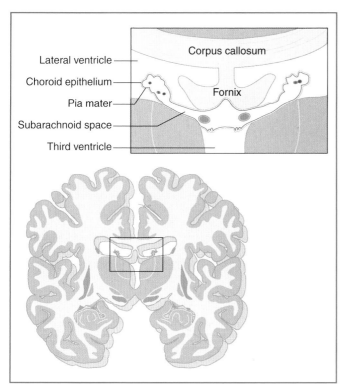

Figure 7-10. Structure of choroid plexus.

If something obstructs this path of circulation, CSF production continues unabated and intracranial pressure rises. If the condition persists, the ventricles expand at the expense of the CNS, and hydrocephalus results. The most common sites of obstruction are places that are already mechanical bottlenecks, such as an interventricular foramen, the aqueduct, or arachnoid villi.

●●● CENTRAL NERVOUS SYSTEM BLOOD SUPPLY

Neurons are extremely active metabolically but have very limited energy stores, so they depend on an abundant, constant blood supply to deliver glucose, oxygen, and other necessities. At about 1400 g, the CNS accounts for only 2% or so of an average human's body weight, but around 15% of the blood pumped by the heart goes there. Interruption of this supply for just a few minutes causes irreversible damage.

ANATOMY & EMBRYOLOGY

An Obstruction to CSF Circulation

Some forms of spina bifida are accompanied by an Arnold-Chiari malformation, in which the most inferior parts of the cerebellum protrude through the foramen magnum. Hydrocephalus can result if the apertures of the fourth ventricle are squeezed shut, blocking the flow of CSF.

PHYSIOLOGY

Control of CNS Blood Flow

Some tissues and organs, including the kidneys and others, are able to regulate their own blood supply. This capacity for autoregulation is well developed in the CNS, where arteriolar smooth muscle contracts or relaxes in responses to increases or decreases in arterial blood pressure. This is the principal mechanism that maintains constant blood flow to the CNS.

Arteries

The blood supply of the entire brain comes from two pairs of arteries: an internal carotid artery and a vertebral artery on each side (Fig. 7-12). The internal carotid and its branches supply most of the cerebrum. The vertebral system supplies the rest of the cerebrum, all of the cerebellum and brainstem, and upper levels of the spinal cord.

Internal Carotid Artery

The internal carotid artery arises from the common carotid, ascends through the base of the skull, passes by the optic

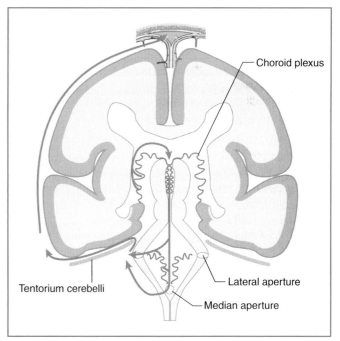

Figure 7-11. Circulation of CSF. Once out of the fourth ventricle, CSF is beneath the tentorium cerebelli and can move downward through the foramen magnum or upward through the subarachnoid space surrounding the brainstem as it passes through the tentorial notch. A relatively small amount moves into the subarachnoid space surrounding the spinal cord; some is reabsorbed through arachnoid villi associated with spinal nerve sheaths and some turns around and moves back up through the foramen magnum. Most CSF, however, passes through the tentorial notch and reaches subarachnoid spaces around the base and lateral surfaces of the brain.

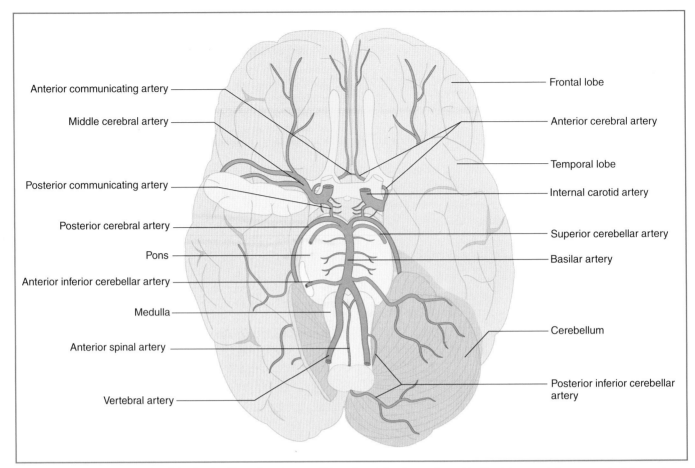

Figure 7-12. Arterial supply of the brain. Note that the carotid and vertebral supplies of both sides are interconnected through the circle of Willis: internal carotid artery → anterior cerebral artery → anterior communicating artery → anterior cerebral artery → internal carotid artery → posterior communicating artery → posterior cerebral artery → posterior cerebral artery → posterior communicating artery → original starting point.

chiasm, and divides into its last two branches, the middle cerebral and anterior cerebral arteries. The middle cerebral artery heads off laterally, reaches the insula, and divides into several branches that collectively supply most of the cerebral cortex on the lateral surface of the hemisphere (Fig. 7-13; also see Fig. 8-2). The anterior cerebral artery moves into the longitudinal fissure between the hemispheres, where it and its branches supply the cingulate gyrus and the medial surface of the frontal and parietal lobes. A short anterior communicating artery interconnects the two anterior cerebral arteries near where they enter the longitudinal fissure.

As they move off toward their major areas of supply, the middle and anterior cerebral arteries give off numerous small branches called ganglionic or perforating arteries that supply nearby deep structures such as the basal ganglia (Fig. 7-14). This is a uniform occurrence in all the arteries around the base of the brain (see Fig. 7-12).

Vertebral Artery

The vertebral arteries ascend through the neck, enter the skull through the foramen magnum, move upward beside the medulla, and fuse at the pontomedullary junction to form the single, midline basilar artery. The basilar artery travels along the anterior surface of the pons, then ends adjacent to the cerebral peduncles by bifurcating into the two posterior cerebral arteries. Each posterior cerebral artery wraps around the midbrain, gives off a series of perforating branches to the thalamus, and travels across the medial and inferior surfaces of the temporal lobe on its way to the medial surface of the occipital lobe (see Fig. 7-13). As it moves laterally around the midbrain, each posterior cerebral gives off a posterior communicating artery that joins the internal carotid. Prior to the basilar bifurcation, the vertebral-basilar system gives rise to three major arteries—the posterior inferior, anterior inferior, and superior cerebellar arteries (see Fig. 7-12)—that supply the cerebellum. Perforating branches of the vertebral and basilar arteries supply medial parts of the brainstem, and similar branches from the three cerebellar arteries and the posterior cerebral artery supply lateral and dorsal parts (Fig. 7-15).

Collateral Circulation

Alternative routes to deliver blood to an area of the CNS can limit the degree of damage if the primary source of supply is blocked. One route of such collateral circulation is a series of end-to-end anastomoses between distal branches of cerebral and cerebellar arteries (see Fig. 7-13). However, these routes

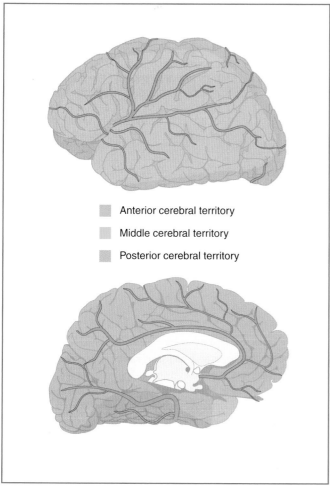

Anterior cerebral territory

Middle cerebral territory

Posterior cerebral territory

Figure 7-13. Cortical territories of the anterior, middle, and posterior cerebral arteries.

PATHOLOGY

Aneurysms and the Circle of Willis

Aneurysms usually develop at arterial branch points, and those affecting the brain are found most commonly at the junctions between different vessels of the circle of Willis. Rupture of an aneurysm causes extensive bleeding into the subarachnoid space.

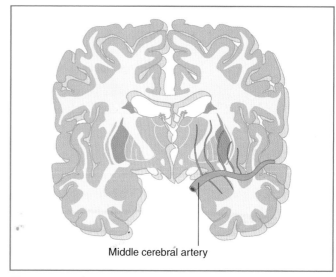

Middle cerebral artery

Figure 7-14. Ganglionic (perforating) arteries leaving the middle cerebral artery to supply parts of the basal ganglia, internal capsule, and diencephalon.

are limited and variable. The major set of collateral connections form the circle of Willis, through which the internal carotid and vertebral-basilar systems of both sides are interconnected (see Fig. 7-12). This potentially allows the territory of both internal carotids, for example, to be supplied by just one of these arteries if the other one becomes occluded.

Arterial Supply of the Spinal Cord

The spinal cord is supplied by the anterior and posterior spinal arteries (see Fig. 7-15), both branches of the vertebral artery. The two anterior spinal arteries fuse to form a single midline artery that supplies the anterior two thirds of the cord; the posterior spinal arteries travel near the lines of

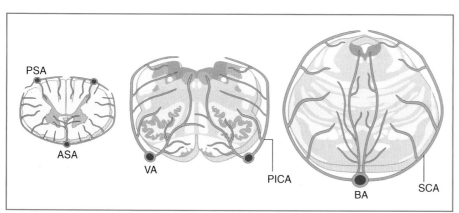

PSA

ASA

VA

PICA

BA

SCA

Figure 7-15. General pattern of blood supply to the spinal cord and brainstem. At each level, perforating branches from the anterior spinal, vertebral, or basilar artery supply medial zones. Perforating branches from circumferential arteries such as the posterior inferior cerebellar, superior cerebellar, and posterior cerebral artery supply lateral and dorsal zones (the posterior spinal artery starts out as a circumferential branch of the vertebral artery). ASA, anterior spinal artery; BA, basilar artery; PICA, posterior inferior cerebellar artery; PSA, posterior spinal artery; SCA, superior cerebellar artery; VA, vertebral artery.

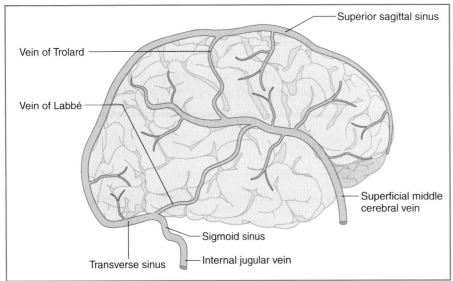

Figure 7-16. The superficial veins form an interconnected, variable network that mostly drains upward into the superior sagittal sinus. Exceptions are the vein of Labbé, which drains downward into the transverse sinus, and the superficial middle cerebral vein, which drains both downward into other sinuses at the base of the brain and upward through the vein of Trolard.

attachment of the dorsal rootlets, and between them supply the posterior third. As they descend along the spinal cord, the anterior and posterior spinal arteries receive repeated infusions of blood from a series of radicular arteries that enter the vertebral canal with spinal nerves.

Veins

The veins that drain the brain fall into two general categories: a variable collection of superficial veins (Fig. 7-16) that carry blood toward the surface of the brain, then mostly upward to the superior sagittal sinus, and a more constant collection of deep veins (Fig. 7-17) that carry blood toward the ventricles, eventually reaching the straight sinus. A series of deep veins in the ventricular walls join each other near the interventricular foramen and turn posteriorly as the internal cerebral vein (see Fig. 8-8). The two internal cerebral veins join to form the thick but short great vein (of Galen), which then empties into the straight sinus.

Barrier Systems

Consistent neuronal functioning requires that the extracellular concentrations of ions and other substances be maintained within narrow limits. This is accomplished, in part, by isolating the extracellular fluids around neurons from other extracellular fluids of the body and transporting things in and out as necessary. The isolation is achieved by three sets of diffusion barriers (Fig. 7-18). The first and most straightforward is a network of tight junctions between the endothelial cells of CNS capillaries. This blood-brain barrier, by itself, would not take care of the isolation job, and additional barriers block other potential points of entry into CNS fluids. A layer of arachnoid cells is also zipped up by tight junctions, forming an arachnoid barrier that prevents diffusion from the dura mater into subarachnoid space. Finally, things that leak out of

choroid plexus capillaries (which have no blood-brain barrier) are stopped by the choroid epithelium.

Similar barriers continue into peripheral nerves, forming a blood-nerve barrier. The arachnoid barrier continues into the perineurium, and capillaries inside the perineurium also have barrier properties.

Circumventricular Organs

There are a few parts of the brain whose business it is to keep track of the concentration of something in the bloodstream,

PHARMACOLOGY

Getting Across the Blood-Brain Barrier

Barrier systems are effective at preventing solutes and infectious agents from reaching CNS neurons, but they can also make it difficult for therapeutic agents to get in. One strategy for circumventing the barriers is to use something lipid soluble, allowing it to move across endothelial cell membranes and bypass the tight junctions. Another strategy is to link a drug to some substance normally transported across the barrier.

MICROBIOLOGY

Pathogens Can Breach the Blood-Nerve Barrier

The blood-brain and blood-nerve barrier systems prevent most pathogens from getting into the nervous system. The blood-nerve barrier ends, however, at the endings of peripheral nerves. Some viruses (e.g., poliovirus, rabies virus) are able to enter at these sites and be transported in retrograde fashion into the CNS.

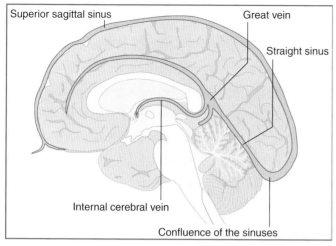

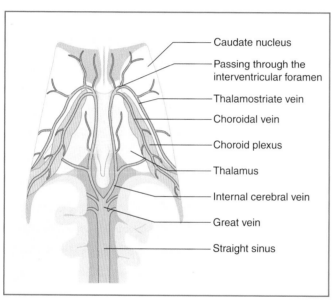

B

Figure 7-17. Deep veins. **A,** The principal deep vein for each cerebral hemisphere is the internal cerebral vein, both of which join to form the great vein, which then proceeds to the straight sinus. **B,** A view downward into a horizontally sectioned brain shows the series of veins in the wall of each lateral ventricle that join to form the internal cerebral vein.

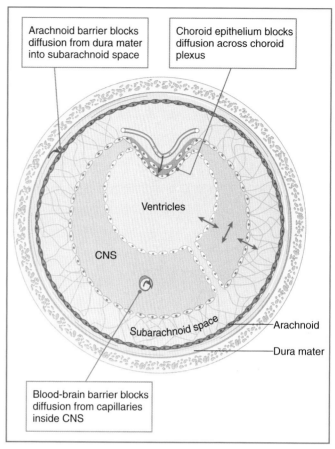

Figure 7-18. The system of barriers that separate the extracellular fluids around neurons from other extracellular fluids of the body.

and at these sites the blood-brain barrier is missing. For example, cells in one part of the hypothalamus monitor blood osmolality, and those in another part monitor hormone concentrations (see Chapter 18). Because all these areas are in the walls of the third or fourth ventricle, collectively they are known as circumventricular organs. Diffusion from the margins of circumventricular organs into the rest of the brain is prevented by tight junctions among special glial cells.

Imaging the Nervous System   8

CONTENTS

The relatively recent ability to peer into the brains of live humans has resulted in dramatic changes in clinical neurology and neurosurgery. The even more recent ability to make images showing various aspects of brain physiology is now providing increased understanding of distinctively human mental functions in health and disease. All of these imaging techniques are based on finding and measuring some kind of contrast, much as standard photographs are based on contrasting amounts of light reflected from different parts of a scene.

Understanding the sources of contrast in a clinical image is critical for interpreting what the image shows.

●●● IMAGING X-RAY DENSITY
Skull Films

The first viable methods for measuring contrast in the head used x-rays, discovered late in the 19th century. Skull films (Fig. 8-1), made by directing x-rays through a person's head and mapping what comes out the other side, provide images with excellent spatial resolution. Unfortunately, they include little information about the CNS, for two reasons. First, Ca^{++} salts, primarily located in bone, account for most of the x-ray density in the head. The densities of gray matter and white matter are similar to each other (i.e., there is little contrast) and much less than that of bone. Hence, most of the contrast in a skull film is that between dense and less dense bone (e.g., the petrous temporal bone vs other parts of the skull); the CNS contributes only a negligible amount of x-ray attenuation. Second, a skull film is a record of all the x-ray density in a three-dimensional structure flattened into a two-

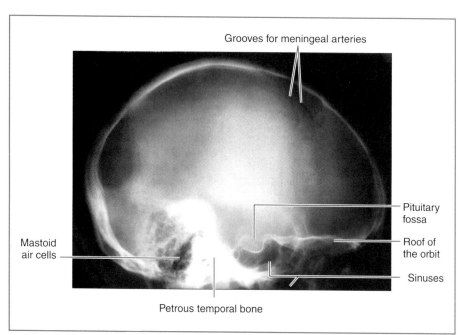

Grooves for meningeal arteries

Mastoid air cells

Petrous temporal bone

Pituitary fossa

Roof of the orbit

Sinuses

Figure 8-1. Normal skull film, lateral view. Many details of bony and air-filled structures can be distinguished easily, although some are superimposed on each other (e.g., the two temporal bones). The CNS, however, cannot be seen. (Courtesy of Dr. Raymond F. Carmody, University of Arizona College of Medicine.)

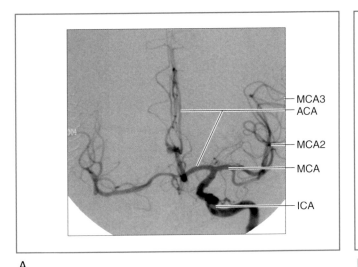

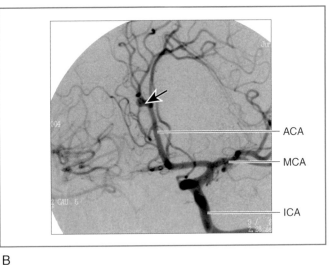

A   B

Figure 8-2. The internal carotid circulation of a 56-year-old man, revealed by injecting an x-ray-dense contrast agent. **A,** An anteroposterior view. **B,** An oblique view makes an aneurysm (*arrow*) at a branch point of the anterior cerebral artery more apparent. ACA, anterior cerebral artery; ICA, internal carotid artery; MCA, middle cerebral artery; MCA2, middle cerebral branches on the surface of the insula; MCA3, middle cerebral emerging from the lateral sulcus. (Courtesy of Dr. Raymond F. Carmody, University of Arizona College of Medicine.)

dimensional map, again ensuring that variations in bone density will account for nearly all the contrast in the image.

During the first half of the 20th century, clinicians had to rely on imaging techniques based on decreasing or increasing the x-ray density of intracranial structures, providing only indirect information about the CNS. Intra-arterial injection of an X-ray-dense contrast agent followed by a rapid series of skull films yields a series of angiograms that demonstrate, first, arteries (Fig. 8-2) and then veins. Because these vessels have a known relationship to CNS structures, displacement of one of them can provide information about underlying processes in the brain (e.g., an expanding tumor). Conversely, air is much less dense than neural tissue, so replacing some cerebrospinal fluid with air creates contrast between those CSF spaces and adjoining parts of the CNS. This can be visualized in a pneumoencephalogram (literally, "a picture of air in the head") (Fig. 8-3). Pneumoencephalography is a painful procedure, because the air causes the brain to float or sag in the remaining CSF, tugging on the meninges; fortunately, it has been completely supplanted by the tomographic techniques described in this chapter.

Computed Tomography

Tomography simply means "taking pictures of slices" and refers to any of a number of techniques for doing so. Optical tomography was first developed in the 1950s by a Dutch medical student as a method for creating cross-sectional images of bone. If an x-ray source and a sheet of x-ray film are oscillated back and forth around a pivot point inside a bone,

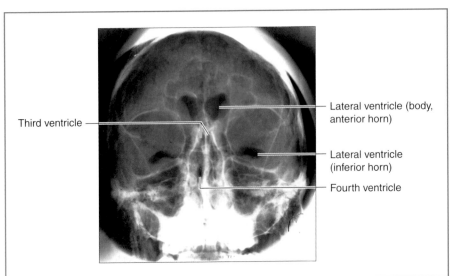

Third ventricle —

— Lateral ventricle (body, anterior horn)

— Lateral ventricle (inferior horn)

— Fourth ventricle

Figure 8-3. A normal pneumo-encephalogram, anteroposterior view. The anterior horn/body and the inferior horn of each lateral ventricle are particularly prominent because in this orientation x-rays travel through most of their (air-filled) longitudinal extent, increasing the contrast between them and their surroundings. (Courtesy of Dr. John Stears, University of Colorado Health Sciences Center.)

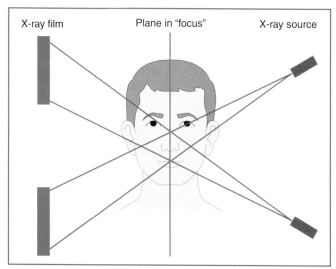

Figure 8-4. The principle of optical tomography. Oscillating an x-ray source between the upper and lower position, while keeping x-ray film coupled to it, results in the recording of a constant pattern of x-ray attenuation from the plane in "focus." Patterns of x-ray attenuation from other planes vary, depending on the angle of the x-ray beam.

then the only constant pattern of x-ray intensities to reach the film will be that passing through a plane containing the pivot point (Fig. 8-4). Variable additional amounts of x-ray attenuation will be added to this constant pattern, depending on the angle of the beam. These will average out, leaving behind an image of the plane containing the pivot point.

Computers became sufficiently powerful in the 1970s to utilize essentially the same logic to construct maps of the x-ray densities in planes through the head (Fig. 8-5). X-ray

computed tomography (usually called simply CT) was the first technique to circumvent the limitations of skull films alluded to above, and it revolutionized neuroradiology. However, an additional trick needs to be applied in order to see brain structures by means of CT. The range of x-ray densities from dense bone to the air in sinuses is about 2000-fold, but the human visual system can discriminate only 200 to 300 shades of gray. Hence, if the gray scale is applied linearly to the entire range of x-ray densities, two things that differ by less than about 0.5% in density (e.g., gray matter and white matter) will wind up being the same shade of gray. A CT image produced in this way (called a bone window setting) demonstrates many details in bony areas but little detail in the CNS (Fig. 8-6A). Resetting the computer so that all shades of gray are distributed through a narrow mid-range of x-ray densities (a soft tissue window) allows gray matter, white matter, and CSF to be distinguished from one another (see Fig. 8-6B). Everything more dense than this mid-range is white and everything less dense is black, so bony detail is lost but calcified intracranial structures stand out (Fig. 8-7).

Because CT makes maps of x-ray density, contrast agents such as those used for angiography make it possible to visualize blood vessels and structures with no blood-brain barrier, such as dural septa and choroid plexus (Fig. 8-8).

●●● MAGNETIC RESONANCE IMAGING

Magnetic resonance imaging (MRI), introduced in the 1980s, is another kind of tomography. Atomic nuclei with an odd number of protons or neutrons act like tiny spinning magnets that can be aligned with each other by a strong external magnetic field. Aligned nuclei absorb radiofrequency electro-

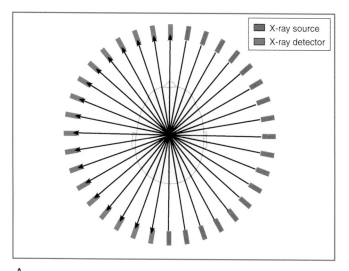

A

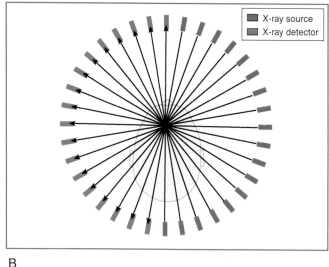

B

Figure 8-5. The principle of x-ray CT. In essence, this is a point-by-point version of the tomography shown in Figure 8-4. **A,** As an x-ray source and x-ray detector rotate around the head, the beam is attenuated by varying amounts, but the x-ray density at the center of rotation is always present. **B,** Changing the center of rotation results in a set of measurements with a different constant value of x-ray attenuation. Combining a large series of such sets of measurements allows the varying attenuations in each set to be subtracted out.

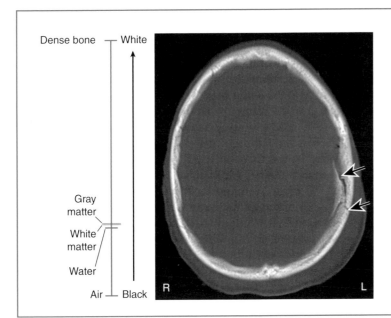

Dense bone — White

Gray matter

White matter

Water

Air — Black

R   L

A

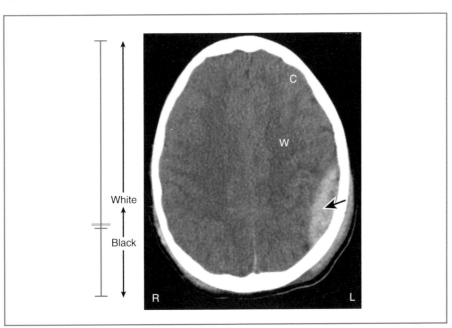

C

W

White

Black

R   L

B

Figure 8-6. CTs of an 11-year-old boy who had been involved in a motor vehicle accident. The scales to the left of each CT show the x-ray densities of air, bone, and some intracranial contents, together with the ranges of x-ray densities set to appear black and white. **A,** With bone window settings, the details of a skull fracture (*arrows*) can be seen easily, but intracranial contents cannot. By convention, the patient's left side is on the right side of the image (as though you were looking up from his feet). **B,** Restricting the gray scale to the range of x-ray densities close to gray matter and white matter makes it possible to discriminate between cerebral cortex (C) and white matter (W), and also reveals an epidural hematoma (*arrow*). (Courtesy of Dr. Raymond F. Carmody, University of Arizona College of Medicine.)

PATHOLOGY

Imaging a Defective Blood-Brain Barrier

X-ray-dense contrast agents are highly polar and unable to cross the blood-brain barrier. However, they leak out into intracranial tumors that lack such a barrier. These include tumors such as meningiomas that arise outside the CNS as well as some types of CNS tumors in which the barrier does not form properly. Hence, contrast-enhanced CT studies can be used not only to indicate the location and extent of some tumors but also to provide diagnostic clues.

magnetic waves at a preferred resonant frequency, determined by the nature of the nuclei and the strength of the external field, making their axis of rotation wobble. They then gradually regain their alignment with the external magnetic field, emitting the absorbed energy. Measuring the emission of these radiofrequency signals can provide the information needed to map the locations and abundance of resonant nuclei. The most common nucleus suitable for such mapping is hydrogen, mostly in water but also in hydrocarbons and other organic molecules. The chemical situation of a given hydrogen nucleus affects the rate at which it emits absorbed energy, so

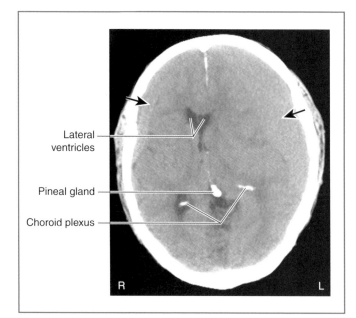

Figure 8-7. CT of an 85-year-old man who had fallen and hit his head. Intracranial structures with significant calcium deposits, such as choroid plexus and the pineal gland, can be seen easily with CT because of their x-ray density. Also revealed in this case are bilateral subdural hematomas (*arrows*). The one on the left is much larger and has pushed the lateral ventricles (and other intracranial structures) to the right. (Courtesy of Dr. Raymond F. Carmody, University of Arizona College of Medicine.)

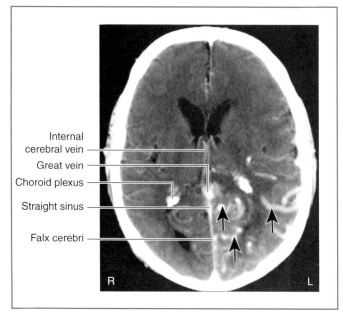

Figure 8-8. Contrast-enhanced CT of a 69-year-old man. The x-ray-dense contrast agent fills blood vessels and also leaks out into structures that lack a blood-brain barrier, making structures such as dural septa and choroid plexus even more prominent. This patient had an arteriovenous malformation, a congenital jumble of dilated arteries and veins (*arrows*) that run directly into each other without intervening capillaries. (Courtesy of Dr. Raymond F. Carmody, University of Arizona College of Medicine.)

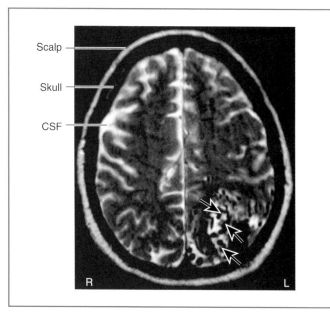

Figure 8-9. T2-weighted MRI (see Fig. 8-10) of the same patient as shown in Figure 8-8. For reasons explained in the text, there is no MRI signal from the skull or from the blood vessels (*arrows*) of the arteriovenous malformation. (Courtesy of Dr. Raymond F. Carmody, University of Arizona College of Medicine.)

by carefully choosing the times at which measurements are made, gray matter, white matter, and CSF can easily be distinguished from each other. Two kinds of areas are notable for their lack of a signal in most MRIs (Fig. 8-9): bone, because of its relative lack of protons, and arteries and veins, because blood keeps moving after absorbing radiofrequency energy and has left the imaging plane by the time the emission signal is measured.

Different time constants of energy emission can be measured, two of which are of particular importance for clinical imaging (Fig. 8-10). T1 is a measure of the rate at which nuclei become realigned with the external field, and T2 is a measure of the rate at which nuclei become desynchronized with each other as they wobble. T2-weighted images are particularly effective for detecting many types of pathology (Fig. 8-11), and T1-weighted images are better for revealing anatomic details (Fig. 8-12).

MRI measurements can be tuned to emphasize flowing blood (Fig. 8-13), and magnetic resonance angiography (MRA), despite its somewhat lower resolution, has largely replaced traditional angiography because it is noninvasive.

FUNCTIONAL IMAGING

CT and especially MRI provide detailed views of structures in and around the CNS but no information about what different parts of the brain are actually doing at any given point in time. Functional imaging techniques, often combined with structural data from CT and MRI, provide this complementary information.

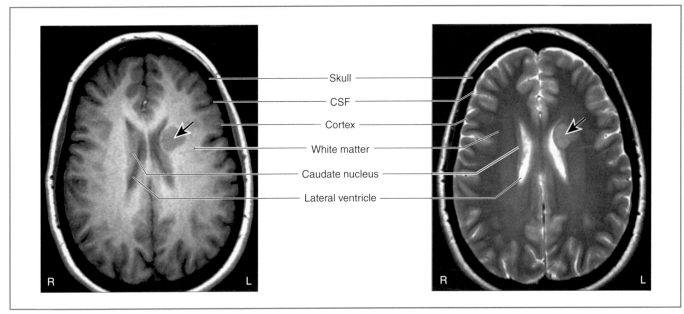

A   B

Figure 8-10. T1-weighted (**A**) and T2-weighted (**B**) MRIs of a 28-year-old woman. In T1-weighted images, gray matter is gray, white matter is white, and CSF is dark (which can make it difficult to discriminate from bone). T2-weighted images are almost the reverse—gray matter is gray, white matter is dark, and CSF is white. This patient had a heterotopia (*arrows*), a developmental defect in which one or more clumps of neurons fail to migrate as far as they should, in this case staying near the lateral ventricle. (Courtesy of Dr. Raymond F. Carmody, University of Arizona College of Medicine.)

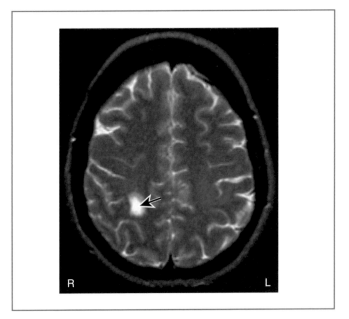

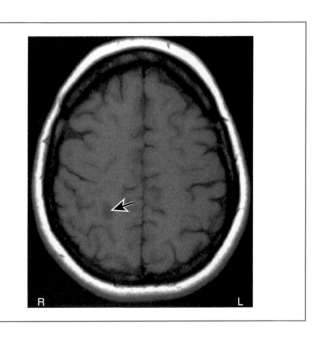

A   B

Figure 8-11. Many types of pathology, in this case a brain tumor, are more easily seen in T2-weighted (**A**) than in T1-weighted (**B**) images. (Courtesy of Dr. Raymond F. Carmody, University of Arizona College of Medicine.)

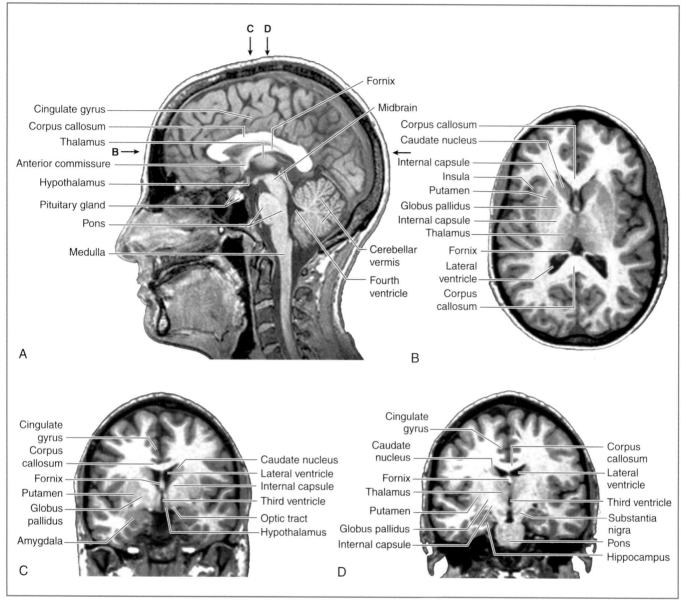

Figure 8-12. Normal brain anatomy, as seen in sagittal (**A**), axial (**B**), and coronal (**C** and **D**) T1-weighted MRIs. The arrows in A indicate the planes in B, C, and D. All of the labeled structures are discussed in various parts of this book. (Courtesy of Dr. Elena Plante, University of Arizona.)

Positron Emission Tomography

Positron emission tomography (PET scanning) uses mathematical analyses like those of CT but in this case to map out the locations of radioisotopes in reconstructed brain slices. Positrons emitted by certain isotopes decay by colliding with a nearby electron, emitting two gamma rays that fly off in opposite directions. Simultaneous hits registered by gamma ray detectors on opposite sides of a person's head indicate a positron source someplace in between the two detectors; the intersection of multiple paths localizes the source (Fig. 8-14). Positron-emitting isotopes can be incorporated into ligands that bind neurotransmitter receptors, into metabolites taken up by active neurons, or, most commonly, into water molecules.

Blood flow increases slightly in proportion to changes in electrical activity in different parts of the CNS, so intravenously injected $H_2^{15}O$ can be used to track blood flow increases and provide an indirect measure of local areas of brain activity.

Functional MRI

Although PET scanning can provide spectacular images of the brain in action, it has some limitations. A positron can travel for a few millimeters before encountering an electron, so its spatial resolution is not very good. In addition, the production of positron-emitting isotopes is demanding and their half-lives are short. For these reasons, the development

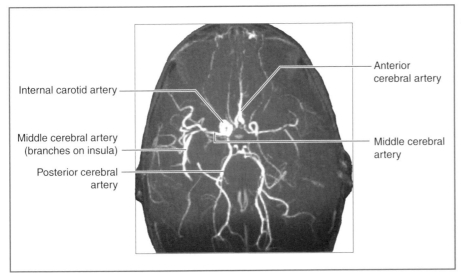

Figure 8-13. Major arteries at the base of the brain, as seen in a magnetic resonance angiogram (MRA). (Courtesy of Dr. Raymond F. Carmody, University of Arizona College of Medicine.)

Internal carotid artery

Anterior cerebral artery

Middle cerebral artery (branches on insula)

Middle cerebral artery

Posterior cerebral artery

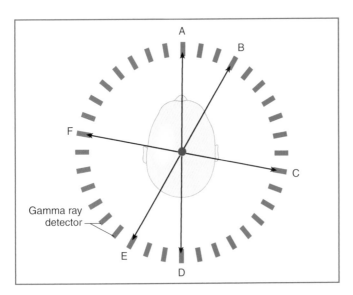

Gamma ray detector

Figure 8-14. The principle of PET scanning. The computations are basically similar to those in CT (see Fig. 8-5), but in this case the signal comes from inside the brain. A series of simultaneous "hits" at detectors A and D, B and E, and C and F would indicate the presence of a positron emitter at the intersection of these three paths.

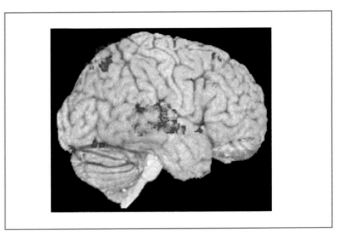

A

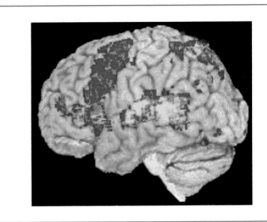

B

Figure 8-15. Functional MRIs showing cortical areas where blood flow increased (yellow and orange areas) as normal adults listened to stories. The activated areas largely correspond to the language-processing network discussed in Chapter 19 (see Fig. 19-13) and are more extensive in the left hemisphere (**B**) than in the right (**A**). (Courtesy of Dr. Elena Plante, University of Arizona.)

of MRI methods for tracking changes in blood flow has been a significant advance.

The increase in blood flow to active areas of the brain is actually even larger than required, so active areas wind up with greater levels of oxygenated hemoglobin than less active areas. Measuring hemoglobin-deoxyhemoglobin ratios with MRI provides a blood oxygen level–dependent (BOLD) signal related to blood flow that is the basis for functional magnetic resonance imaging (fMRI). Functional MRI can be used to map blood flow changes with greater temporal and spatial resolution than PET scanning (Fig. 8-15), without the need for radioisotopes.

Somatosensory System 9

CONTENTS

Sensory receptors of different types, as indicated in Chapter 4, are specialized in distinctive ways but also have some common organizing principles. The same is true of the CNS systems to which these receptors provide information, so this chapter reviews not just the specific properties of the somatosensory system, but also the ways in which it resembles or differs from the other sensory systems discussed in the four subsequent chapters.

●●● SOMATOSENSORY RECEPTORS

We use the somatosensory system as the basis for perceiving a variety of modalities and submodalities—touch, texture, the position of body parts, pain, temperature, tickle, itch, and others—by combining the information provided by multiple kinds of receptors. With one possible exception, all of them are receptors with long axons. In general, those for touch and position have large-diameter, heavily myelinated axons, and those for pain and temperature have small-diameter, thinly myelinated or unmyelinated axons.

The receptive endings of large-diameter fibers are mechanoreceptors that typically have either connective tissue capsules or accessory structures that filter mechanical stimuli in some way (Table 9-1). The receptive endings of small-diameter fibers, in contrast, are typically free nerve endings with no obvious anatomic specializations, even though some of them respond selectively to painful stimuli, others to innocuous temperature changes or light touch.

Cutaneous and Subcutaneous Receptors

Touch Receptors

The receptors that provide the information we use for the discriminative aspects of touch—assessing the shape and texture of objects, and the direction of movement across the skin—all have large-diameter axons and encapsulated endings or endings with accessory structures. Prominent examples of this category are Meissner corpuscles, pacinian corpuscles, and Merkel endings (Fig. 9-1). The packing density of receptors like this, especially the Meissner corpuscles and Merkel endings, determines the tactile acuity of a given area of skin. This varies quite a bit, from the fingertips and lips, where we

Ending Type	Receptor Type	Location	Responds to	Axon Type
Free nerve endings		Ubiquitous	Pain, temperature, light touch	Aδ, C
Encapsulated endings	Meissner corpuscles	Glabrous skin	Changing touch	Aβ
	Pacinian corpuscles	Skin, joints, deep connective tissue	Vibration	Aβ
	Muscle spindles	Skeletal muscle	Muscle stretch	Ia, Aβ
	Golgi tendon organs	Muscle-tendon junction	Muscle tension	Ib
Endings with accessory structures	Merkel endings	Glabrous and hairy skin	Touch	Aβ
	Endings around hairs	Hairy skin	Touch	Various

TABLE 9-1. Major Somatosensory Receptor Types

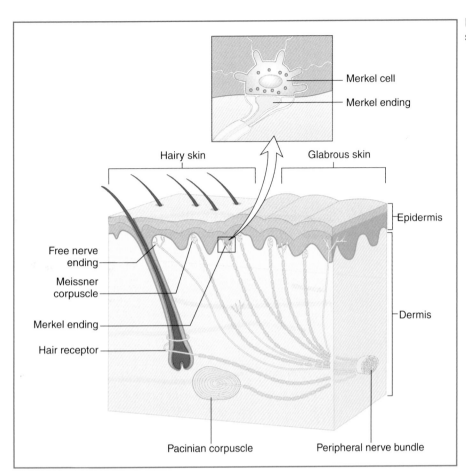

Figure 9-1. Major cutaneous and subcutaneous receptors.

can distinguish between two small objects separated by only a few millimeters, to the skin of the legs and trunk, where objects can be separated by a few cm and still feel like a single object.

Meissner corpuscles, found in the dermal papillae of glabrous (hairless) skin, are encapsulated structures containing flattened disks of Schwann cell cytoplasm piled up like a stack of pancakes. One or more large-diameter axons enter the capsule and wind back and forth between the Schwann cell disks. Pushing on the skin compresses the receptive ending, but the Schwann cells and capsule filter out sustained indentations, making this a rapidly adapting receptor. Meissner corpuscles are important for detecting the details of things moving across the skin. They come into play when we move our fingertips across something, or when something in our grasp begins to slip and distorts the skin.

Pacinian corpuscles, widespread in subcutaneous connective tissue, have a multilayered capsule shaped like an onion in cross-section. The layers act as a mechanical filter (see Fig. 4-9A), making this a very rapidly adapting receptor that responds briefly at the beginning and end of a mechanical stimulus. This makes pacinian corpuscles good at detecting rapidly changing stimuli, such as vibrations.

Merkel endings, abundant in both glabrous and hairy skin, are the flattened sensory terminals of large-diameter axons applied to Merkel cells in the basal layer of the epidermis. Merkel endings are sensitive, slowly adapting receptors

important for detecting the shape and texture of stationary objects touching the skin. Merkel cells are thought by some to be the actual receptor cells because they make what look like synaptic contacts on Merkel endings, but definitive evidence is lacking.

Other receptors involved in detecting tactile stimuli include sensory endings wrapped around the bases of hairs, and a recently discovered population of unmyelinated (C) fibers with free nerve endings in hairy skin that respond best to slow, gentle brushing of the skin. The C-fiber touch receptors are probably more important for the pleasurable feelings associated with this kind of touch than for its explicit detection (see Chapter 18).

Receptors for Coolness and Warmth

The receptors for conscious awareness of innocuous temperature changes are all free nerve endings. Those for cooling have thinly myelinated (Aδ) axons, and those for warming have unmyelinated (C) axons. These are different receptors from those that detect painful heat and cold (see Fig. 4-4).

Nociceptors

Receptors that detect events that damage or threaten to damage tissue are grouped together as nociceptors. One might imagine that the receptors for painful stimuli would have the largest, most rapidly conducting axons, but in fact the need for speed is greater in the receptors used to coordinate escape, and nociceptors have small-diameter axons. Some are thinly myelinated (Aδ) fibers, and others are C fibers. These two groups of nociceptors correspond to everyone's experience with pain as a two-part sensation. A physically painful event (e.g., touching a very hot pot, missing a nail and hitting a finger with the hammer) elicits first a sensation of sharp, well-localized fast pain followed by a dull, poorly localized, aching sensation of slow pain. Fast pain is initiated by firing of Aδ nociceptors, and the delayed onset of slow pain is directly related to the slower conduction velocity of the C fibers that mediate it.

Tissue damage is more complicated than something like skin indentation or muscle stretch. Multiple things can cause it, and once it occurs a series of chemical changes in the damaged tissue ensue. Correspondingly, nociceptors transduce multiple aspects of painful stimuli. Aδ nociceptors respond specifically to intense mechanical stimulation (e.g., pinprick), to painful heat or cold, or to both. C-fiber nociceptors respond to all of these, as well as to a variety of substances released in damaged tissue; for this reason, they are also referred to as polymodal nociceptors.

Muscle Receptors

Skeletal muscles, like other tissues, contain free nerve endings; some of these detect muscle pain, and others probably keep track of the metabolic status of the muscle. They also contain muscle spindles and Golgi tendon organs (Fig. 9-2), encapsulated receptors that monitor the length and tension of a muscle, respectively.

Muscle spindles are small, cigar-shaped organs consisting of a few slender, intrafusal ("inside the spindle") muscle fibers enclosed in a capsular continuation of the perineurium. They are found in nearly all skeletal muscles; just as the packing density of cutaneous receptors is related to the tactile acuity of an area of skin, the number of spindles in a muscle is related to the degree of fine control we have over its contraction. Each intrafusal fiber has a central, nucleated, noncontractile zone with sensory endings wrapped around it, flanked by contractile zones. Both ends of the spindle are anchored in the muscle among the extrafusal ("outside the spindle") muscle fibers, so stretching the muscle also stretches the central zones of the intrafusal fibers and distorts the mechanosensory endings. The contractile portions of the intrafusal fibers are innervated by gamma motor neurons (so called because their

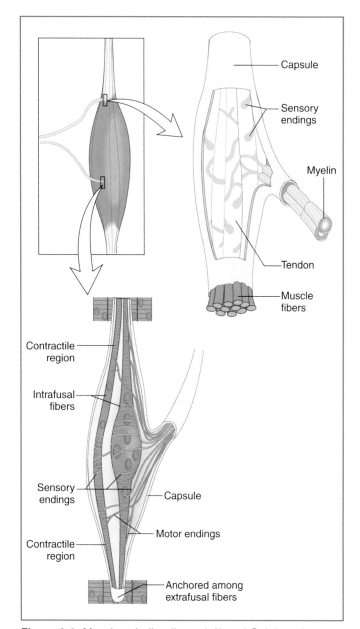

Figure 9-2. Muscle spindles (*lower left*) and Golgi tendon organs (*upper right*), the major encapsulated receptors of skeletal muscle.

axons are in the Aγ category), but are too small to generate a significant amount of force. Instead, the power of a muscle is produced by contraction of the extrafusal fibers, and contraction of the intrafusal fibers stretches their sensory region, thereby regulating their sensitivity (see Fig. 4-7A). This provides an elegant mechanism for maintaining constant sensitivity of a spindle during contraction and relaxation of a muscle. Muscle spindles monitor changes in the length of muscles as a person moves about, providing information important for the coordination of movement and awareness of changes in position.

Golgi tendon organs are encapsulated regions of myotendinous junctions in which large-diameter sensory axons enter the perineurial capsule and divide into branches that are

---

PHARMACOLOGY

Relieving Pain by Suppressing Nociceptors

As the membranes of damaged cells begin to break down, arachidonic acid is released. Its conversion to prostaglandins by cyclooxygenase contributes to the inflammation following tissue damage, because prostaglandins lower the threshold of nociceptive endings. Aspirin and NSAIDs such as ibuprofen help alleviate inflammatory pain by blocking cyclooxygenase.

interdigitated with the collagen bundles there. Contracting a muscle against resistance squeezes the endings between the collagen bundles, allowing Golgi tendon organs to monitor the tension in a muscle, something that muscle spindles cannot provide much information about.

Position Sense

Movement at a joint stimulates receptors in the joint itself, changes the length of muscles that insert around the joint, and distorts the skin and subcutaneous tissues surrounding the joint. The CNS uses all of this information both to coordinate movements and for conscious awareness of the position of our parts in space (proprioception). The importance of specific receptor types varies at different joints, but in general muscle spindles play a major role and joint receptors, surprisingly, are the least important.

●●● DISTRIBUTION OF SOMATOSENSORY INFORMATION IN THE CENTRAL NERVOUS SYSTEM

Each vertebrate sensory system has one collection of receptors that are used for multiple functions—at the very least, feeding into pathways to the cerebral cortex (conscious awareness), into reflex circuitry, and in most or all cases into pathways to the cerebellum as well. As in the somatosensory system (Fig. 9-3), this is accomplished by primary afferents that branch repeatedly and make synapses on multiple sets of interneurons on the ipsilateral side of the CNS.

Although no one knows exactly why, somatosensory pathways to the cerebral cortex cross the midline (i.e., something touching the left hand causes electrical activity in the right postcentral gyrus). Because both primary afferents and thalamocortical neurons terminate without crossing, at least one additional neuron with an axon that does cross the midline must be involved. With the exception of olfaction, the pathways that convey other kinds of sensory information to the cerebral cortex also involve at least three neurons, but they do not all cross the midline as somatosensory pathways do. Some project bilaterally (e.g., vision, hearing), and others are largely uncrossed (e.g., taste). The olfactory bulb is an outgrowth of the telencephalon, and the axons of olfactory receptors project directly to ipsilateral olfactory cortex, bypassing the thalamus.

Pathways to the cerebellum do not include a stop in the thalamus, so only two neurons need to be involved (see Fig. 9-3) although, as discussed in Chapter 16, many involve more than two. In addition, the cerebellum affects the ipsilateral side of the body (see Fig. 5-24), so most spinocerebellar neurons are uncrossed.

Reflexes

Reflexes are automatic responses to sensory inputs, such as pupillary constriction in response to bright light and salivation in response to something appetizing. Important reflexes

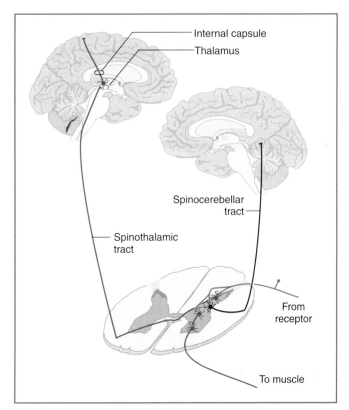

Figure 9-3. Distribution pattern of somatosensory information in the CNS. Note that primary afferents terminate without crossing, and that projections to the thalamus cross and those to the cerebellum do not. Not all somatosensory projections to the thalamus travel through the spinothalamic tract (see text for details), and there are multiple spinocerebellar tracts (see Chapter 16).

involving somatosensory afferents include the stretch reflex (see Figs. 2-23 through 2-25) and the flexor reflex, one that we all know from common experience—it withdraws a body part from a painful stimulus. The stretch reflex is as simple as a reflex can be, involving a large-diameter primary afferent from a muscle spindle and a motor neuron that projects back to the same muscle. All other reflexes involve one or more interneurons, generally because they affect multiple muscles. Withdrawing an entire limb through a flexor reflex, for example, requires contacting motor neurons in several spinal segments (Fig. 9-4).

●●● TOUCH AND POSITION: POSTERIOR COLUMN–MEDIAL LEMNISCUS PATHWAY

Sensory axons of all sizes are intermingled in spinal nerves, but as dorsal rootlets approach the spinal cord the large- and small-diameter fibers separate from each other. The large-diameter axons move medially, enter the ipsilateral posterior funiculus (also called the posterior column), and give off numerous branches (see Fig. 9-3). One of these branches continues rostrally through the spinal cord, forming the first leg of the major pathway that conveys touch and position

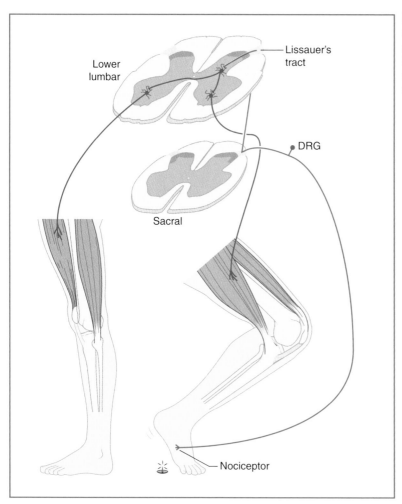

Figure 9-4. Circuitry of the flexor reflex (also known as the withdrawal reflex because of its function). Although only one lumbar segment is shown here to keep the diagram simple, the motor neurons for leg and hip flexors on one side and leg extensors on the other side are spread over several segments.

information to somatosensory cortex (Fig. 9-5). Those from the lower extremity form a fasciculus gracilis ("slender bundle"), which moves progressively more medially as it ascends the spinal cord, displaced by similar fibers that enter in more rostral segments and form a fasciculus cuneatus ("wedge-shaped bundle"). These two sets of axons then synapse on the second neuron in the pathway, located in nucleus gracilis and nucleus cuneatus (the posterior column nuclei) in the medulla. Their axons in turn cross the midline in the medulla, forming the medial lemniscus. (The medial lemniscus ["ribbon"] was so named because it starts out near the midline and is shaped like a ribbon cut in cross-section.) The medial lemniscus ascends through the brainstem and terminates in the ventral posterior nucleus of the thalamus (in a lateral part called the ventral posterolateral nucleus, or VPL), which in turn projects through the posterior limb of the internal capsule to somatosensory cortex in the postcentral gyrus. Comparable information from the face arrives in the trigeminal nerve and terminates at a midpontine level in the main sensory nucleus of the trigeminal nerve (also referred to as the chief sensory or principal sensory nucleus of the trigeminal). Axons arising in the main sensory nucleus cross the midline, join the medial lemniscus, and terminate in the medial part of the ventral posterior nucleus (the ventral posteromedial nucleus, or VPM).

The face and body are represented systematically in the postcentral gyrus in a distorted somatotopic map. The area devoted to any part is related to the packing density of receptors there, so the somatosensory homunculus (a figurative "little person") has disproportionately large fingers and lips. This mapping starts way back in the spinal cord, where lower extremity fibers are situated medial to upper extremity fibers, and continues into the medial lemniscus and the pattern of its terminations in the thalamus. Systematic, distorted maps are a common feature of sensory systems. Visual cortex, for example, has a retinotopic map with an enlarged area devoted to the central part of the visual field; different levels of the auditory system contain tonotopic maps with speech frequencies emphasized.

●●● PAIN AND TEMPERATURE: ANTEROLATERAL PATHWAY

Pain is different from touch and position in that it has not only a discriminative aspect but also a powerful emotional and motivational component. The discriminative aspect (judging the location, nature, and intensity of a painful stimulus) is similar in all of us and fairly consistent from day to day. The emotional and motivational component (how

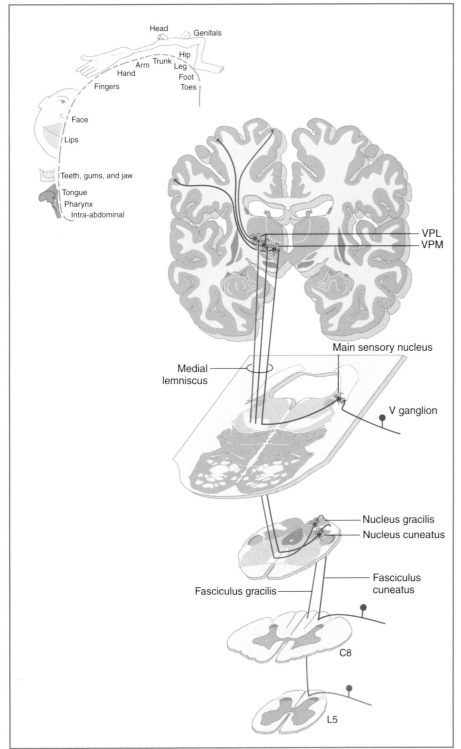

Figure 9-5. The posterior column–medial lemniscus pathway.

unpleasant the pain is, autonomic responses to it) varies from person to person and from one behavioral situation to another. The anatomic substrate for these dual components is a more widespread distribution of pain information than of touch and position information in the CNS. Warm and cool stimuli, even when innocuous, often feel pleasant or unpleasant and motivate a person to persist in a behavior or change

it. This is reflected by a similar distribution of pain and temperature information in the CNS.

Pain and temperature pathways begin with small-diameter primary afferent fibers that separate from large-diameter fibers as the dorsal rootlets join the spinal cord. The Aδ and C fibers enter the cord lateral to the larger fibers, join Lissauer's tract, and divide into ascending and descending branches that

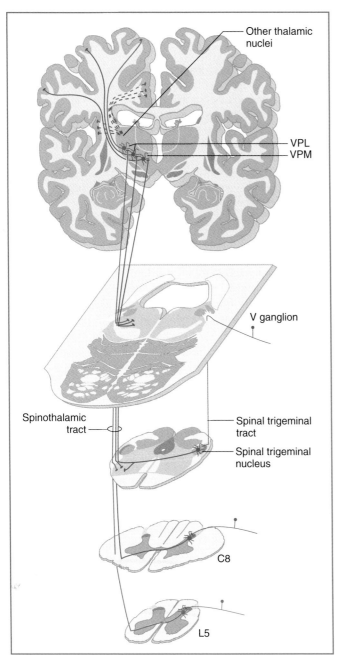

Figure 9-6. The anterolateral pathway. VPM, ventral posteromedial nucleus.

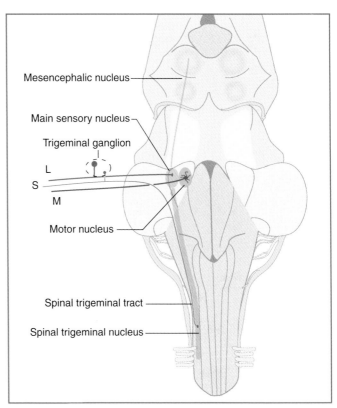

Figure 9-7. Trigeminal nuclei in the brainstem. L, S, and M are large-diameter afferents, small-diameter afferents, and motor axons to muscles of mastication.

distribute synapses to neurons in the posterior horn over several segments. Some of these are interneurons in flexor reflex arcs, others are tract cells that project to the cerebellum, but many are tract cells with axons that cross the midline in the spinal cord to form the anterolateral pathway (Fig. 9-6). The anterolateral pathway, so called because of its location in the anterior part of the lateral funiculus, is actually a composite of several tracts, all conveying pain and temperature information. Some constitute the spinothalamic tract, axons that project all the way to VPL and other thalamic nuclei. Others, as well as branches of spinothalamic axons, project to the reticular formation (to get the attention of a person in

discomfort), to autonomic centers in the brainstem and spinal cord, and to a distinctive area of gray matter surrounding the cerebral aqueduct (the periaqueductal gray). VPL then relays some of this information to somatosensory cortex, subserving the discriminative aspects of pain and temperature sensation. Other thalamic nuclei project to limbic areas of cortex such as the cingulate gyrus and insula, subserving the emotional and motivational aspects.

The trigeminal nerve also contributes to this pathway, bringing information about pain and temperature in the face and head. The primary afferents take an unexpected course (see Fig. 9-6). There are four trigeminal nuclei in the brainstem (Fig. 9-7)—one motor and three sensory. The trigeminal motor nucleus is a collection of motor neurons for the muscles of mastication. The mesencephalic trigeminal nucleus (so named because it extends all the way into the midbrain) is notable more for its anatomic weirdness than for its functional importance: it is a slender collection of pseudounipolar primary afferent neurons that by rights should live in the trigeminal ganglion. The peripheral branches of these neurons innervate mechanoreceptors in and around the temporomandibular joint, and the central branches terminate in the same places as other large-diameter trigeminal afferents. The main sensory nucleus (see Fig. 9-5) is the trigeminal's equivalent of a posterior column nucleus. Finally, the spinal trigeminal nucleus extends from the level of the main sensory nucleus

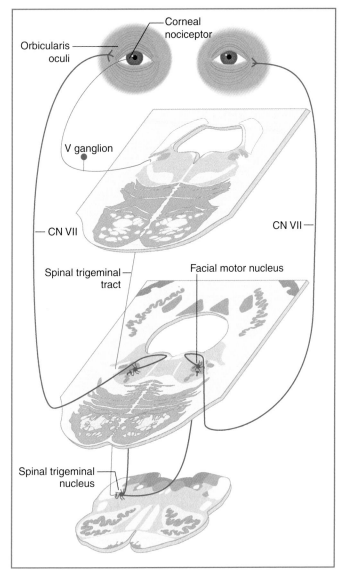

Figure 9-8. Circuitry of the blink reflex. The facial motor nucleus contains the motor neurons for the muscles of facial expression (the peculiar course taken by axons leaving this nucleus is discussed in Chapter 14).

all the way to the cervical spinal cord, where it merges with the posterior horn. Small-diameter trigeminal afferents enter the brainstem at a midpontine level with the rest of the trigeminal nerve, descend through the spinal trigeminal tract and synapse on the trigeminal's equivalent of spinothalamic tract cells in the part of the spinal nucleus in the caudal medulla.[1] The reason for this seemingly odd location of second-order neurons is that it completes a somatotopic pain and temperature map that unfolds through progressively more rostral levels of the spinal posterior horn and continues

[1]Pain and temperature information from the vicinity of the outer ear is conveyed to the CNS in part by cranial nerves VII, IX, and X, but once these fibers reach the brainstem they behave like trigeminal afferents and enter the spinal trigeminal tract.

PHARMACOLOGY & CLINICAL MEDICINE

Trigeminal Neuralgia

Trigeminal neuralgia is characterized by brief episodes of intense pain in trigeminal territory, usually in one division on one side. Although the mechanism is not known with certainty, many cases are thought to start with abnormal activity in a branch of the trigeminal nerve caused by a pulsating artery impinging on it, followed over time by the development of seizure-like hyperactivity of the spinal trigeminal nucleus. Consistent with this mechanism, trigeminal neuralgia is most commonly and successfully treated with anticonvulsant agents such as carbamazepine.

into the spinal trigeminal nucleus. Parts of the spinal trigeminal nucleus in the rostral medulla and caudal pons take care of the remaining spinal-cord-like functions, such as relaying trigeminal information to the cerebellum and housing interneurons for the blink reflex (Fig. 9-8). This is the trigeminal's equivalent of a flexor reflex and results in both eyes blinking in response to something touching either cornea.

Control of Pain Transmission

The CNS controls the sensitivity of all of its sensory systems, but perhaps nowhere is this more apparent than with pain. Pain serves functions crucial for survival, warning of damage and convincing an animal to protect injured tissues, but in some situations pain could actually impede survival-related activities. For example, limping slowly away from a threatening situation might not be healthy. To address situations like this (and the reverse, lowering the pain threshold when possible pain is anticipated), the nervous system has multiple mechanisms for adjusting the sensitivity of the spinothalamic tract. The best known is a descending pain-control pathway that originates in the periaqueductal gray (Fig. 9-9). This area

PHARMACOLOGY

Opiates and Pain Relief

Morphine and other opiate analgesics produce their effects by mimicking the actions of opioid peptides (enkephalin, endorphin, dynorphin) manufactured by neurons and used as neurotransmitters. Opioid receptors are widespread in pain-related parts of the CNS (and in others parts of the CNS and other parts of the body). Opioid peptides have inhibitory postsynaptic effects and are used by interneurons in the substantia gelatinosa to inhibit transmission from nociceptors to spinothalamic tract cells. They inhibit a tonic inhibition of periaqueductal gray pain-suppression neurons, thereby activating this system. They even work in the periphery, by acting on opioid receptors borne by cells of the immune system.

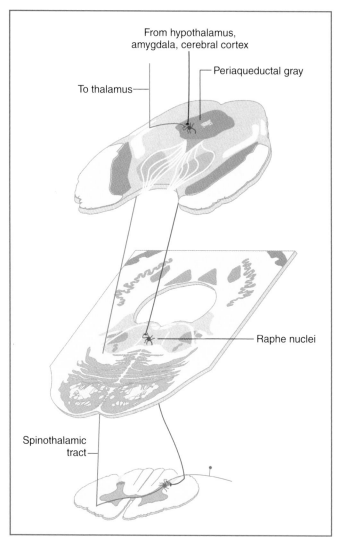

From hypothalamus,
amygdala, cerebral cortex

Periaqueductal gray

To thalamus

Raphe nuclei

Spinothalamic
tract

Figure 9-9. Mediation of descending pain control by the periaqueductal gray (PAG). Although only a projection to the raphe nuclei is shown, the PAG actually projects to several areas of the reticular formation that in turn project to the spinal cord and suppress pain transmission. Other reticular projections (not shown) enhance pain transmission in other situations.

of the midbrain receives converging inputs from the anterolateral pathway, from the hypothalamus, and from other parts of the limbic system. In situations when pain suppression is appropriate, the periaqueductal gray projects to medullary raphe nuclei and other parts of the reticular formation, which in turn project to the spinal cord and inhibit the transmission of information from pain and temperature afferents to spinothalamic tract cells.

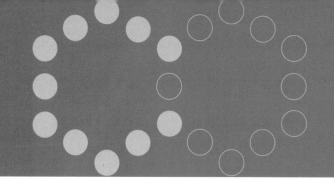

Auditory System

CONTENTS

The sensory systems of animals typically are stunning achievements of compactness and efficiency, but in many ways the auditory system stands out among them. Beginning with the capture by the eardrum of the energy in movements of atomic dimensions, continuing through a frequency analyzer (the cochlea) the size of a few grains of rice, using a relatively minuscule number of receptors and sensory neurons, the human ear is able to analyze a seemingly limitless variety of sounds. One consequence of the specialized components and connections involved in these feats is that distinctive deficits result from damage to them.

●●● THE NATURE OF SOUND

Pushing against a resistive medium such as air or water causes a local increase in pressure. This in turn pushes against neighboring areas of the medium, resulting in a shell of compression that moves through the medium in three dimensions; the air or water doesn't move much, but rather the wave of compression moves through it. Similarly, pulling back on the interface causes a wave of rarefaction to move through the medium. Alternating between the two, as an oscillating speaker cone does, causes successive waves of compression and rarefaction with a frequency dictated by the frequency of oscillation and an amplitude (i.e., degree of compression and rarefaction)

related to the magnitude of the oscillation. The job of the auditory system is to capture the energy of such waves in the environment, convert it into electrical signals that the nervous system can use, and then interpret these signals.

Range of Audible Frequencies

Strictly speaking, *sound* refers to the range of frequencies that cause electrical changes in the auditory system of a given species. For humans (Fig. 10-1), this range is from about 20 to 20,000 Hz (1 Hz = 1 hertz = 1 cycle per second). Physical waves in the environment cover a wide range of frequencies, however, and other animals have audible spectra displaced toward lower frequencies (elephants, 5 Hz to 12 kHz) or higher frequencies (bats, 2 kHz to 110 kHz). Sensitivity is not uniform across the audible spectrum. Largely because of the mechanical properties of the outer ear (see below), humans are most sensitive in the lower mid-frequency range, peaking around 3 kHz (see Fig. 10-1). Not coincidentally, this range of maximum sensitivity is the range that is most important for perception of speech.

Decibel Scale

The range of sound pressure levels over which humans have meaningful hearing ability is remarkable. From threshold at

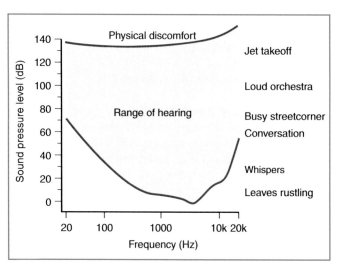

Figure 10-1. Frequency and intensity range of human hearing.

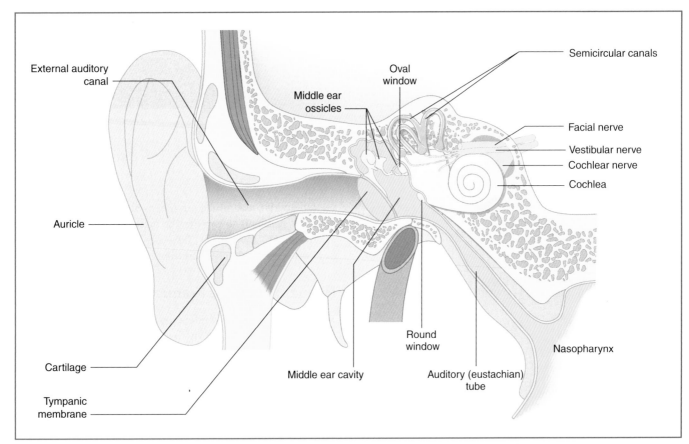

Figure 10-2. Outer, middle, and inner ear, showing the bony labyrinth embedded in the temporal bone.

3 kHz, at which the system almost allows us to hear the Brownian motion of air molecules banging against the tympanic membrane, our hearing extends over a 10 million–fold range of pressure levels until sound causes physical discomfort. Action potential rates cannot change nearly enough to effectively code this great a range in a proportional way, and so the nervous system codes sound intensity logarithmically: each 10-fold jump in sound intensity causes the same linear step increase in perceived loudness. Auditory stimuli and thresholds are also quantified using a logarithmic scale (see Fig. 10-1), one in which the units are decibels:

$$\text{decibels (dB)} = 20 \log P/P_0$$

where P is the sound pressure level and P_0 is a reference level (usually the threshold for normal hearing at the best frequency). Thus, a threshold stimulus is at 0 dB ($\log P_0/P_0 = 0$) and the loudest comfortable sound pressure level is 140 dB ($\log 10^7 P_0/P_0 = 7$).

●●● OUTER, MIDDLE, AND INNER EAR

Fish have a relatively easy time of it when it comes to hearing, because sounds have little trouble moving from the water surrounding them into the fluids in which their auditory receptor cells (like virtually all parts of all nervous systems) are bathed. Terrestrial vertebrates, in contrast, must somehow transfer the energy of airborne sound vibrations into the fluids surrounding receptor cells in the inner ear. This is a problem, since the density of water makes it hard to move (relative to air) and 99.9% of the sound incident on a simple air-water interface is simply reflected. This problem is addressed by two air-filled components—the outer and middle ears (Fig. 10-2). The outer ear funnels airborne vibrations to the middle ear, emphasizing certain frequencies along the way, and the middle ear effectively transfers this vibratory energy to the fluid-filled inner ear.

Outer Ear

The outer ear is the direct air connection through which sounds enter the auditory apparatus. Its major components are the auricle (or pinna) and the external auditory canal (ear canal) into which it leads. It ends at the tympanic membrane (eardrum), the boundary between the outer and middle ears.

The auricle is a cartilaginous plate with a series of elevations and depressions. The most important of these for the overall function of the outer ear is the concha ("sea shell"), the depression that funnels into the ear canal. The concha and ear canal resonate at certain frequencies, with the result that sound pressure in a broad mid-frequency range peaking at

Innervation of the Auricle

The skin of the outer ear is at the junction between spinal nerve territory (the back of the head) and cranial nerve territory. As a result, it has an odd, overlapping innervation pattern, with contributions from the trigeminal, facial, glossopharyngeal, and vagus nerves, as well as C2 and C3 dorsal roots. Pathology affecting any of these nerves can cause symptoms involving the ear, and stimulation of the ear can cause autonomic responses through central connections of cranial nerves IX and X.

Measuring How Well the Tympanic Membrane Works

The tympanic membrane is most free to move when the air pressure in the middle ear cavity is the same as that in the ear canal (as is normally the case). Middle ear pathology can block the eustachian (auditory) tube and result in decreased or increased pressure in the middle ear cavity, impeding vibration of the tympanic membrane. This can be assessed qualitatively with an otoscope or quantitatively with a tympanometer, by determining whether increased or decreased pressure in the ear canal improves the ability of the tympanic membrane to move.

about 3 kHz is amplified by up to 20 dB by the time it reaches the tympanic membrane.

The asymmetric arrangement of the auricle's corrugations is the basis for its second major function, that of helping in the localization of sound. Because of these asymmetries, high frequencies coming from different directions are absorbed by different amounts. Remarkably, humans and other animals learn these distortion patterns and use them unconsciously to help decide the direction of a sound source (especially for sources in or near the sagittal plane, as explained below).

Middle Ear

The middle ear, an air-filled cavity in the temporal bone, functions as a mechanical transformer that largely overcomes the air-water interface problem. The tympanic membrane forms its lateral wall, part of the periosteal surface of the temporal bone forms its medial wall, and an air connection to the pharynx (the eustachian, or auditory, tube) maintains the same atmos-

pheric pressure in the middle ear cavity as in the ear canal. The cavity is bridged by a series of three tiny bones, or ossicles (Fig. 10-3). The malleus ("hammer") is attached to the medial surface of the tympanic membrane and to the incus ("anvil"). The incus in turn is attached to the stapes ("stirrup"), whose oval footplate occupies a hole in the temporal bone (the oval window). On the other side of the oval window are the fluids of the inner ear. The stapes acts somewhat like a piston, so that inward and outward movements of the tympanic membrane result in pushes and pulls on the footplate. Because fluids are relatively incompressible, these pushes and pulls would result in no fluid movement unless something else moved out and in to accommodate them. This is accomplished by reciprocal movements of the membrane covering a second hole in the temporal bone (the round window).

The malleus and incus function as a lever system with a slight mechanical advantage, resulting in a small force increase at the stapes footplate. More importantly, the area of

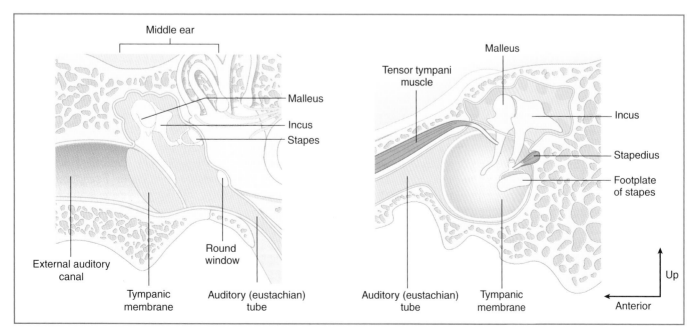

Figure 10-3. Middle ear cavity and its contents, as seen in a coronal (*left*) and parasaggital (*right*) section.

the tympanic membrane is nearly 20 times that of the oval window (like the arrangement of a big piston and a small piston in a hydraulic jack). The combined result is that just as an electrical transformer, without adding any energy, converts one voltage and current to a higher (or lower) voltage and lower (or higher) current, the middle ear system converts the relatively large-amplitude but low-force vibrations at the tympanic membrane into vibrations of smaller amplitude but force sufficient to move the inner ear fluids. At the most effective frequency (about 1 kHz), energy is transferred nearly perfectly, with a loss of only 3 dB or so.

Middle Ear Muscles

Tiny muscles attached to two of the middle ear ossicles (see Fig. 10-3) can dampen the transmission of vibrations into the inner ear fluids. The tensor tympani, innervated by the trigeminal nerve, extends from a small canal above the auditory tube to the handle of the malleus. When it contracts, it pulls in on the tympanic membrane (hence, the name of the muscle), diminishing its ability to vibrate. The stapedius, innervated by the facial nerve, occupies a small cavity in the temporal bone; its tendon emerges from the cavity and attaches to the malleus. Contraction of the stapedius pulls the stapes sideways, diminishing the ability of its footplate to move in the oval window.

The functional significance of these muscles has been the subject of much debate. The stapedius contracts in response to loud sounds, as part of a clinically useful reflex (see below). However, the threshold of this reflex is about 85 dB—louder than most sounds encountered in nature—casting doubt on the traditional hypothesis that it has a protective role. The tensor tympani contracts in response to almost painfully loud sounds, but one or both muscles also contract in conjunction with normal activities such as swallowing and speaking. Both muscles selectively decrease the transmission of low-frequency sounds, and they may be more important for enhancing the intelligibility of high-frequency environmental sounds during these normal activities.

Middle Ear Dysfunction

A variety of pathologic conditions can impede the transfer of energy through the middle ear apparatus (e.g., infections [otitis media], trauma, bony growths [otosclerosis] that fix the stapes footplate in the oval window), resulting in conductive hearing loss. At their worst, such conditions might be expected to cause the inner ear to behave like a simple air-water interface, absorbing only 0.1% of the incident sound (i.e., a 30 dB loss). In fact, the hearing loss can be as much as 60 dB, in large part because airborne sound would then simultaneously impinge on both the oval window and the round window, trying unsuccessfully at both locations to compress an incompressible fluid. Regardless of the severity of middle ear damage, however, there would be little change in the effectiveness of vibrations delivered directly to the fluids of the inner ear. This can be tested by applying a vibrating probe to the temporal bone, typically to the bony prominence behind the ear (the mastoid process), stimulating hearing by

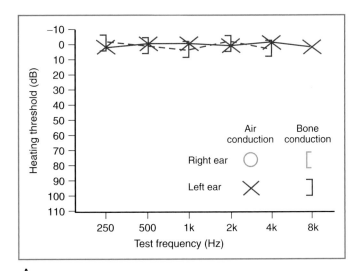

A

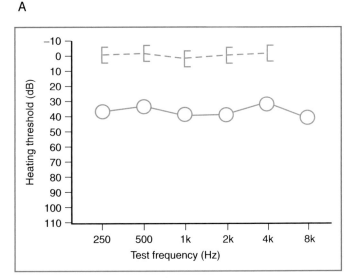

B

Figure 10-4. Audiograms of a normal left ear (**A**) and a right ear with a conductive hearing loss (**B**), such as might result from otitis media.

bone conduction (in contrast to the usual route of hearing by air conduction).

Hearing by air conduction and by bone conduction can be assessed quantitatively by using an audiometer to construct a pure-tone audiogram. A series of brief single-frequency tones that cover part of the audible spectrum (typically from 250 Hz to 8 kHz) are delivered through either headphones or a vibrating probe, and the intensity of each is gradually increased until it is just audible. The audiometer automatically compensates for irregularities in sensitivity (see Fig. 10-1) and for the greater efficiency of air conduction, so that for an individual with normal hearing the threshold is plotted as 0 dB at all frequencies. For a patient with hearing loss caused by outer ear obstruction or middle ear damage (i.e., conductive hearing loss), the audiogram will therefore indicate a hearing loss by air conduction but not by bone conduction (Fig. 10-4).

Inner Ear

The inner ear, a tortuous system of fluid-filled channels also called the labyrinth (Fig. 10-5), contains the receptor cells of both auditory and vestibular systems. The labyrinth is actually two systems of channels, one inside the other: the bony labyrinth is the cavity in the temporal bone and the membranous labyrinth is suspended within it. The two are generally parallel to each other, with one exception. The semicircular canals and cochlea of the bony labyrinth house the semicircular ducts and cochlear duct, but the vestibule houses two distinct components of the membranous labyrinth, the utricle and the saccule. The cochlea is the sensory organ for hearing; the remaining components of the labyrinth are considered in more detail in Chapter 11.

As spatially complex as the bony and membranous labyrinths appear, each is nevertheless a continuous space. The two contain distinctly different fluids, however, and diffusion barriers in the walls of the membranous labyrinth separate one from the other. The bony labyrinth is filled with perilymph, which has a composition typical of extracellular fluids elsewhere (high [Na⁺], low [K⁺]) and is in fact continuous with the CSF around the base of the brain through a small channel in the temporal bone. The membranous labyrinth, in contrast, is filled with endolymph, a peculiar fluid with an ionic composition more like that of cytoplasm (i.e., low [Na⁺], high [K⁺]). Endolymph is produced by secretory cells in the walls of the membranous labyrinth and continuously eliminated; much as in the case of CSF circulation and reabsorption, disruption of endolymph flow is thought to underlie some forms of labyrinthine pathology.

Hair Cells

Each subdivision of the membranous labyrinth includes in its wall a discrete collection of hair cells, modified epithelial cells

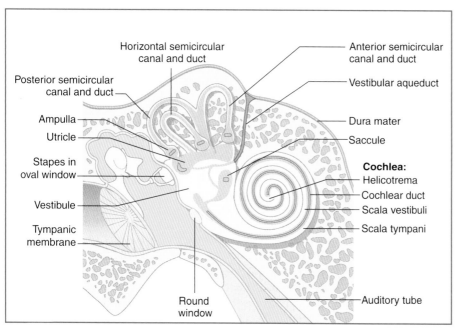

Figure 10-5. Lateral view of the right membranous labyrinth, seen inside the bony labyrinth. The purple areas indicate the locations of patches and strips of hair cells in each of the labyrinthine receptor organs.

Horizontal semicircular canal and duct

Posterior semicircular canal and duct

Ampulla

Utricle

Stapes in oval window

Vestibule

Tympanic membrane

Round window

Anterior semicircular canal and duct

Vestibular aqueduct

Dura mater

Saccule

Cochlea:
Helicotrema
Cochlear duct
Scala vestibuli
Scala tympani

Auditory tube

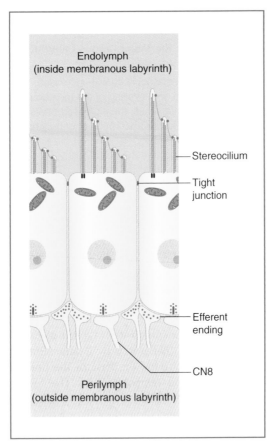

Figure 10-6. Schematic view of a typical hair cell of the labyrinth. The tight junctions near the stereociliary end are part of the functional wall of the membranous labyrinth, helping separate the endolymph bathing the stereocilia from the perilymph bathing the rest of the hair cell, which is effectively outside the membranous labyrinth.

that are the characteristic receptors of the labyrinth (Fig. 10-6). The "hairs" for which these cells were named are actually actin-filled microvilli, oddly but traditionally called stereocilia, arranged in a graduated array according to height. (During development, each also contains a kinocilium, a true cilium positioned near the tallest stereocilia, but this degenerates in adult cochlear hair cells.) With one apparent exception (cochlear inner hair cells; see below), at least the tallest stereocilia are attached to an overlying gelatinous mass of one sort or another; movement of the gelatinous mass causes deflection of the stereocilia. Their actin core makes stereocilia relatively rigid, like little baseball bats that pivot only at the point where each inserts into the hair cell, and cross-links between them ensure that the hair bundle moves as a unit.

The transduction mechanism used by hair cells is strikingly simple and extremely fast (Fig. 10-7). Filamentous proteins called tip links join each stereocilium to its next tallest neighbor, attaching at one or both ends to a mechanosensitive cation channel. Deflecting a hair bundle in the direction of the tallest stereocilia increases the tension on the tip links and opens the channels, allowing K^+ influx that depolarizes the hair cells. (Increased K^+ permeability is not usually associated with depolarization, but in this case the interior of the membranous labyrinth is electrically positive, creating a large voltage gradient that drives K^+ ions into the hair cells despite the lack of a concentration gradient.) Deflection of the hair bundle away from the tallest stereocilia relieves some resting tip link tension, causing hyperpolarization, whereas deflection parallel to the rows of stereocilia has little effect. Depolarizing and hyperpolarizing receptor potentials are converted to increased and decreased glutamate release at the hair cell synapse, resulting in increases and decreases in the resting firing rate of eighth nerve fibers.

COCHLEA

The pea-sized cochlea (Latin, "snail shell") curves through 2½ turns of a tapering spiral surrounding a bony core (the modiolus). Despite its orientation with the narrow end of the spiral pointing anteriorly and laterally (see Figs. 10-2 and 11-6), it is customarily described as having a base and an apex, oriented with the apex (the narrow end of the spiral) pointing superiorly (Fig. 10-8). The osseous spiral lamina, a shelf-like bony extension of the modiolus, spirals around with the cochlea, partially subdividing each turn into two perilymph-filled compartments: scala vestibuli and scala tympani. Scala vestibuli opens into the vestibule (hence, its name), scala tympani ends blindly at the round window membrane (also called the secondary tympanic membrane), and the two scalae communicate with each other through a small aperture at the apex of the cochlea (the helicotrema; literally, the "hole in the helix"). The separation of scala vestibuli from scala tympani through most of the cochlea is completed by the cochlear duct (scala media), which extends from the osseous spiral lamina to the wall of the cochlea. The cochlear duct is triangular in cross-section (Fig. 10-9)—one side is attached to the wall of the cochlea while the other two (Reissner's membrane and the basilar membrane) separate the endolymph of the cochlear duct from the perilymph of scala vestibuli and scala tympani, respectively. The organ of Corti, containing the cochlear hair cells, spirals around with the basilar membrane. The net result is that oscillations of the stapes footplate cause waves of compression and rarefaction that move through the cochlear perilymph, ultimately reaching the round window membrane. Very low (subaudible) frequencies move all the way up scala vestibuli, through the helicotrema, and down scala tympani. Audible frequencies, however, cut across the cochlear duct, deflecting the basilar membrane and stimulating cochlear hair cells (Fig. 10-10).

Basilar Membrane

Reissner's membrane is only two cell layers thick and serves mainly as a diffusion barrier between scala vestibuli and scala media. The basilar membrane, in contrast, is thicker and collagenous. Its mechanical properties vary smoothly from the base of the cochlea, where it is stiff and narrow, to the apex, where it is floppier and 10 times wider. This allows it to function as a miniature frequency analyzer that begins the

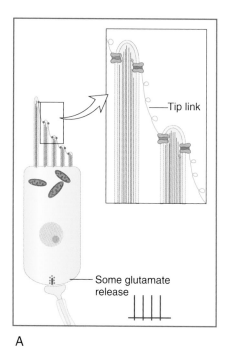 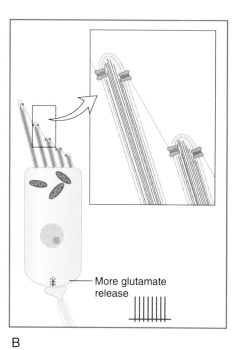 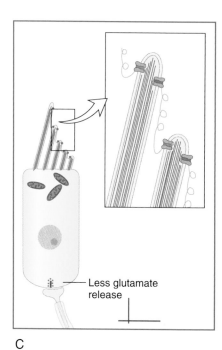

Tip link

Some glutamate release

More glutamate release

Less glutamate release

A

B

C

Figure 10-7. Transduction in hair cells, and transmission of information from hair cells to eighth nerve fibers. **A,** In the absence of stimulation, some transduction channels are open; the hair cell is moderately depolarized, some glutamate is released, and eighth nerve fibers have a "resting" firing rate. **B,** Deflecting the hair bundle toward the tallest stereocilia stretches the tip links and opens more cation channels near the tips of the stereocilia, allowing entry of K^+ and depolarization of the hair cell. This in turn increases the release of excitatory neurotransmitter onto the endings of eighth nerve fibers and increases their firing rate. **C,** Deflecting the hair bundle away from the tallest stereocilia relaxes tension on the tip links and has an opposite effect from that seen in **B**.

Figure 10-8. Cochlea split down the middle and turned so that it sits on its base, with the path of sound waves indicated.

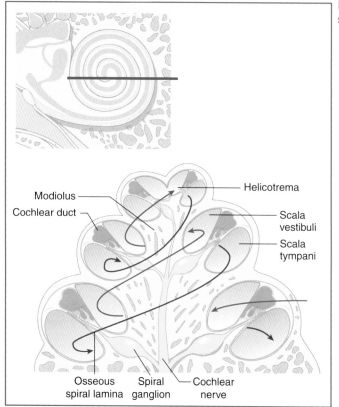

Modiolus

Cochlear duct

Helicotrema

Scala vestibuli

Scala tympani

Osseous spiral lamina

Spiral ganglion

Cochlear nerve

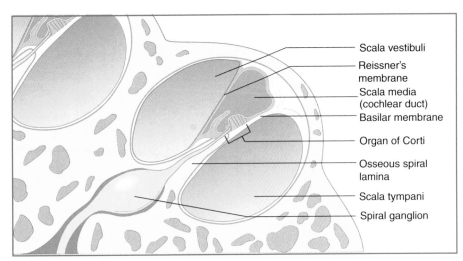

Figure 10-9. Cross-section through one turn of the cochlea, indicating its chambers and the location of the organ of Corti.

Scala vestibuli

Reissner's membrane

Scala media (cochlear duct)

Basilar membrane

Organ of Corti

Osseous spiral lamina

Scala tympani

Spiral ganglion

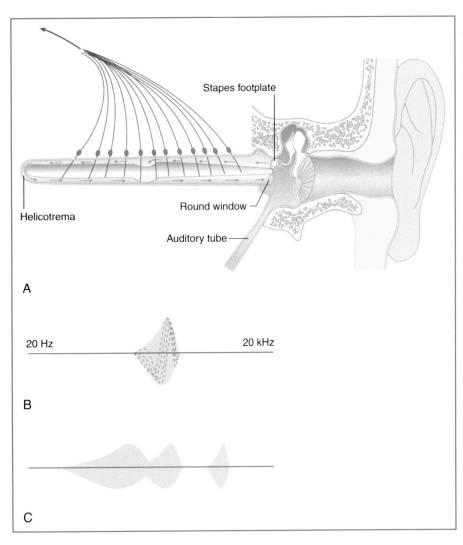

Stapes footplate

Round window

Auditory tube

Helicotrema

A

20 Hz   20 kHz

B

C

Figure 10-10. A, Schematic longitudinal section through an unrolled cochlea, showing the path of very low frequencies through the helicotrema and other frequencies across the cochlear duct. **B,** The traveling wave in the basilar membrane in response to a 10 kHz sound at four different instants in time; the envelope of the traveling wave shows maximum deflection at one location on the basilar membrane. **C,** Multiple points of deflection in response to a complex tone. The patterns of vibration in B and C represent the passive properties of the basilar membrane, without the amplification normally contributed by the outer hair cells (see Fig. 10-13).

deconstruction of complex sounds into their component tones: oscillations in the perilymph cause traveling waves of basilar membrane deformation that reach a maximum at longitudinal levels that depend on the frequency of the oscillations (see Fig. 10-10). Consistent with the varying mechanical properties of the basilar membrane, the audible spectrum is mapped out from low to high frequencies in going from the apex to the base of the cochlea. This is the beginning of a tonotopic mapping of sound frequencies that recurs throughout most of the auditory system.

Although these passive mechanical properties underlie part of the frequency analysis performed by the cochlea, they

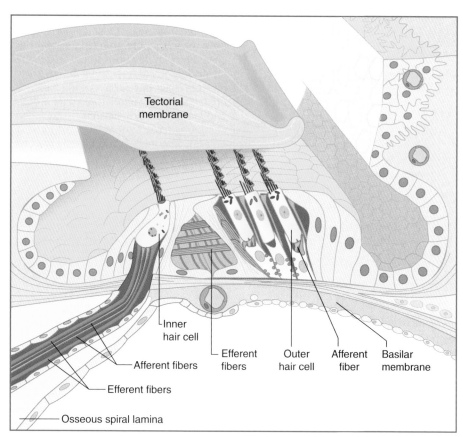

Figure 10-11. Cross-section of the organ of Corti.

Tectorial membrane

Inner hair cell

Afferent fibers

Efferent fibers

Osseous spiral lamina

Efferent fibers

Outer hair cell

Afferent fiber

Basilar membrane

are inadequate to fully explain either its sensitivity or its frequency selectivity, indicating that some additional source of energy must be added to the cochlea to augment that provided by incoming sound. This cochlear amplifier is now known to reside in the organ of Corti.

Organ of Corti

Cochlear hair cells of two different types, together with a variety of unique supporting cells, spiral around on the surface of the basilar membrane as the organ of Corti (Fig. 10-11). The flask-shaped inner hair cells, numbering about 3500, form a strip a single cell wide situated just above the edge of the osseous spiral lamina. The more numerous outer hair cells (about 12,000) form a strip 3 to 5 cells wide suspended above the basilar membrane by supporting cells. The stereocilia of outer hair cells are inserted into the overlying, gelatinous, tectorial membrane. The tectorial and basilar membranes have different pivot points, so vibration of the basilar membrane causes deflection of these stereociliary bundles. The stereocilia of inner hair cells, in contrast, extend across the narrow cleft between the organ of Corti and the tectorial membrane but apparently are not attached to the membrane; they probably are stimulated by endolymph squirting back and forth through this cleft as the basilar membrane vibrates.

The inner and outer hair cells have entirely different roles in hearing: inner hair cells provide the information about sound stimuli that gets conveyed to the CNS by CN VIII fibers, and outer hair cells power the cochlear amplifier. This difference is hinted at by their pattern of innervation (Fig. 10-12). A spiral channel within the modiolus houses the spiral ganglion, the surprisingly small collection (about 30,000) of auditory primary afferent cell bodies; their peripheral processes end at the bases of cochlear hair cells, and their central processes travel through the vestibulocochlear nerve to reach second-order neurons in the brainstem. About 95% of these spiral ganglion cells receive their input from single inner hair cells. Each of the remaining 5% receives inputs from numerous outer hair cells; their role in providing auditory information to the CNS is unclear but probably minor. The critical role of the outer hair cells in hearing arises from their ability to lengthen and shorten in response to membrane potential changes. Length changes in response to receptor potentials in these cells amplify the vibration of the particular part of the basilar membrane to which they are

CLINICAL MEDICINE

Sounds from the Cochlea

Basilar membrane vibration caused by length changes of outer hair cells propagates backward along the middle ear ossicles, turning the tympanic membrane into a tiny loudspeaker. The resulting otoacoustic emissions can be detected by a sensitive microphone in the ear canal, and used as the basis of a test of outer hair cell function in individuals who cannot cooperate in the production of an audiogram (e.g., infants).

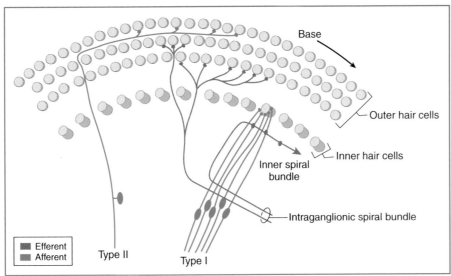

Figure 10-12. Innervation pattern of inner and outer hair cells. Most spiral ganglion cells receive inputs from single inner hair cells; each spiral ganglion cell in a small second population receives inputs from multiple outer hair cells. CN VIII also contains efferent fibers that spiral around and innervate hair cells in a complementary pattern (see text for details), with most going directly to outer hair cells.

attached, increasing the level of stimulation of nearby inner hair cells. This increases the threshold sensitivity of eighth nerve fibers by as much as 50 dB and, because the amplification is spatially focused, also increases the frequency selectivity of each small area of the basilar membrane (Fig. 10-13).

PHARMACOLOGY & MICROBIOLOGY

Drugs That Damage Outer Hair Cells

A variety of medications, including aspirin, aminoglycoside antibiotics, quinine, and some diuretics, are toxic to hair cells (i.e., ototoxic). Most preferentially affect outer hair cells, compromising the cochlear amplifier and causing a sensorineural loss of up to 50 dB.

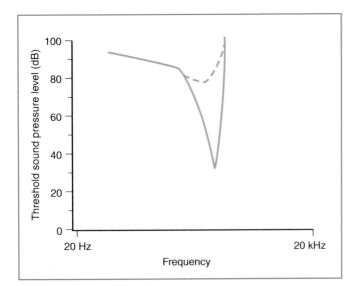

Figure 10-13. Typical threshold vs frequency curve for a cochlear nerve fiber with (solid line) and without (dashed line) the amplification of basilar membrane vibration provided by outer hair cells.

Cochlear Dysfunction

Damage to either cochlear hair cells or the eighth nerve causes an ipsilateral sensorineural hearing loss. In this situation, hearing is impaired by *both* air conduction and bone conduction (Fig. 10-14; compare with Fig. 10-4).

●●● AUDITORY CONNECTIONS IN THE CENTRAL NERVOUS SYSTEM

As in other sensory systems, the auditory parts of the CNS have the task of figuring out the identity and location of stimuli. Deciphering the identity of a sound is largely based on analyzing the frequencies that make it up, using two different kinds of information. Because different parts of the basilar membrane are tuned to different frequencies, the identities of active cochlear nerve fibers form the basis of a place code for frequency. In addition, many cochlear nerve fibers are more likely to fire during a particular part of each cycle of a sound wave (Fig. 10-15); this forms the basis of a time code for frequency. Place coding is more important for higher frequencies and time coding for lower frequencies.

Unlike the case for some other senses such as somatic sensation and vision, where a great deal of information about the location of a stimulus is provided by its position on the skin or retina, the auditory system must construct a map of

PATHOLOGY

Tumors of the Eighth Nerve

Acoustic neuromas account for about 8% of intracranial tumors. These benign tumors are more properly called vestibular schwannomas, because nearly all of them involve Schwann cells of the vestibular branch of cranial nerve VIII. They grow slowly enough that the contralateral vestibular nerve can compensate, but they also compress the cochlear nerve and cause ipsilateral sensorineural hearing loss.

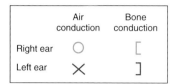

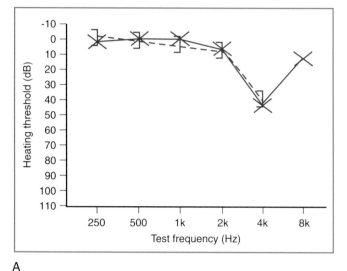

A

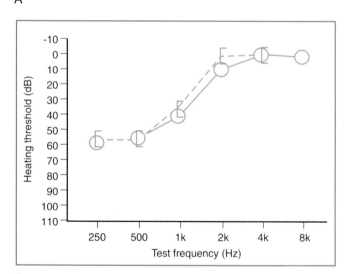

B

Figure 10-14. Audiograms showing sensorineural deficits (comparable losses by both air and bone conduction) typical of noise-induced hearing loss (**A**) and Ménière's disease (**B**). Because of the amplification provided by the outer ear at about 3 kHz, noise-induced hearing loss is greatest in this frequency range. In contrast, the increased endolymphatic pressure in Ménière's disease is thought to result in the greatest stretching and damage in the widest, least tense part of the basilar membrane, where sensitivity to low frequencies is maximal.

auditory space. This process begins in the brainstem, using three different kinds of information. A sound originating from one side or the other will reach the ipsilateral ear slightly sooner than the contralateral ear, and it will be slightly louder in the ipsilateral ear because some energy will be absorbed or reflected by the head before it reaches the contralateral ear. Comparison of time of arrival and intensity differences

between the two ears can therefore be used for localization. This will obviously not work well for sound sources near the sagittal plane, and in this case the auricle distortion patterns referred to earlier have a more important role.

Subcortical Auditory Connections

Cochlear nerve fibers terminate in the ipsilateral cochlear nuclei, a band of gray matter draped across the inferior cerebellar peduncle at the pontomedullary junction. The cochlear nuclei then project bilaterally to a host of brainstem nuclei, the most important being the superior olivary nucleus and the inferior colliculus (Fig. 10-16). Because these projections are bilateral, hearing loss strictly confined to one ear almost always indicates pathology in the ipsilateral peripheral auditory apparatus or CN VIII (or, more rarely, cochlear nuclei).

Some neurons of the cochlear nuclei, primarily conveying information about the frequency and duration of sounds, project to both inferior colliculi (mainly the contralateral one) through the lateral lemniscus, the principal ascending auditory pathway of the brainstem.

Other neurons of the cochlear nuclei project bilaterally to the nearby superior olivary nuclei; those axons that cross the midline do so in the trapezoid body. The superior olivary nucleus is the first CNS location where information from both ears converges, allowing initial processing of sound localization information. Olivary neurons tuned to particular small interaural time and intensity differences then project bilaterally through the lateral lemniscus to the inferior colliculus.

The inferior colliculus combines information from lower brainstem levels to construct maps of auditory space and signals about combinations of frequencies and frequency changes. It then projects to the medial geniculate nucleus, the auditory system's piece of the thalamus, through the brachium of the inferior colliculus.

Acoustic Reflex

The superior olivary nucleus does more than process sound-localization data. Some of its neurons project back to cochlear hair cells in a differential pattern related to the roles of inner and outer hair cells (see Fig. 10-12). Efferents to

CLINICAL MEDICINE

Recording Activity in the Central Auditory Pathway

Brief sounds cause electrical signals that can be recorded far away on the scalp but are so small that the responses to many repetitions must be averaged in order to retrieve the signals from the background noise. These brainstem auditory evoked responses have the form of a series of waves with predictable latencies, representing activity in successive levels of the auditory pathway, and so they can be helpful in determining the location of damage in this pathway.

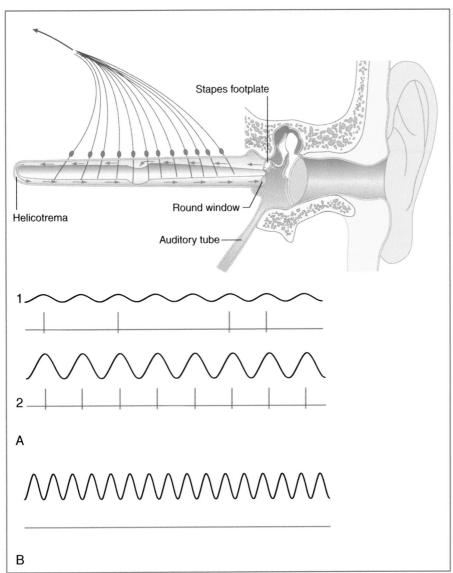

Figure 10-15. Coding of frequency and amplitude by cochlear nerve fibers. Upper trace of each pair (black), stimulus; lower trace (red), firing of a typical cochlear nerve fiber innervating the indented region of the cochlear duct. The fiber responds selectively to sounds of one frequency (**A** vs **B**); i.e., the region of the cochlear duct innervated by the fiber is the basis for a place code indicating the stimulus frequency. In addition, the firing occurs during a particular part of the stimulus waveform, occasionally in response to a faint sound (A, upper traces) and during every cycle in response to a loud sound (A, lower traces).

outer hair cells are more numerous, ending directly on the hair cells and modulating their contractile abilities. Efferents to inner hair cells, in contrast, end mostly on the sensory endings of cochlear nerve fibers, modulating their transmission of information to the brainstem. In neither case do the efferents play a major role in normal hearing.

Other olivary neurons participate in the clinically useful acoustic middle ear reflex (Fig. 10-17). Neurons of the cochlear nuclei project bilaterally to the superior olivary nucleus, which in turn projects (again, bilaterally) to the facial motor nucleus. As a result, the stapedius contracts in both middle ears in response to loud sound delivered to either ear (just as both eyes blink when something touches either cornea, and both pupils constrict in response to illumination of either retina). The reflex is usually assessed indirectly by using a small microphone in the ear canal to measure how much of a test tone is reflected back from the tympanic membrane; the stiffening of the ossicular chain caused by stapedial contraction decreases the transmission of sound and increases the amount reflected.

Auditory Cortex and Beyond

The medial geniculate nucleus projects through the sublenticular part of the internal capsule to primary auditory cortex (see Fig. 10-16), hidden from view on the superior surface of the temporal lobe in the transverse temporal gyri (Heschl's gyri; Fig. 10-18). Primary auditory cortex is organized in a manner reminiscent of somatosensory and visual cortex

ANATOMY & CLINICAL MEDICINE

Paralysis of the Stapedius

Compression of the facial nerve as it traverses the temporal bone on its way to the stylomastoid foramen, e.g., by inflammatory swelling, causes ipsilateral facial weakness (Bell's palsy). If the damage is high in the facial canal, before the branch to the stapedius has emerged, the patient will experience loud sounds as abnormally loud (hyperacusis).

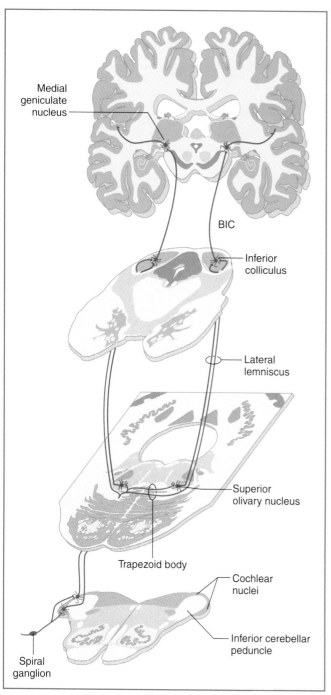

Figure 10-16. Ascending auditory pathway. BIC, brachium of the inferior colliculus.

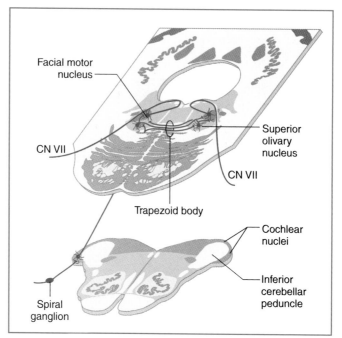

Figure 10 17. Pathway of the acoustic middle ear reflex. Loud sounds in one ear result in increased activity bilaterally in the facial motor neurons that innervate the stapedius. (See Chapter 14 for more information about the facial motor nucleus and the peculiar course of the fibers that leave it.)

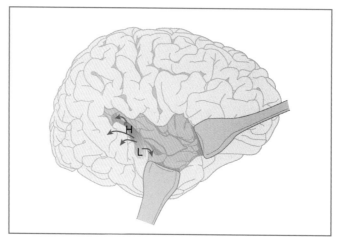

Figure 10-18. Primary auditory cortex and its projections to adjacent auditory association areas. H and L indicate the high- and low-frequency areas in the tonotopic map in primary auditory cortex.

(see Chapters 9 and 12). Sound frequencies are represented in an orderly tonotopic map, and superimposed on this map is a series of columns in which neurons respond to various combinations of inputs from the two ears at that frequency. Because of the extensive bilaterality of auditory CNS connections, unilateral damage to this area does not cause major deficits. Primary auditory cortex, like other primary sensory cortices, then projects to nearby areas of auditory association cortex (see Fig. 10-18), some of which are particularly important for the interpretation of spoken language. In this case, unilateral damage typically does cause substantial deficits (see Chapter 19).

Vestibular System 11

Animals need to keep track of which end is up, i.e., how they are oriented relative to the rest of the world. Vision can help with this and in many ways is the dominant sense for this task in primates (including humans). Vision by itself, however, cannot distinguish between movement of an animal and movement of the outside world, because either would make images of the outside world move across the retina. This is where the vestibular part of the eighth nerve comes in. Every head movement starts as some combination of linear and angular acceleration, and the vestibular part of the labyrinth contains sets of receptors that can detect either of these, in any direction.

●●● VESTIBULAR LABYRINTH

The vestibule of the bony labyrinth houses two expansions of the membranous labyrinth (Fig. 11-1)—a saccule continuous with the cochlear duct, and a utricle that is continuous with the saccule through a narrow tube. Each of the three semicircular canals contains a semicircular duct continuous at each of its ends with the utricle. These five parts make up the vestibular part of the labyrinth. The utricle and saccule, together called the otolithic organs for reasons explained below, detect linear acceleration. The semicircular ducts detect angular acceleration.

The vestibular labyrinth contains populations of hair cells basically similar to those of the cochlea (see Fig. 10-6), with stereocilia embedded in a gelatinous mass. Differences in the physical arrangement of the gelatinous masses determine the specific mechanical sensitivity of different parts of the labyrinth.

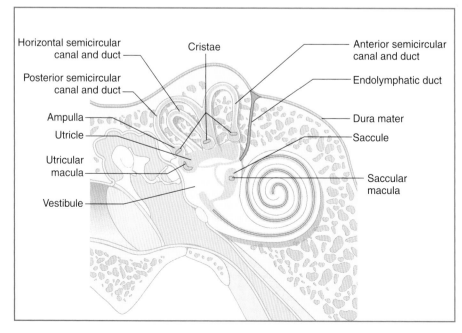

Figure 11-1. Lateral view of the right membranous labyrinth, seen inside the bony labyrinth. The locations of patches of hair cells in the vestibular part of the labyrinth are indicated.

Horizontal semicircular canal and duct

Cristae

Anterior semicircular canal and duct

Posterior semicircular canal and duct

Endolymphatic duct

Ampulla

Dura mater

Utricle

Saccule

Utricular macula

Saccular macula

Vestibule

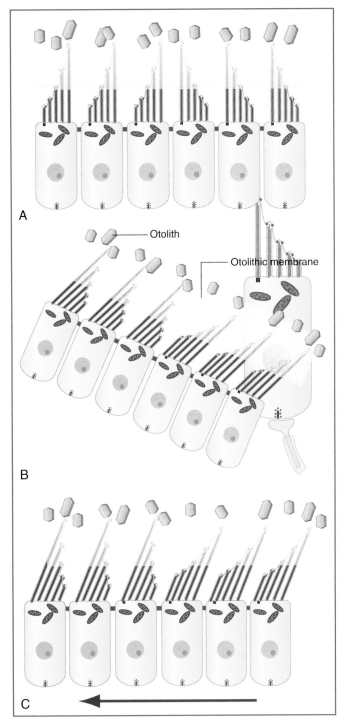

Figure 11-2. A, Arrangement of hair cells in the utricle and saccule. The otolithic membrane is denser than endolymph, so it moves relative to the stereociliary bundles in response to changes in orientation (**B**) or to linear acceleration (**C**).

Otolithic Organs and Linear Acceleration

A curved patch in the floor of the utricle and another in the medial wall of the saccule, each called a macula ("spot"), contain the hair cells of the otolithic organs. Their stereocilia are inserted into an otolithic membrane, a gelatinous membrane with small crystals of calcium carbonate (otoliths, "ear stones") embedded in it (Fig. 11-2). Otolithic membranes are denser than endolymph, making them responsive to gravity.

PHARMACOLOGY

Ototoxicity

Many substances, including aminoglycoside and some other antibiotics, some chemotherapeutic agents, and even aspirin, are toxic to hair cells. Some are relatively selective for cochlear or vestibular hair cells and can cause permanent hearing loss or loss of vestibular function.

If a macula is oriented so that its rigid stereocilia point upward, not much happens (think about pushing your hand down on the bristles of a hairbrush). Tilts starting from such a stereocilia-vertical orientation, however, would allow the otolithic membrane to sink a little, slipping across the surface of the macula and deflecting the stereocilia (think about sliding your hand laterally while in contact with the bristles of a hairbrush). Because of the way the maculas are situated, the utricular macula is most sensitive to tilts starting from a head-upright position and the saccular macula is most sensitive to those starting from a head-sideways position. Each macula has hair cells with multiple orientations (Fig. 11-3), so between them the utricle and saccule can signal tilts in any direction.

The density of otolithic membranes also makes them sensitive to linear acceleration (see Fig. 11-2). Again, because of the way the maculas are situated, the utricular macula is most sensitive to linear acceleration in horizontal planes (forward-backward, side to side) and the saccular macula is most sensitive to those in sagittal planes (forward-backward, up-down). In our normal head-upright position, the stereocilia of saccular hair cells are tonically deflected, but hair

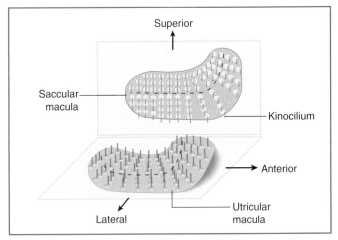

Figure 11-3. Orientation of the hair cells in the right utricle and saccule. In the normal head-upright position, the utricular stereocilia mostly point upward and the saccular stereocilia mostly point laterally, accounting for the directions of acceleration to which each is most sensitive. The kinocilium (adjacent to the tallest stereocilia), defining the axis of maximum sensitivity, is indicated on the top of each hair cell. This axis varies systematically in each macula and reverses abruptly (dotted line) in each. The result is that any tilt or linear acceleration sets up a unique pattern of depolarizations and hyperpolarizations among various hair cells.

cells adapt to whatever position they are in (see Fig. 4-9B), so even starting from this position they are sensitive to acceleration in sagittal planes.

Semicircular Canals and Angular Acceleration

Semicircular ducts use a different strategy to tune their mechanical sensitivity (Fig. 11-4). At one end of each is a dilatation (an ampulla, "little flask") with a partition extending across its lumen. The partition is formed partly by a crista, a transversely oriented ridge studded with hair cells, and completed by a gelatinous flap (a cupula). The cupula is isodense with endolymph, so gravity has no effect on it. However, at the beginning of a rotation in the plane of a semicircular duct, its endolymph lags behind a little bit because of inertia and pushes on the cupula, deflecting the hair cells (Fig. 11-5). If the rotation continues at a constant angular velocity, the endolymph catches up after 10 seconds or so. At the end of rotation, again because of inertia, the endolymph keeps going and pushes the cupula in the opposite direction. Hence, semicircular ducts are sensitive to changes in angular velocity, i.e., angular acceleration. Because the three semicircular ducts on each side are in orthogonal planes (Fig. 11-6), angular acceleration in any direction will cause endolymph movement in at least one duct. (Linear acceleration would also cause inertial forces in the endolymph, but these would be the same in both legs of a semicircular duct and no endolymph movement would ensue.)

CLINICAL MEDICINE

Making a Semicircular Canal Gravity-Sensitive

The most common affliction of the peripheral vestibular system is benign paroxysmal positional vertigo, in which fragments of an otolithic membrane become detached and enter one of the semicircular ducts (usually the posterior duct). Once there, these fragments can respond to gravity and bump up against the cupula, causing vertigo and nystagmus. Most cases can be treated by positioning the head so that the otolithic fragments leave the affected canal and return to the utricle.

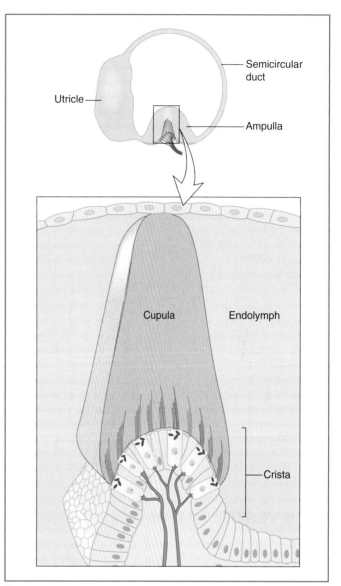

Figure 11-4. Arrangement of hair cells in a semicircular duct. Unlike the situation in the maculas, the hair cells in a given crista are oriented in the same direction, so all respond similarly to deflection of the cupula.

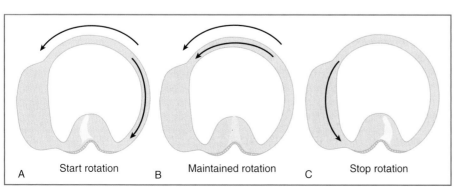

Figure 11-5. Responses of hair cells in a semicircular duct to angular acceleration. **A,** At the beginning of rotation (= positive angular acceleration), endolymph lags behind, deflecting the cupula. **B,** After 10 seconds or so, the endolymph catches up (= no angular acceleration), and as far as the semicircular canal is concerned, there is no movement. **C,** At the end of rotation (= negative angular acceleration), endolymph keeps moving, deflecting the cupula in the opposite direction.

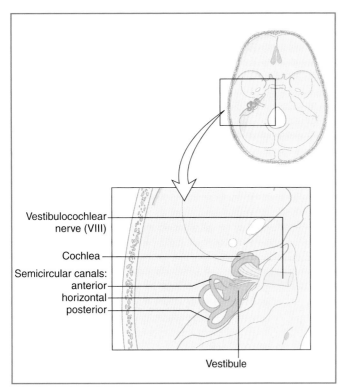

Figure 11-6. Orientation of the labyrinth within the temporal bone. The horizontal (lateral) semicircular canals are actually tilted backward about 30 degrees. The anterior and posterior semicircular canals are oriented at about 45 degrees to the midsagittal plane, so each anterior canal is in a plane parallel to that of the contralateral posterior canal and acts in concert with it.

●●● VESTIBULAR PATHWAYS

Vestibular signals about changes in orientation contribute to conscious awareness of orientation but are more important for the production of postural adjustments and eye movements in response to such changes. CNS vestibular pathways reflect these functions.

Vestibular Nuclei and Their Connections

The primary afferents of the vestibular branch of CN VIII terminate in the CNS in a set of vestibular nuclei (Fig. 11-7). These are largest near the pontomedullary junction, where the eighth nerve enters the brainstem, and like other sensory nuclei of cranial nerves, they have a lateral location (see Fig. 6-12). The vestibular nuclei then project to the thalamus, the spinal cord, and the nuclei of cranial nerves III, IV, and VI (Figs. 11-7 and 11-8). In addition, the cerebellum is involved in the coordination of both trunk movements and eye movements (see Chapter 16), and there are substantial interconnections between the vestibular nuclei and the cerebellum.

Vestibular Projections to Cerebral Cortex

Conscious awareness of vestibular stimuli is mediated by a pathway from the vestibular nuclei to a part of the thalamus near the ventral posterolateral and posteromedial nuclei

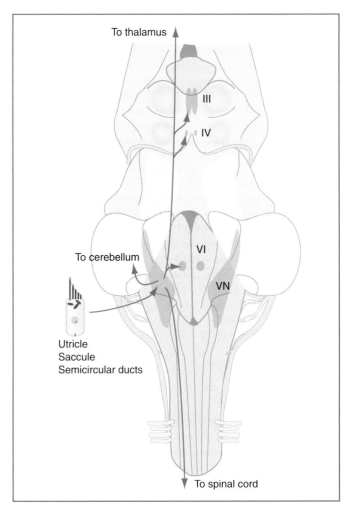

Figure 11-7. Location of the vestibular nuclei in the brainstem, and the general pattern of connections of these nuclei. Projections from the vestibular nuclei are shown on one side only, although some are bilateral. III, IV, VI, and VN indicate the oculomotor, trochlear, abducens, and vestibular nuclei. (More information about the oculomotor, trochlear, and abducens nuclei is provided in Chapter 17, but note their relatively medial location in the brainstem.)

(VPL/VPM). The thalamus then projects vestibular information to several cortical areas, including a posterior part of the insula and parietal areas near the representation of the head in somatosensory cortex.

Vestibulospinal Tracts

The vestibular nuclei project to the spinal cord through the lateral and medial vestibulospinal tracts. The lateral vestibulospinal tract, an uncrossed pathway to motor neurons for extensor muscles, extends to all levels of the spinal cord and is the principal pathway mediating postural adjustments. The medial vestibulospinal tract is a bilateral projection to motor neurons for neck muscles that helps stabilize the position of the head. It travels through the medial longitudinal fasciculus (commonly referred to as the MLF), a longitudinal bundle that extends throughout the brainstem, helping coordinate head movements and eye movements.

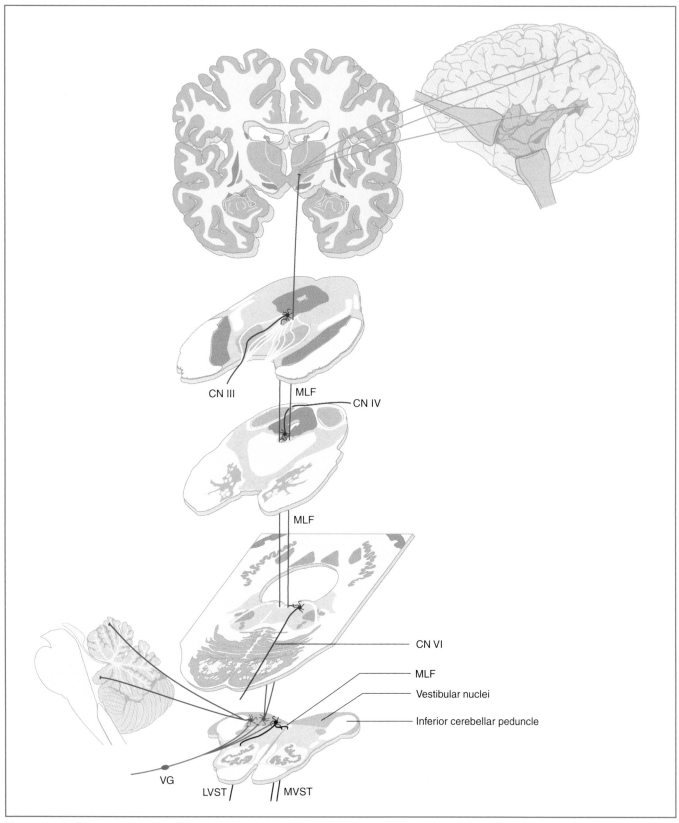

Figure 11-8. Connections of the vestibular nuclei. To simplify the drawing, some connections that are actually bilateral (e.g., from the vestibular nuclei to the thalamus) are shown as one-sided, and all the ascending connections of the vestibular nuclei are shown as traveling through the MLF, even though some take other routes as well. The vestibular system projects to medial parts of the cerebellum (the vermis and nearby regions), as discussed further in Chapter 16. LVST, lateral vestibulospinal tract; MLF, medial longitudinal fasciculus; MVST, medial vestibulospinal tract; VG, vestibular ganglion.

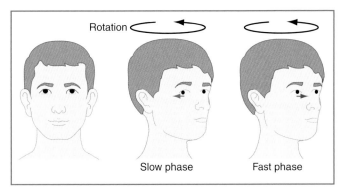

Figure 11-9. Rotatory nystagmus consists of a slow phase (the VOR) in the direction opposite the rotation, which keeps the image of the outside world stationary on the retina. This is interrupted by fast phases in the direction of the rotation, allowing the retina to acquire a new image.

Vestibulo-ocular Reflex

For reasons discussed in Chapters 12 and 17, it is critical to keep images from moving too quickly across the retina. (Basically, photoreceptors are sensitive but slow, so images that move quickly cannot be perceived clearly.) As animals locomote, their heads bob around, which would cause images of the outside world to move quickly across the retina unless the eyes moved in a way that precisely compensated for the head movements. The compensatory movements are produced by the vestibulo-ocular reflex (VOR), a fast, simple, three-neuron reflex arc (see Fig. 11-8). The afferent limb is vestibular primary afferents; interneurons in the vestibular nuclei project through the MLF and the reticular formation to motor neurons in the abducens, trochlear, and oculomotor nuclei.

Nystagmus

The VOR can compensate for relatively small head movements but by itself cannot take care of large movements (e.g., spinning around in a desk chair). Faced with a sustained rotation like this, the VOR that compensates for the rotation (by moving the eyes in the opposite direction) is periodically interrupted by quick eye movements in the direction of rotation (Fig. 11-9). These back and forth eye movements are called nystagmus, whose net effect is that images are stabilized on the retina for most of the rotation. If the rotation continues for a while in the dark (not likely to happen in routine living), the endolymph catches up and the nystagmus stops (see Fig. 11-5). (If the lights are on, the nystagmus continues even after the endolymph catches up. Even though vestibular stimulation has ceased, the slow phase of nystagmus is sustained by the visual pursuit mechanisms described in Chapter 17; optokinetic nystagmus, caused by the sight of moving visual stimuli, replaces the rotatory nystagmus.) At the end of the rotation, the endolymph keeps going, and nystagmus resumes but now in the opposite direction.

Because the neural circuitry for rotation-induced nystagmus involves the eighth nerve and a substantial longitudinal

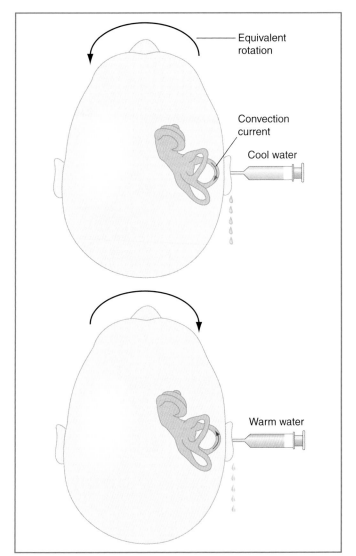

Figure 11-10. Caloric nystagmus. The most lateral part of the horizontal semicircular canal is the part closest to the middle ear cavity, so cool or warm water instilled into the ear canal causes convection currents (in opposite directions) in the endolymph of this canal. Warm water in the right ear, for example, causes the same endolymph motion in the right horizontal duct as would rotation to the right. This in turn is sufficient to cause nystagmus with its fast phase to the right. Conversely, cool water in the right ear (or warm water in the left) would cause nystagmus with its fast phase to the left.

extent of the brainstem, studying it clinically can yield useful diagnostic information. This can be done simply by irrigating an ear with warm or cool water, setting up convection currents in the endolymph that fool the vestibular system into thinking that the head is rotating, eliciting caloric nystagmus (Fig. 11-10).

Nystagmus is a normal response designed to keep images stable on the retina most of the time, but damage to the vestibular system (or to other parts of the brainstem or the cerebellum) can cause pathologic nystagmus of various distinctive types.

PHYSIOLOGY

Ethanol and Vestibular Symptoms

Anything that changes the relative densities of cupula and endolymph can be expected to make the semicircular ducts gravity-sensitive, and this is one of the mechanisms by which overindulgence in ethanol causes its effects. Ethanol first moves from the labyrinthine circulation into the cupulae, making them less dense than endolymph. As the blood alcohol level declines, ethanol leaches out of the cupulae into the endolymph, now making the endolymph less dense than the cupulae. As a result, holding the head in various positions stimulates one or more semicircular ducts, causing nystagmus and vertigo. Predictably, the direction of the nystagmus reverses during the later stage, when the cupulae become denser than endolymph.

CLINICAL MEDICINE

Romberg's Sign

Closing your eyes removes one of the three systems contributing to equilibrium, so standing upright with feet close together and eyes closed requires that proprioception and vestibular function be intact. Romberg's sign (swaying or falling that becomes substantially worse with eyes closed) is an indication of defective proprioception or vestibular function.

●●● COMBINING MULTIPLE SOURCES OF POSITION INFORMATION

Hair cells adapt to maintained positions, and the semicircular canals stop working during constant rotation, so the vestibular system by itself is inadequate to provide complete information about changes in orientation. Combining visual and vestibular information can compensate for the shortcomings of each, but only for specifying the orientation and motion of the head. To develop a sense of the orientation of your entire self, you also need to factor in somatosensory information about the position of the parts of your body relative to your head. All of this is accomplished at multiple levels. Neurons in the vestibular nuclei, for example, receive some visual inputs as well as somatosensory inputs from the spinal cord, and vestibular cortical areas receive visual and somatosensory inputs as well. Damage to any of these three sensory systems can cause disturbances of equilibrium, and mismatches between any of the three can cause illusions of movement. For example, if you are stationary and some large object in your peripheral vision starts to move, you are likely to have a compelling feeling that *you* are moving.

Visual System

12

CONTENTS

All sensory systems are important, but for primates the visual system is one of the most important. Partly for this reason and partly because of its *relatively* simple organization, it is also one of the most studied and best understood. In addition, the precise retinotopic mapping at different levels of the visual system make it a fairly straightforward task to predict the consequences of damage at various locations.

●●● EYE

There are two complementary ways to consider the eye. On the one hand, the retina is an outgrowth of the CNS, and so in addition to its neural properties it is surrounded by structures that are outgrowths of the meninges and are built similarly. On the other hand, the eye is often compared to a camera, with these various tissues in different roles as camera parts. The camera analogy is emphasized in the first section of this chapter because it helps make functional sense of the parts of the eye.

Tissue Layers of the Eye

The eye is basically a three-layered structure (Fig. 12-1) with a lens suspended inside it. The outermost layer is a thick,

collagenous continuation of the dura mater, and it accounts for most of the eye's mechanical strength. The anterior sixth of this layer is the transparent cornea, which continues posteriorly as the white sclera over the rest of the eye.

The middle layer, called the uveal tract, is a pigmented, vascular continuation of the arachnoid and pia mater. It consists of the choroid lining of the sclera and continues anteriorly as the bulk of the ciliary body and the iris. The lens (itself not a part of any of the three tissue layers) is suspended from the ciliary body by strands of connective tissue called zonules. The iris separates the space between the cornea and the lens into an anterior chamber and a posterior chamber.

The innermost layer is actually a double layer, owing to its development as a cup-shaped outgrowth from the diencephalon (Fig. 12-2). The outer of the two layers is a one-cell-thick sheet of retinal pigment epithelium, adjacent to the choroid, that extends all the way from the optic disc (exit of the optic nerve) to the edge of the pupil. The inner layer forms the photoreceptive neural retina in the posterior part of the eye; anteriorly it continues over the ciliary body and iris as a second epithelial layer accompanying the pigment epithelium.

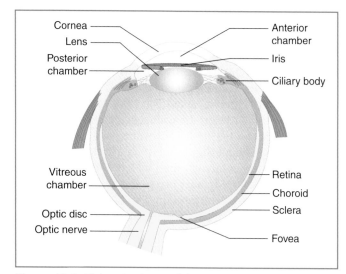

Figure 12-1. Major structures of the eye.

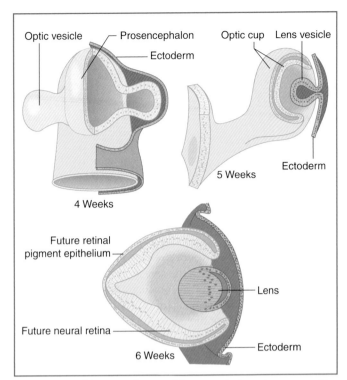

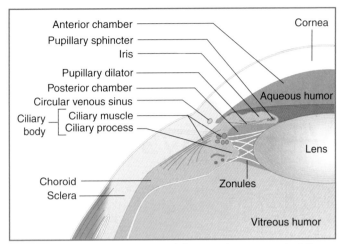

Figure 12-2. The neural part of the eye starts out as a roughly spherical outpouching from the diencephalic part of the neural tube. It subsequently folds in on itself (imagine pushing your fist into an inflated balloon) to form a double-layered, cup-shaped structure. Posteriorly, the outer layer develops into the retinal pigment epithelium and the inner layer into the neural retina. Both layers curve around anteriorly as parts of the ciliary body and iris.

Figure 12-3. Major structures of the anterior segment of the eye. Part of the ciliary body is responsible for the formation of aqueous humor, and part contains the ciliary muscle.

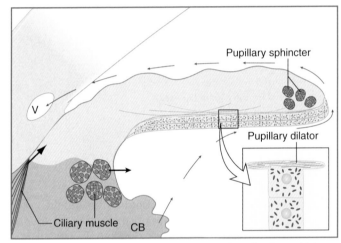

Figure 12-4. Functional anatomy of the ciliary body and iris. The ciliary muscle includes fibers oriented parallel to the sclera and fibers arranged circumferentially, like a sphincter. Together, they pull the scleral anchor points of the zonules anteriorly and toward the center of the pupil, relieving tension on the lens capsule and letting its anterior surface bulge forward. The pupillary sphincter appears to be embedded in the choroidal part of the iris but is actually derived from the posterior pigment epithelial layer (the layer that continues as the neural retina). The path of flow of aqueous humor from the ciliary body (CB) to the circular venous sinus (canal of Schlemm, V) is indicated by colored arrows.

Functional Parts of the Eye

Camera Body

Cameras have rigid metal or plastic bodies designed to keep the photosensitive element in a stable position relative to incoming light. In the eye, the sclera and cornea provide the rigid mechanical support for the retina. Unlike a metal camera body, however, the shape is maintained by keeping the eyeball pumped up under fluid pressure. The ciliary body is a loose connective tissue structure covered by a double-layered epithelial continuation of the optic cup, and it functions as a bit of choroid plexus (Fig. 12-3). Water and solutes leak out of capillaries in the connective tissue core and are transported across the epithelial covering and into the posterior chamber as aqueous humor ("watery fluid"). Aqueous humor then moves through the pupil and into the anterior chamber and is forced under pressure into a circular venous sinus at the corneoscleral junction (Fig. 12-4). (The interior of the eyeball behind the lens is filled with a gel called vitreous humor ["glassy fluid"]. Its composition is similar to that of aqueous humor, except for the presence of hyaluronic acid and some scattered collagen fibrils.) Besides providing mechanical rigidity, the sclera also provides a smooth surface upon which the eyeball can rotate in its fascial socket, and it provides insertion points for the extraocular muscles.

PHYSIOLOGY & PHARMACOLOGY

Blockage of Aqueous Humor Circulation

Just as obstruction of CSF flow causes increased intracranial pressure and hydrocephalus, obstruction of aqueous humor circulation causes increased intraocular pressure. Glaucoma results, with increased intraocular pressure, pain, and visual losses. Autonomic innervation of the arterioles in the ciliary body regulates the rate of aqueous humor secretion, making it possible to use β-blockers to reduce intraocular pressure in the treatment of glaucoma.

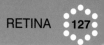

Focusing

The cornea is fundamentally similar to the sclera but has some structural specializations that make it transparent. The collagen fibers are more highly organized, arranged into sheets in which all the fibers are parallel and precisely spaced. Epithelial layers covering the front and back of the cornea keep it in a relatively dehydrated state; this in turn maintains the close spacing of fibers, which is crucial for transparency. There are no blood vessels in the cornea—another concession for transparency. However, there are many trigeminal nerve endings, which account for its irritability and for the afferent limb of the blink reflex (see Fig. 9-8). The cornea has a refractive index similar to that of water, so the air-cornea interface is able to do most of the refracting for the eyes of terrestrial animals such as humans. The lens is mostly water and sits in watery aqueous humor, but it provides the rest of the refractive power.

Adjusting the Focus

Different species use nearly any imaginable mechanism to adjust the focus of their eyes when viewing near and far objects. Some have muscles that change the shape of the cornea, adjusting its refractive power. Others have muscles that move the lens back and forth in front of the retina (like a camera lens). Arthropods have lenses fixed in their exoskeletons and cannot use this strategy, but some have muscles that move the retina back and forth behind the lens. Terrestrial vertebrates use a ciliary muscle to change the shape of the lens and thereby accommodate to near objects.

The ciliary muscle is a smooth muscle embedded in the loose connective tissue core of the ciliary body. At rest, with the eye's optics focused at infinity, the lens is flattened out in a connective tissue capsule held under radial tension by the zonules, which are arranged somewhat like spokes surrounding a fat central hub. Contraction of the ciliary muscle relieves some of this tension (see Fig. 12-3), so the lens gets fatter under its own elasticity and focuses the eye on nearer objects. Innervation of the ciliary muscle is parasympathetic: oculomotor nucleus → oculomotor nerve (CN III) → ciliary ganglion → short ciliary nerves → ciliary muscle. It is an autofocus system—you decide what you want to look at, and your brain takes it from there.

Regulation of Light

The iris is similar to the iris diaphragm in a camera and regulates the amount of light that gets in (although functionally this is much less important than the automatic regulation of sensitivity that happens at various levels of the nervous system). The iris is a three-layered structure, with an anterior layer of loose connective tissue continuous with the choroid and a double-layered epithelium continuous with the neural retina + pigment epithelium. The anterior layer has lots of pigment in brown-eyed individuals but not much pigment in blue-eyed individuals. Both layers of the double-layered pigment epithelium are always pigmented (otherwise the iris could not do its job). Two muscles that arise from the pigment epithelial layers control the size of the pupil (see Fig. 12-4). The pupillary sphincter, the stronger of the two, constricts it and the radially arranged fibers of the pupillary dilator widen it. Innervation of the sphincter is parasympathetic: oculomotor nucleus → oculomotor nerve (CN III) → ciliary ganglion → short ciliary nerves → sphincter. Innervation of the dilator is sympathetic: spinal cord → superior cervical ganglion → long ciliary nerves → dilator. (So parasympathetic damage on one side causes an ipsilateral dilated pupil that does not constrict in response to light. In contrast, sympathetic damage on one side causes an ipsilateral constricted pupil that constricts further in response to light.)

Antireflection Lining

The choroid, which lines the inner surface of the sclera, is a layer of pigmented, spongy, vascular connective tissue with three main functions. The pigment (melanin) helps keep light from bouncing around inside the eyeball, just like the flat black interior of a camera does. The choroid also contains an extensive capillary bed (the choriocapillaris) at its inner margin; these capillaries supply the retinal pigment epithelium and part of the photoreceptors themselves. Finally, the choroid provides a physical route through which nerves and blood vessels can spread out over the eyeball once they have made it through the sclera (just like the route provided by the subarachnoid space around the CNS).

Film

Here, the camera analogy starts to break down. Retinal images are self-developing, like some films used to be. The retina is erasable and reusable, like videotape and the photosensitive chip of a digital camera. But it is not silicon- or polyester-based and, as described below, is designed *not* to record patterns of light accurately.

●●● RETINA

Photographic film and the sensors in digital cameras are designed to more or less duplicate the appearance of the outside world. The retina, in contrast, takes the information landing on its array of more than 100 million photoreceptors and begins to extract its most important features, funneling this into a pattern of action potentials in about 1 million optic nerve axons. Interposed between the photoreceptor layer and the layer of ganglion cells (whose axons form the optic nerve) is a layer containing three kinds of interneurons (Fig. 12-5). Bipolar cells convey signals straight across this layer, receiving inputs from photoreceptors and synapsing on ganglion cells. Horizontal cells spread laterally in the outer synaptic layer, affecting transmission from photoreceptors to bipolar cells. Amacrine cells have a similar role in the inner synaptic layer, affecting transmission from bipolar to ganglion cells. Retinal photoreceptors develop close to the extension of the neural tube cavity into the optic cup (see Fig. 12-2), and as a result vertebrate retinas have a seemingly illogical orientation: the last part of the retina reached by light is the photosensitive parts of the rod and cone cells, embedded in processes of pigment epithelial cells.

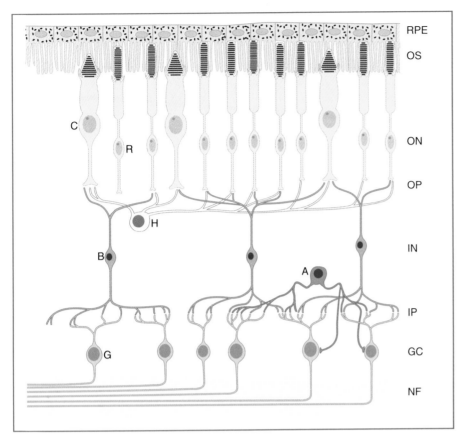

Figure 12-5. Cell types and layers in a typical vertebrate retina. Abbreviations for cell types: A, amacrine cell; B, bipolar cell; C, cone; G, ganglion cell; H, horizontal cell; R, rod. Abbreviations for retinal layers: RPE, retinal pigment epithelium; OS, outer segments (photosensitive regions) of rods and cones; ON, outer nuclear layer (cell bodies of rods and cones); OP, outer plexiform layer (first synaptic layer, where photoreceptors synapse on bipolar and horizontal cells); IN, inner nuclear layer (cell bodies of retinal interneurons); IP, inner plexiform layer (second synaptic layer, where bipolar cells synapse on amacrine and ganglion cells); GC, ganglion cell layer; NF, nerve fiber layer (ganglion cell axons on their way to the optic nerve).

Distinctive Areas of the Retina

A second consequence of the inside-out orientation of the retina is that ganglion cell axons travel along its vitreal surface, so they need to cross the retina, choroid, and sclera in order to leave the eye in the optic nerve. This happens at the optic disc (see Fig. 12-1), where all the axons converge and collect into groups that leave the eye through small holes in the sclera. The sclera continues over the optic nerve as a sheath continuous with the dura mater, much as the spinal dura continues as the epineurium of spinal nerves. The normal layers of the retina are absent at the optic disc, which results in a blind spot in the visual field of each eye, about

the size of a golf ball half a meter away. The optic nerve heads off medially toward the optic chiasm, and the optic disc is a few millimeters medial to the retinal intersection of the optic axis (the line passing through the center of the cornea and lens). Because the cornea and lens reverse everything (side to side and top to bottom), this means the blind spot is a little bit lateral to the center of the visual field.

There are no neurons at all in the optic disc, and in other parts of the retina neurons are distributed nonuniformly. All mammals have two kinds of photoreceptors, named for the shapes of their photosensitive outer segments (see Fig. 12-5). Rods have long, cylindrical outer segments containing a large amount of photopigment and can produce a significant recep-

---

ANATOMY & EMBRYOLOGY

Opening up the Space Between the Neural Retina and the Retinal Pigment Epithelium

Photoreceptors interact metabolically with the retinal pigment epithelium, and normally photoreceptor outer segments are interdigitated with processes of pigment epithelial cells, filling up the space between the two layers of the embryonic optic cup. Under certain conditions, however, liquefied vitreous humor or extracellular fluids from the choroid can ooze into this potential subretinal space, causing retinal detachment.

CLINICAL MEDICINE

Increased Pressure Around the Optic Nerve

The scleral/dural sheath of the optic nerve is lined with continuations of the arachnoid and pia, along with a circumferential slit of subarachnoid space. Increases in intracranial pressure spread through subarachnoid space and can compress veins leaving the eye in the optic nerve. The resulting venous engorgement and edema can be seen as papilledema, or swelling of the optic disc.

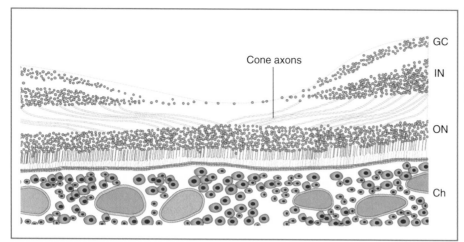

Figure 12-6. Arrangement of cells in and around the fovea. All the ganglion cells and retinal interneurons are pushed to the sides, so the axons of foveal cones take a slanted course to reach them. Ch, choroid; see Fig. 12-5 for other abbreviations.

GC
IN
ON
Ch

Cone axons

tor potential in response to absorption of a single photon. Cones have shorter, tapered outer segments and are less sensitive to light. A human retina contains about 100 million rods and 5 million cones, each type with a distinctive distribution. At the center of the retina (where the optic axis intersects it) is the fovea (Fig. 12-6), a small depression in the center of a yellowish pigmented zone called the macula lutea ("yellow spot"). The macula, and especially the fovea, is specialized for vision of the highest spatial acuity. The fovea contains no rods—only tightly packed, particularly slender cones—and all other neurons that might interfere with the transmission of light are pushed off to the sides. The packing density of cones falls off rapidly outside the fovea, quickly reaching a value less than 5% as great. The distribution of rods is largely complementary, going from zero in the fovea to a maximum value outside the fovea, then declining toward the peripheral retina. The numbers of bipolar cells and ganglion cells also diminish progressively in more peripheral parts of the retina, where there is more convergence. Putting all this together, it means that the fovea is specialized for daytime vision of the highest spatial acuity, that night vision has its highest acuity just outside the fovea, and that ganglion cell receptive fields get bigger and bigger as they become more peripheral.

Rod and Cone Function

The outer segments of both rods and cones are filled with stacked-up membranous discs (Fig. 12-7) that start out as invaginations of the surface membrane. Rod outer segments are longer and have more of them, most of them completely pinched off from the surface membrane. The discs of cone outer segments are smaller and fewer, and they stay attached to the surface membrane.

Vertebrate photoreception is based on a series of closely related opsin proteins, all of them similar to a G protein–coupled norepinephrine receptor. Instead of binding norepinephrine, opsin binds 11-*cis* retinal (the 11-*cis* isomer of vitamin A aldehyde), which gives it light-absorbing properties. Slight differences in the amino acid sequence of different opsins determine the wavelength that a given opsin/retinal complex absorbs best. Absorption of a photon causes the 11-*cis* retinal to photoisomerize into its all-*trans* form, which changes the conformation of opsin, allowing it to activate nearby G proteins. This in turn activates an enzyme (phosphodiesterase) that hydrolyzes cyclic GMP (cGMP), and cGMP-gated cation channels close. So in the dark, photoreceptors have open cation channels, are depolarized, and continuously release neurotransmitter (glutamate) onto bipolar cells. Light causes some of the channels to close, the

---

CLINICAL MEDICINE

Loss of Central Vision

Age-related macular degeneration is a common cause of visual loss in older individuals, affecting as many as a quarter of those older than age 75. Although the cause is still unknown, the consequences are consistent with the organization of the macula: decreased visual acuity and color vision, difficulty reading, and in advanced cases, functional near-blindness.

BIOCHEMISTRY

Night Blindness

Vitamin A is involved in multiple physiologic and developmental functions, but its role as the precursor of 11-*cis* retinal makes it essential for photoreceptor function. One of the earliest signs of vitamin A deficiency is an inability to completely replenish the rhodopsin in retinal rods during dark adaptation, resulting in difficulty seeing in dim light.

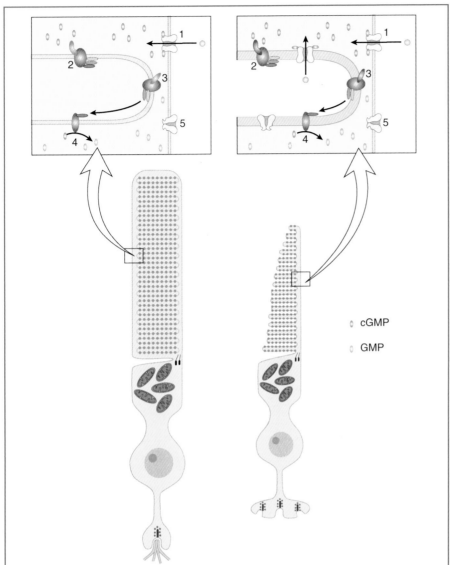

Figure 12-7. Mechanism of phototransduction in rods (*left*) and cones (*right*). The surface membranes of both contain cyclic GMP-gated cation channels (1) that are open in the dark. Absorption of a photon by a photopigment molecule (2) causes a conformational change in its attached retinal (3) and activation of nearby G proteins, which in turn activates phosphodiesterase. Phosphodiesterase hydrolyzes cyclic GMP (4), and some percentage of the cation channels close (5), hyperpolarizing the photoreceptor and decreasing its rate of glutamate release.

cGMP

GMP

membrane to hyperpolarize, and the rate of transmitter release to decline. This multistep transduction process makes photoreceptors highly sensitive (rods can respond to single photons) but slow. In contrast to receptors with directly gated channels (e.g., hair cells), which can begin to respond within microseconds of a stimulus, rod and cone receptor potentials have latencies of milliseconds.

The only role of photons in this entire process is to trigger the conversion of 11-*cis* to all-*trans* retinal, so an individual photoreceptor can tell only that one of these events has occurred, not the wavelength of the photon that caused it. All the rods of a given species have the same opsin, leading to the same visual pigment (rhodopsin). Rhodopsin absorbs blue-green light around 500 nm best, so rods cannot tell whether they are being illuminated by dim green light or brighter orange or violet light. As a result, there is no color vision in light so dim that only rods are functional. However, some vertebrates, including humans, have multiple populations of

cones (Fig. 12-8), each with a different opsin. A single population of cones cannot distinguish colors any better than rods can, but comparing the outputs of multiple populations makes color vision possible. Because of its densely packed cones, the fovea is specialized not just for the highest spatial acuity but also for color vision.

Receptive Fields of Retinal Neurons

The receptive field of a neuron in the visual system is the area of the outside world (or the part of the retina where its image falls) where changes in illumination cause a change in the neuron's electrical activity. The receptive field of a rod or cone is straightforward—it is simply a spot whose image covers the receptor and causes it to hyperpolarize. Making the stimulus larger than the receptor does not have much additional effect. Ganglion cells, in contrast, have receptive fields with different properties. Most fall into two broad

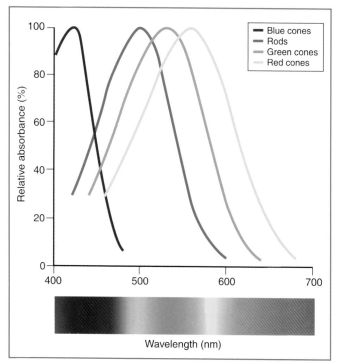

Figure 12-8. Absorption spectra of human rods and cones. (Red, green, and blue cones are so named because of the importance of each for distinguishing colors in that part of the spectrum, not for the peaks of their absorption spectra; this is especially apparent for red cones, which actually absorb yellow light best.)

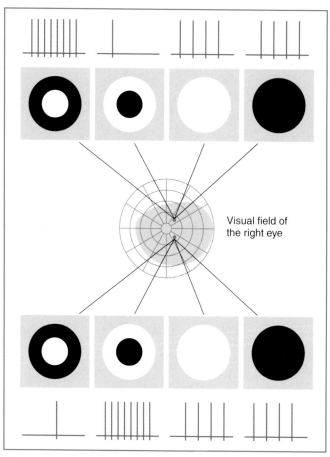

Figure 12-9. Response patterns of an ON-center (*upper row*) and an OFF-center (*lower row*) ganglion cell in the right retina. Each responds to changes in illumination in a small circular area (its receptive field) in that eye's visual field, but only when the illumination is nonuniform (i.e., there is contrast within the receptive field).

GENETICS

Color Blindness

All mammals have at least two types of cones, one that absorbs maximally in the blue or ultraviolet and another in the yellow-green range, thereby allowing a level of color vision. Humans and some other primates improve on this by having blue-absorbing cones and two kinds of long-wavelength cones. The genes for both long-wavelength opsins are on the X chromosome, and as a result, red-green color blindness is a sex-linked condition. The gene for the short-wavelength opsin, in contrast, is located on chromosome 7, so blue color blindness has a low but equal incidence in both males and females.

classes, with complementary center-surround characteristics (Fig. 12-9). The first kind, called ON-center cells, fire faster when light falls on the center of the field, fire slower when light falls on the periphery of the field, and do not do much in response to diffuse illumination (because the two parts of the field cancel each other out). OFF-center cells fire slower when light falls on the center of the field, fire faster when light falls on the periphery of the field, and do not do much in response to diffuse illumination. (Looked at from a different perspective, OFF-center cells fire faster when illumination of the center of their field *decreases*.)

Consequently, (1) the message carried by most fibers in the optic nerve is related not so much to the brightness of things but rather to the contrast between different parts of the visual world (so the retina detects edges and does not waste impulses signaling areas of uniform brightness) and (2) some ganglion cell will fire faster whether the light intensity in any small part of the visual field increases (ON-center cells) or decreases (OFF-center cells). (That is probably why there are both ON-center cells and OFF-center cells—so that something fires faster no matter which way light intensity changes.)

The centers of foveal ganglion cell receptive fields are tiny— the same size as that of a single foveal cone. The centers of receptive fields in the peripheral retina, on the other hand, are much larger, reflecting the convergence of the outputs of hundreds of rods or cones onto single bipolar cells. This leads to a situation analogous to that in the somatosensory system, in which fingertips have many receptors, high acuity, and a disproportionately large representation in somatosensory cortex.

Bipolar cells have a similar center-surround organization and come in ON-center and OFF-center varieties. Bipolar

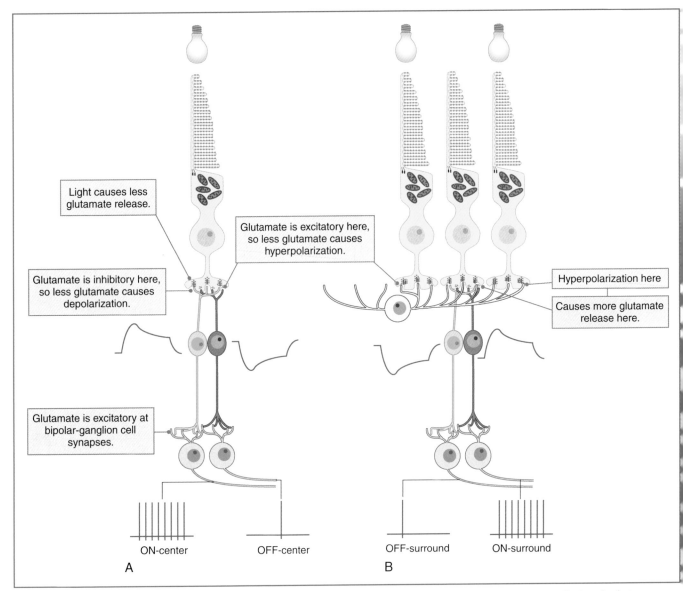

Light causes less glutamate release.

Glutamate is excitatory here, so less glutamate causes hyperpolarization.

Glutamate is inhibitory here, so less glutamate causes depolarization.

Hyperpolarization here

Causes more glutamate release here.

Glutamate is excitatory at bipolar-ganglion cell synapses.

ON-center   OFF-center   OFF-surround   ON-surround

A   B

Figure 12-10. Formation of center-surround receptive fields. Light shone on a given photoreceptor causes its terminals to release less glutamate (**A**); light shone on neighboring photoreceptors causes it (through horizontal cell connections) to release *more* glutamate (**B**). Hence, a maximal change in glutamate release can be realized by simultaneously changing the intensity of illumination of a photoreceptor in one direction and changing the intensity of illumination of its neighbors in the opposite direction (i.e., introducing contrast).

cells do not make action potentials, but these receptive field properties are expressed as slow potential changes. The receptive field center is a reflection of direct photoreceptor input to the bipolar cell. Since rods and cones all hyperpolarize and release less transmitter (glutamate) in response to light, the 2 opposite polarities of bipolar responses mean that glutamate must excite OFF-center bipolar cells and inhibit ON-center bipolar cells (Fig. 12-10). Foveal bipolar cells have tiny receptive field centers because they receive inputs from single cones; they then synapse on single ganglion cells, maintaining the small size of the receptive field center.

Although the exact mechanism is still disputed, horizontal cells are the key elements that convey antagonistic surround information (see Fig. 12-10). Photoreceptors release glutamate in the dark onto both bipolar cells and horizontal cells. Glutamate depolarizes horizontal cells, whose laterally spreading processes then suppress the release of glutamate from the terminals of neighboring photoreceptors. Thus, shining light on photoreceptors in the center of a bipolar cell's receptive field causes less glutamate release on that bipolar cell, and shining light on photoreceptors in the surrounding area has the opposite effect.

●●● CENTRAL VISUAL PATHWAYS

Axons of retinal ganglion cells project to a variety of places: the superior colliculus, to help direct visual attention; other midbrain sites, for things like the pupillary light reflex; the

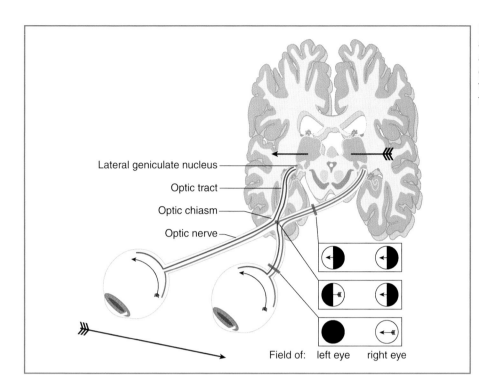

Figure 12-11. Course of ganglion cell axons through the optic nerve, chiasm, and tract on their way to the lateral geniculate nucleus. Qualitatively different visual field deficits result from damage to the nerve, chiasm, and tract.

Lateral geniculate nucleus

Optic tract

Optic chiasm

Optic nerve

Field of: left eye   right eye

hypothalamus, to help regulate circadian rhythms; but mostly to the thalamus, for conscious awareness of visual stimuli. Optic nerve fibers convey all the information we will ever get about the shape, color, location, and movement of objects in the outside world. Different classes of ganglion cells emphasize different properties of a visual stimulus, and these different properties begin to be sorted out in the six-layered lateral geniculate nucleus of the thalamus. Different layers of the lateral geniculate then project differentially to primary visual cortex above and below the calcarine sulcus (also known as striate cortex because of a stripe of myelinated fibers that run through one of its middle layers). Primary visual cortex then picks apart these attributes a little more and parcels them out semiselectively to distinct areas of visual association cortex in the occipital and temporal lobes.

Optic Nerve, Chiasm, and Tract

Just as somatosensory information from one arm or leg gets projected to the contralateral postcentral gyrus, visual information from one side of the world winds up in the contralateral occipital lobe. Because of our frontally directed eyes, each eye looks at most of the right and left half of the total visual field. As a result, half of the output of each retina needs to cross in the optic chiasm, and half needs to stay uncrossed (Fig. 12-11); the crossed and uncrossed fibers representing one half of the visual field emerge from the chiasm as an optic tract. Hence, damage in front of the optic chiasm can cause, at most, complete blindness of the ipsilateral eye, whereas damage to one optic tract (or any part of the visual system behind the chiasm) can cause, at most, loss of the contralateral half of the visual field of both eyes. The

ANATOMY & EMBRYOLOGY

Compression of the Optic Chiasm

The pituitary gland is located just inferior to the optic chiasm, and pituitary tumors are the most common cause of damage to the chiasm. Because fibers from the nasal half of each retina cross in the optic chiasm, compression by a pituitary tumor causes deficits in roughly mirror-image parts of the temporal fields of both eyes (see Fig. 12-11). Fibers from the inferior part of each nasal retina cross in the inferior part of the chiasm, so a pituitary tumor pressing from below causes losses that are often worse in the superior part of each temporal field.

latter deficit has the tongue-twisting name of homonymous hemianopia ("blindness in the same half of both visual fields"). Damage to the optic chiasm typically causes loss of parts of the visual field of both eyes, but different parts.

Getting to Primary Visual Cortex

Optic tract fibers end in a precise retinotopic pattern in the lateral geniculate nucleus. Because the thalamus does relatively little information processing (see Chapter 5), the receptive fields of geniculate neurons are similar to those of ganglion cells—input from only one eye, center-surround antagonism, some receptive fields concerned with color and others with black-white contrast, and a lot of representation of small foveal receptive fields. Lateral geniculate neurons then project to striate cortex, and thereafter things change.

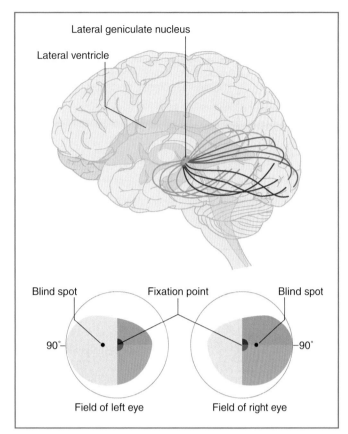

Figure 12-12. Optic radiation, traveling from the lateral geniculate nucleus to primary visual cortex.

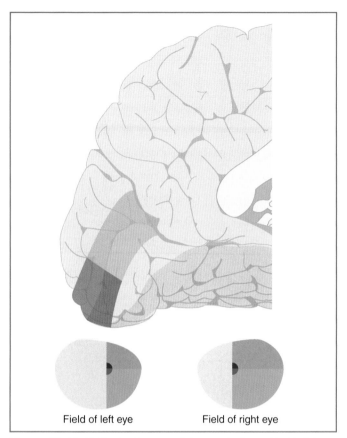

Figure 12-13. Retinotopic map of the contralateral half of the visual field of both eyes in primary visual cortex.

Geniculate axons exit through the retrolenticular and sublenticular parts of the internal capsule and form the optic radiation (Fig. 12-12), a sheet of fibers that sweep backward to the occipital lobe; those from the sublenticular part swing anteriorly through the temporal lobe for a short distance before turning backward. Axons representing inferior visual fields are in the upper half of the optic radiation, and those from the superior fields are in the lower half. Axons representing the fovea occupy a middle zone, with peripheral parts of the field above and below. The optic radiation then terminates in a systematic map in striate cortex (Fig. 12-13), with a large representation of the fovea toward the occipital pole, the superior and inferior parts of the field below and above the calcarine sulcus, and the peripheral part of the field most anterior. The foveal representation near the occipital pole is at a location where territories of the posterior and middle cerebral arteries meet and overlap (see Fig. 7-13). One result is that occlusion of one posterior cerebral artery commonly results in contralateral homonymous hemianopia that is not quite complete, because there is some macular sparing (see Fig. 12-13).

Primary Visual Cortex

The cortical cells most sensitive to contrast have receptive fields that come in a variety of formats, but they generally have a few things in common (Fig. 12-14). Like ganglion cells, they do not respond much to diffuse illumination because there are excitatory and inhibitory regions in their receptive fields that can cancel each other out. Unlike ganglion cells, the receptive fields are not circular, and they do not respond well to small spots of light. Instead, they respond to stripes or edges with a particular orientation. The simplest kinds of contrast-sensitive cortical neurons (often called simple cells) have excitatory and inhibitory regions in the shape of oriented bars. Other, more complex ones may respond only to oriented lines of a particular length. These properties are just what you need to begin to analyze the shape of an object.

Other neurons in area 17 are more concerned with color than with black-white contrast. They have circular receptive fields with antagonistic center-surround color properties. Still others pay attention to motion, or to the small disparities between the images seen by the two retinas that can be used for depth perception.

The whole retinotopic map is divided into a large series of repeating functional units (Fig. 12-15), each one sitting under an area of cortical surface about 1 mm by 1 mm. Within each of these hypercolumns, all aspects of the information coming from a particular part of the contralateral visual field are sorted out, worked on a little bit, and shipped along to other visual areas. This sorting out results in one of the physiologically best-understood examples of the columnar

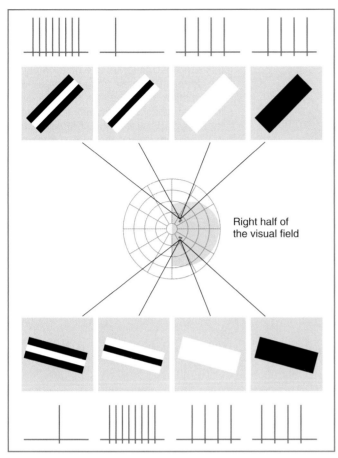

Figure 12-14. Receptive fields of two typical contrast-sensitive neurons in primary visual cortex of the left occipital lobe.

organization of cerebral cortex. Each hypercolumn includes two complete sets of orientation columns, each about 50 μm by 500 μm, through which all stimulus orientations are mapped out systematically for both eyes. Interspersed among these orientation columns are cylinders of color-sensitive neurons reporting on the same part of the visual field. Other aspects of visual stimuli are presumably mapped out systematically within these same hypercolumns in ways that are not as well understood.

Since all hypercolumns are about the same size, and since the fovea occupies so much of the cortical map, it follows that foveal hypercolumns correspond to small areas of the visual field and peripheral hypercolumns to much larger areas. The central part of the receptive field of a simple cell that represents part of the fovea may be only as wide as the receptive field of a single cone.

Beyond Primary Visual Cortex

Once the attributes of a visual stimulus have been partially fractionated in striate cortex, a series of projections convey this information to numerous visual association areas in the occipital and inferior temporal lobes (Fig. 12-16). Although

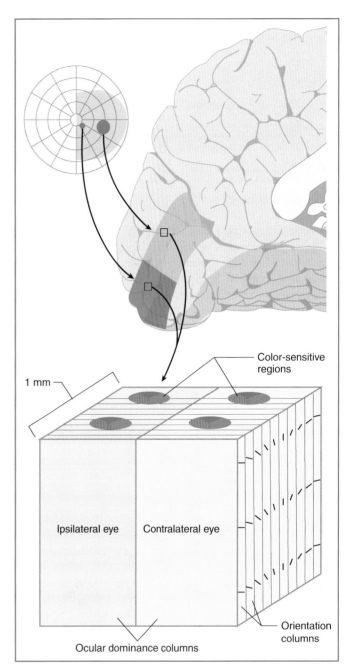

Figure 12-15. Under each square millimeter of primary visual cortex is an assemblage of smaller cortical columns specialized for different functions—analyzing contrast, color, motion, retinal disparities, and other factors. Collectively these components of a hypercolumn dissect all the visual properties of some localized area of the contralateral visual field, preparing them for shipment to appropriate visual association areas. Hypercolumns in the foveal part of the map in visual cortex analyze a smaller area of the visual field than do those in the peripheral retina part of the map.

there is a lot of overlap, further analysis of form and color is largely carried out in ventral parts of the occipital and temporal lobes, and further analysis of location and motion takes place more dorsally, around the junction of the occipital, parietal, and temporal lobes. As a result, damage to

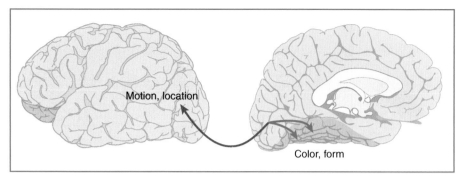

Figure 12-16. General pattern of projections from primary visual cortex to visual association cortex. Although the two streams are not as independent as this simplified diagram seems to imply, the dorsal stream reaching the area near the junction of the parietal, occipital, and temporal lobes is particularly important for analyzing the location and movement of visual stimuli, and the ventral stream reaching the occipitotemporal gyrus is particularly important for analyzing colors and shapes.

the occipitotemporal gyrus can cause deficits in recognizing things visually despite visual fields being intact. The deficits can be fairly selective depending on which part of the occipitotemporal gyrus is damaged (e.g., cortical color blindness [achromatopsia] or difficulty recognizing faces [prosopagnosia]). Conversely, damage near the junction of the parietal, occipital, and temporal lobes can cause difficulties in perceiving the motion of objects or in "stitching together" multiple objects in different locations into a unified scene.

●●● VISUAL REFLEXES

Like most cameras, the eye has autoexposure and autofocus mechanisms, in this case mediated by CNS control of the pupil and ciliary muscle.

Pupillary Light Reflex

Just as touching one cornea causes reflex blinking of both eyes, and loud sound in one ear causes the stapedius to contract bilaterally, light shone in one eye elicits a pupillary light reflex (Fig. 12-17) that causes both the ipsilateral and the contralateral pupil to constrict (the direct and consensual reflex, respectively). Interestingly, this reflex does not depend on the presence of retinal rods or cones. Instead, a special subset of intrinsically photosensitive ganglion cells provide the afferent limb, with axons that distribute bilaterally in the optic chiasm and terminate in the pretectal area (at the junction between the superior colliculus and the diencephalon, so called because the superior and inferior colliculi together are referred to as the tectum). The pretectal area projects bilaterally to the Edinger-Westphal nucleus (the preganglionic parasympathetic component of the oculomotor nucleus). Because light in either eye causes both the ipsilateral and the contralateral pupil to constrict (direct and consensual reflexes, respectively), both pupils ordinarily will be pretty much the same size under any given condition of illumination; if they are not, there likely is a problem with the autonomic innervation or with the iris itself.

Accommodation Reflex

When animals with frontally directed eyes, such as humans, look at something nearby, two of the things that need to

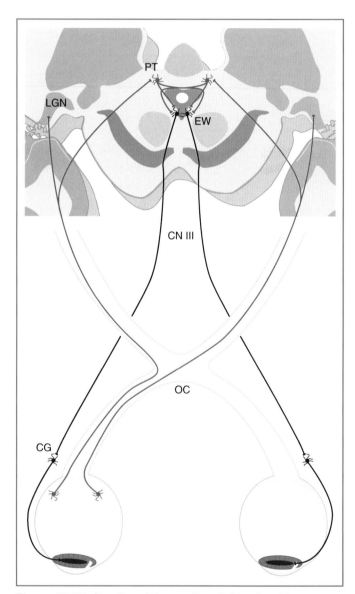

Figure 12-17. Circuitry of the pupillary light reflex. The ganglion cells of one retina project to the pretectal area of both sides because of the optic chiasm. In addition, pretectal neurons project bilaterally to the Edinger-Westphal nucleus. As a result, light in one eye affects both Edinger-Westphal nuclei equally. CG, ciliary ganglion; CN III, oculomotor nerve; EW, Edinger-Westphal nucleus (part of the oculomotor nucleus); LGN, lateral geniculate nucleus (no role in this reflex); OC, optic chiasm; PT, pretectal area.

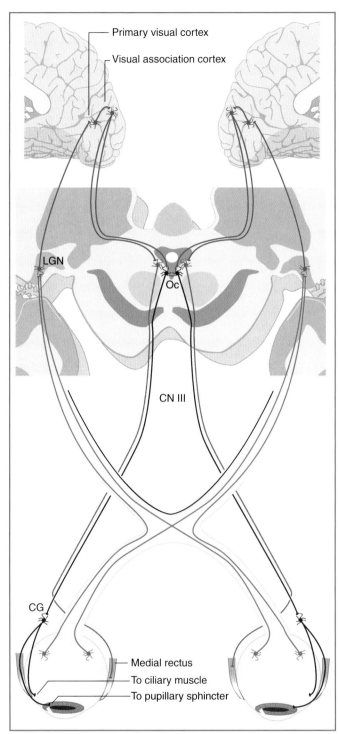

Figure 12-18. Circuitry of the accommodation (near) reflex. CG, ciliary ganglion; CN III, oculomotor nerve; LGN, lateral geniculate nucleus; Oc, oculomotor nucleus.

Primary visual cortex

Visual association cortex

LGN

Oc

CN III

CG

Medial rectus

To ciliary muscle

To pupillary sphincter

happen are fairly obvious: (1) the eyes converge, so that the image of the object lands on both foveae, and (2) the eyes refocus on the near object. A third, less obvious, response is that the pupil constricts, bringing more things at different distances into focus (i.e., the depth of focus improves). All three things happen automatically as parts of the accommodation reflex (or near reflex; Fig. 12-18). The response normally involves a conscious look at something close, and the afferent limb is the usual pathway from retina to lateral geniculate to striate cortex. Striate cortex then projects to visual association cortex, which completes the loop by projecting to the efferent components in the oculomotor nucleus (medial rectus motor neurons and preganglionic parasympathetics for the ciliary muscle and pupillary sphincter).

The pupillary constriction that accompanies the accommodation reflex provides another nice example of the remarkable things the CNS does in the background. Making the pupil smaller improves the eye's optical performance, but it also reduces the amount of light that reaches the retina. The brain automatically figures out the pupil size that provides the best tradeoff between acuity and intensity, and that is the size that is used.

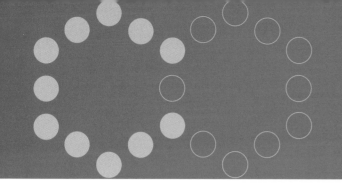

Chemical Senses

13

CONTENTS

All cells are chemical engines that need to be chemosensitive in various ways, at a minimum metabolizing selected chemicals. Some have more specific chemosensitivities (e.g., responding to hormones or neurotransmitters). Multicellular organisms have systems of chemoreceptors specifically designed to detect favored food sources and avoid ingesting things that might be harmful.

●●● TASTE, SMELL, AND FLAVOR

A first impulse is to consider the flavor of something to be based solely on information provided by taste buds on the tongue. Taste buds, however, respond to a relatively limited repertoire of chemicals, and the totality of something's flavor reflects an integration of gustatory inputs from taste buds, olfactory input, trigeminal input, the visceral chemoreceptors that we usually think of as working outside the realm of consciousness, and even visual input.

Trigeminal, visceral, and visual inputs, although not considered in any detail in this chapter, make important

CLINICAL MEDICINE

Testing Taste

Selective testing of gustation requires the application of substances such as sucrose, NaCl, weak acids, or quinine in some odorless format. Drops of a solution or bits of soaked filter paper, for example, can be applied to specific areas of the tongue.

contributions to the perception of flavor. Most trigeminal endings convey somatosensory information (think about how much better some things "taste" when hot or cold, tender or chewy, smooth or granular), but some are themselves chemosensory and respond to spicy or pungent aspects of foods and odors (e.g., the heat of chili peppers or the unpleasant sharpness of ammonia). Visceral chemoreceptors keep track of our internal concentration of glucose and other nutrients (see Chapter 18) and make major contributions to feelings of hunger and thirst. (Think about how good food and beverages taste when you are hungry or thirsty, or how relatively unappetizing even a favorite food can be after a big meal.) Finally, we learn to associate the visual appearance of foods with their taste (e.g., judging the ripeness of fruit by its color, salivating at the sight of a favorite food).

●●● GUSTATORY SYSTEM

Taste is the major arbiter of whether something in the mouth should be consumed; the other contributors to flavor perception help determine how much it should be relished. As monitors of nutrient intake, taste cells (gustatory receptor cells) detect the general constituents of food and beverages and lead to taste sensations of sweet, salty, sour, and bitter. Amino acids lead to a fifth taste, generally referred to as "umami" (Japanese, "delicious"), that accounts for the flavor-enhancing properties of monosodium glutamate. Most taste cells differ from other receptors in being relatively insensitive, responding only when tastant concentrations exceed 1–10 mmol/L (presumably so that things with low nutrient content will not be particularly enjoyable to eat). The exception is bitter receptors, which have thresholds in the micromolar range. Many plant toxins taste bitter, and bitter receptors help prevent the consumption of potentially injurious substances (although, of course, many learn to enjoy some bitter things such as coffee, beer, and tonic water).

Taste Buds

Each taste bud (Fig. 13-1) is an encapsulated cluster of 50 to 100 taste cells and a smaller number of basal (precursor) cells. Taste cells are elongated, modified epithelial cells with microvilli at one end that protrude through an opening (the taste pore) at the surface of the taste bud, where they are exposed to tastants dissolved in saliva. At the deep end

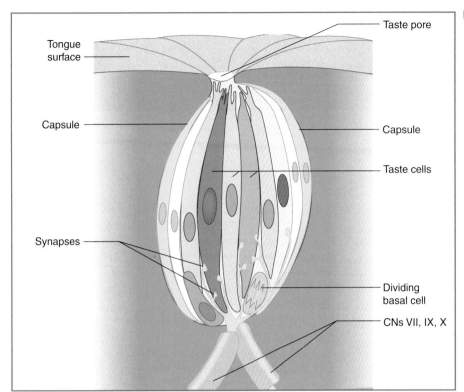

Figure 13-1. Structure of a taste bud.

Tongue surface

Capsule

Synapses

Taste pore

Capsule

Taste cells

Dividing basal cell

CNs VII, IX, X

of the taste bud, taste cells synapse on peripheral endings of gustatory primary afferents. Like other epithelial cells, taste cells are replaced throughout life. Each lasts 10 days or so before dying and being replaced by differentiation of basal cells.

Taste buds are widely distributed in the oral cavity, but most of the approximately 5000 of them are located on the tongue, in some of the bumps and folds (papillae) that cover its upper and lateral surface (Fig. 13-2). Fungiform papillae on the anterior two thirds of the tongue, innervated by the facial nerve, contain about a quarter of the taste buds. Foliate papillae on the posterolateral surface, innervated mostly by the glossopharyngeal nerve, contain another quarter. Each of the approximately nine circumvallate (or vallate) papillae, also innervated by the glossopharyngeal nerve, contains hundreds of taste buds; collectively, they account for about half of the total population. The vagus nerve innervates the small population of taste buds in the epiglottis and esophagus. Some of the taste cells in all these papillae respond to each of the basic tastants, so the whole spectrum of tastes can be experienced using any part of the tongue. There is, however, some regional specialization, so that the tip is *relatively* more sensitive to sweet substances and amino acids, the lateral surfaces to salty and sour stimuli, and the circumvallate papillae to bitter substances.

Transduction by Taste Cells

Taste cells are in most ways typical short receptors (see Fig. 4-2), producing depolarizing receptor potentials in response to exposure to an appropriate tastant and increasing

their rate of transmitter release onto the peripheral endings of primary afferents. Both ionotropic and metabotropic mechanisms are used to produce these depolarizing receptor potentials (Fig. 13-3). The salt transduction mechanism is as simple as it can be: high concentrations of NaCl result in an

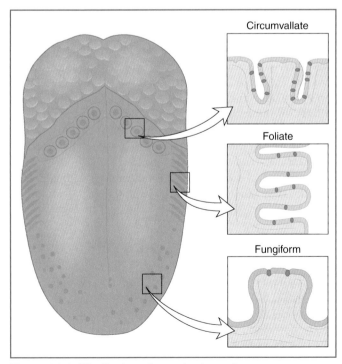

Circumvallate

Foliate

Fungiform

Figure 13-2. Distribution of taste buds on the tongue.

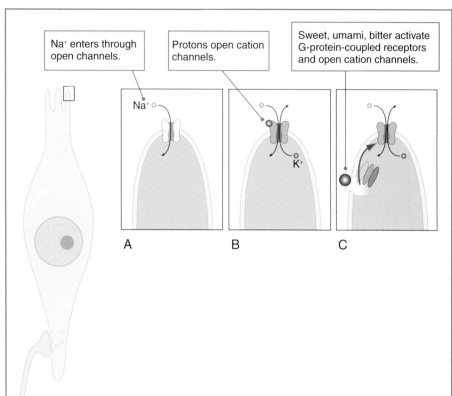

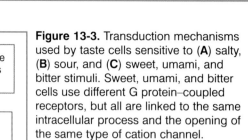

Figure 13-3. Transduction mechanisms used by taste cells sensitive to (**A**) salty, (**B**) sour, and (**C**) sweet, umami, and bitter stimuli. Sweet, umami, and bitter cells use different G protein–coupled receptors, but all are linked to the same intracellular process and the opening of the same type of cation channel.

influx of Na$^+$ through open channels. Acidic substances taste sour, and the receptor potential of sour-sensitive taste cells is produced via pH-sensitive cation channels. Sweet-, umami-, and bitter-sensitive taste cells all use different G protein–coupled receptors that lead to the opening of the same type of cation channel. (It's a dangerous world out there, and there are about 30 different bitter receptors, allowing the detection of a wide range of potentially harmful chemicals.)

Gustatory Connections in the Central Nervous System

Fibers of cranial nerves VII, IX, and X convey signals not just from taste buds but also from glands and organs of the head, thorax, and abdomen. These primary afferents then enter the brainstem and travel rostrally or caudally in the solitary tract before synapsing in the surrounding nucleus of the solitary tract (Fig. 13-4). The nucleus of the solitary tract, the major visceral sensory nucleus of the brainstem, is located just lateral to the sulcus limitans (see Fig. 6-12) and is systematically organized, with subdivisions at different medullary levels dealing with gustatory, cardiovascular, respiratory, and alimentary functions. The solitary tract is the highway through which different categories of primary afferents reach the appropriate subdivision of the nucleus.

The lateral part of the rostral end of the nucleus of the solitary tract is its gustatory subdivision. Neurons here project (Fig. 13-5) to the reticular formation (for taste-related reflexes such as salivation), to the hypothalamus and amygdala (contributing to feelings of hunger, satiety, and pleasure),

and to the thalamus (leading to conscious awareness of taste). The pathway to the thalamus ascends through the reticular formation and terminates in the most medial part of VPM, which then projects to primary gustatory cortex in the anterior insula. Unlike most other sensory pathways, this one is largely uncrossed. The olfactory system is also uncrossed (see below), so both sets of chemosensory data wind up on the same side of the CNS.

●●● OLFACTORY SYSTEM

The olfactory system has a much broader role than the gustatory system, participating not just in the selection and enjoyment of food and beverages but also in the general experience of the environment (e.g., the scent of flowers or a pine forest) and in social interactions (e.g., the fragrance industry). Its role in the appreciation of flavor (e.g., the complexity of a glass of wine), however, is very substantial and in many ways surpasses that of the gustatory system. Indeed, most patients who complain of a "taste" disorder actually have an olfactory impairment.

Olfactory Epithelium

Humans, compared with many other animals, have a relatively impoverished olfactory sense, but still it is quite extraordinary. Human noses have about 5 million olfactory receptor neurons (more than 10 times the total complement of taste receptors) on each side, in an olfactory epithelium (Fig. 13-6) in the roof and upper walls of the nasal cavity.

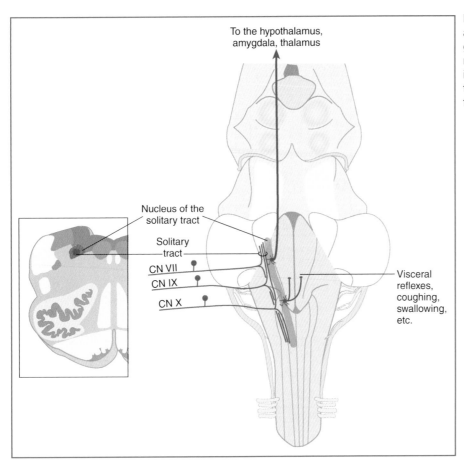

Figure 13-4. Location of the solitary tract and its nucleus in the brainstem, and the general pattern of connections of the nucleus. (See Chapter 18 for more information on the role of the nucleus of the solitary tract in autonomic control functions.)

Each olfactory receptor is a bipolar neuron with a very thin axon emerging from one side of the cell body and a single dendrite extending from the other side toward the surface of the epithelium. The dendrite ends as a small, bulbous expansion from which a couple of dozen chemosensitive cilia emerge and spread out in the mucous layer covering the epithelium. Like taste cells, olfactory receptor neurons are continually replaced throughout life; each lasts a month or two before being replaced by division of stem cells deep in the olfactory epithelium. This makes new olfactory receptors one of the few neuronal types to appear after birth (see Chapter 20). The chemosensitive microvilli of taste cells and cilia of olfactory receptors, unlike almost all other parts of the nervous system, are exposed to the outside world rather than being sheltered behind a barrier (see Fig. 7-18). It is thought that enough wear and tear results to necessitate the regular replacement of these cells.

Olfactory Transduction

Olfactory receptor neurons are long receptors. Like other long receptors they produce depolarizing receptor potentials that, if large enough, trigger trains of action potentials. Although there are many subtly different types of olfactory receptor neurons (see below), all have the same morphology and use the same G protein–coupled transduction mechanism (Fig. 13-7). Binding of an odorant by the G protein–coupled receptor results in activation of adenylate cyclase, an increase in the intraciliary cAMP concentration, and the opening of cAMP-gated cation channels. This is followed by an additional amplification step unique to olfactory receptors. The cAMP-gated cation channels are even more permeable to Ca^{++} than to Na^+, and the Ca^{++} influx through these channels causes Ca^{++}-gated Cl^- channels to open. Olfactory receptor neurons maintain a relatively high intracellular Cl^- concentration, about the same as the extracellular concentration, so the Cl^- equilibrium potential (see Equation 2-2) is about 0 mV. As a result, opening Cl^- channels in these neurons has the unusual result of causing additional depolarization.

Just as it is impossible to discriminate among colors using a single population of photoreceptors (see Chapter 12), it

---

MICROBIOLOGY

Respiratory Infections and Olfactory Epithelium

Odorants have easy access to olfactory receptor cells, but viruses and bacteria have relatively easy access too. The most common cause of loss of olfaction in adults is a severe upper respiratory infection, which is sometimes followed by death of most or all olfactory receptor cells. This occurs more frequently in older individuals, whose ability to generate new receptor cells is diminished.

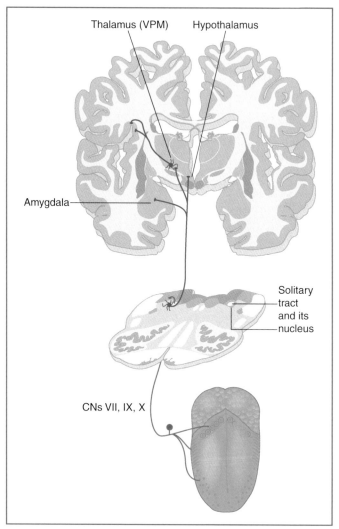

Figure 13-5. Projections of gustatory information in the CNS. Although the gustatory projections of the nucleus of the solitary tract are shown for simplicity as direct and uncrossed, some may involve relays in other brainstem nuclei and some may be bilateral.

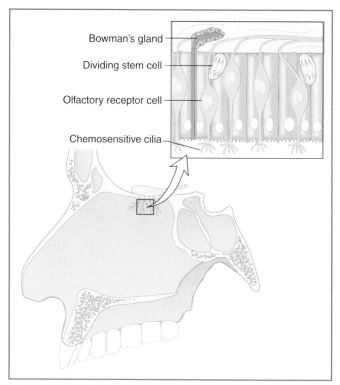

Figure 13-6. Olfactory epithelium. Receptors are interspersed with supporting cells and the ducts of Bowman's glands (which secrete the mucous layer in which the chemosensitive cilia of the receptor cells spread out).

would be impossible to discriminate among odorants using a single population of olfactory receptors. The problem is exacerbated in the olfactory system, because even humans can discriminate among thousands of odors (versus a hundred or so wavelengths). This is addressed by having a very large number of different olfactory receptor molecules and putting a single type in each receptor neuron, in effect resulting in the olfactory equivalent of many different cone populations. In fact, the genes coding olfactory receptor molecules make up the largest known gene family. More than 300 such genes are active in humans; some other mammals have more than a thousand.

Olfactory Connections in the Central Nervous System

The axons of olfactory receptor neurons collect into small bundles—collectively forming CN I—that pass upward

through holes in the cribriform plate of the ethmoid bone and terminate in spherical synaptic zones called glomeruli in the ipsilateral olfactory bulb (Fig. 13-8). The termination pattern is a remarkable feat of sorting and convergence, again unique to the olfactory system. All of the tens of thousands of axons from receptors that express a given olfactory receptor molecule manage to find each other and converge on just one or two glomeruli; each glomerulus receives afferent inputs from a single receptor type. Dendrites of a relatively small number of olfactory bulb output neurons (mostly mitral cells), together with processes of olfactory bulb interneurons, also enter each glomerulus. The thousand-to-one convergence from receptors to mitral cells enhances the sensitivity of the olfactory system, and the selective mapping of receptor types onto

ANATOMY & EMBRYOLOGY

Trauma and the Olfactory System

A blow to the head can shear off the bundles of axons of olfactory receptor cells as they pass through the cribriform plate, resulting in posttraumatic anosmia. Even though the receptors can regenerate, the anosmia is often permanent because scarring covers the small holes and prevents regrowth.

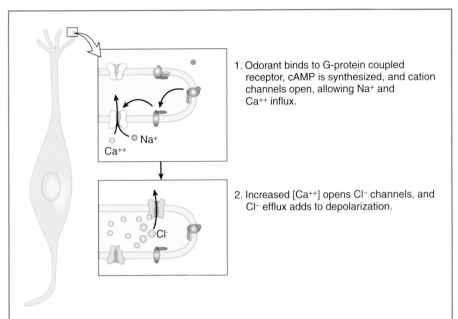

Figure 13-7. Transduction by olfactory receptor neurons.

1. Odorant binds to G-protein coupled receptor, cAMP is synthesized, and cation channels open, allowing Na^+ and Ca^{++} influx.

2. Increased $[Ca^{++}]$ opens Cl^- channels, and Cl^- efflux adds to depolarization.

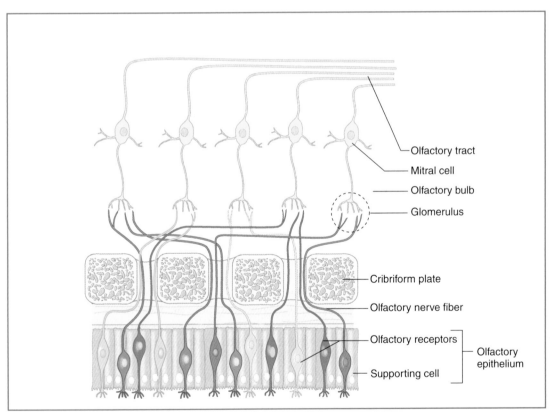

Figure 13-8. Termination of olfactory receptor axons in glomeruli of the olfactory bulb. The colors of different receptors and axons are meant to indicate the presence of a particular type of olfactory receptor molecule.

- Olfactory tract
- Mitral cell
- Olfactory bulb
- Glomerulus
- Cribriform plate
- Olfactory nerve fiber
- Olfactory receptors
- Supporting cell
- Olfactory epithelium

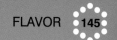

EMBRYOLOGY & GENETICS

Congenital Anosmia

The olfactory epithelium develops from a placode of neural crest–like cells whose axons grow into the surface of the telencephalon and induce the formation of the olfactory bulb. The same placode also gives rise to neuroblasts that subsequently migrate along olfactory nerve fibers, reach the hypothalamus, and become the neurons that produce gonadotropin-releasing hormone; these are the only known examples of CNS neurons that migrate in from outside. The X-linked form of Kallmann syndrome involves a defect in a guidance molecule that is normally produced by the telencephalon and attracts olfactory receptor axons. As a result, the olfactory bulbs fail to form and affected individuals are anosmic. In addition, the neurons that produce gonadotropin-releasing hormone are unable to migrate into the CNS, so affected individuals also suffer from hypogonadism.

CLINICAL MEDICINE

Olfactory Auras Before Seizures

Seizures originating from the medial temporal lobe near the uncus may be preceded by an olfactory hallucination (usually an unpleasant one). Because of their origin, these are still referred to as uncinate seizures.

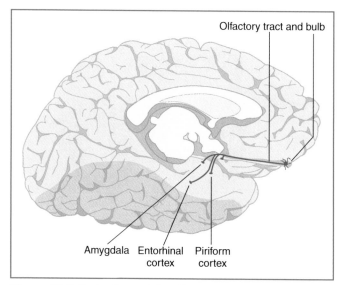

Figure 13-9. Projections of the olfactory tract to the ipsilateral cerebral hemisphere. Piriform cortex is three-layered, one of the few non-neocortical areas of cerebral cortex. It is continuous with neocortex through intervening transitional areas.

particular glomeruli plays an important role in discriminating odorants.

Mitral cell axons travel posteriorly through the olfactory tract and reach the base of the brain, where some terminate; those remaining curve laterally as the lateral olfactory tract (Fig. 13-9). Each olfactory bulb develops as a direct outgrowth of a cerebral hemisphere, and as a result axons of the olfactory tract bypass the thalamus and terminate directly in primary olfactory cortex (piriform cortex), the amygdala, and anterior parahippocampal cortex (entorhinal cortex) on the ipsilateral side.

Pheromones

Animals use not just sounds and visual displays to communicate with each other but also chemicals. Sometimes the chemical signals and the responses to them are obvious, as in marking territory, but others are more subtle. Pheromones are chemicals that are released by animals and produce behavioral changes in others of the same species, typically by changes in motivation rather than a particular perception of an odorant. Pheromonal communication in most mammals is largely mediated by a separate set of chemoreceptors in the vomeronasal organ, a small tubular structure in the nasal

septum, but its importance varies widely among species. Rodents, for example, have a hundred or more types of vomeronasal receptors, whereas canines have only a few. The vomeronasal organ of adult humans appears to be mostly vestigial, with few or no functional receptors. Nevertheless, some level of pheromonal communication persists in humans, apparently mediated by the olfactory system. The most clearly demonstrated example is the synchronization of the menstrual cycles of women living together, which is based on variations in axillary secretions having no apparent odor, but a variety of other pheromonal effects on mood or behavior have been suggested.

●●● FLAVOR

Neurons in primary gustatory cortex faithfully record the properties of intraoral contents, with individual cells responding to various combinations of tastants, temperatures, and textures. Their responses change little with changes in appetite. However, gustatory cortex projects to a part of orbital cortex that serves as association cortex for the chemical senses, analogous to the unimodal association areas of other senses. The same orbital area receives converging inputs (Fig. 13-10) not just from gustatory cortex, but also from olfactory cortex, from visual and somatosensory areas, and from limbic structures such as the amygdala. Neurons here respond to multiple attributes of foods, and their responsiveness is modulated in a way that reflects how hungry an animal is and thus how good a particular food is likely to taste.

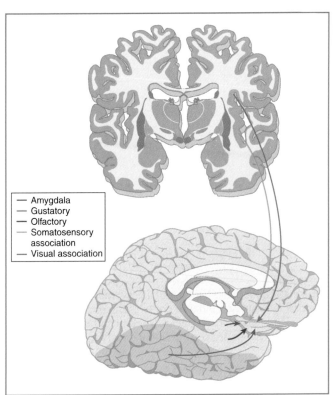

Amygdala
Gustatory
Olfactory
Somatosensory
association
Visual association

Figure 13-10. Convergence in orbital cortex of information from multiple sources, in a pattern that supports the perception and appreciation of flavor.

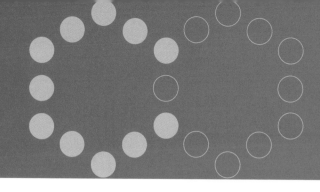

Motor Neurons and Motor Units

14

Humans somehow manage to do all sorts of complicated things by having the CNS direct the patterns of contraction of a few hundred muscles, using just a million or so neurons (lower motor neurons) with axons that leave the CNS and terminate on skeletal muscle fibers (Fig. 14-1). Some of these movements, such as reflexes, are mostly automatic; others vary widely and may be uniquely suited for particular situations. Movements that are more automatic are implemented by instructions to lower motor neurons from spinal cord or brainstem circuitry, whereas less automatic movements require input from the cerebral cortex, acting in collaboration with the basal ganglia and cerebellum. However, there is a lot of overlap; higher centers tap into spinal cord and brainstem circuitry as appropriate, instead of reinventing the wheel for every movement.

●●●● SKELETAL MUSCLE

The basic force-producing unit of skeletal muscle is an individual muscle fiber—an elongated, multinucleated cell packed full of contractile myofibrils. The surface membrane of muscle fibers is excitable, and depolarization to threshold causes an action potential that spreads over the surface of the fiber and into its interior, causing a release of Ca^{++} from intracellular stores. The transient increase in Ca^{++} concentration (until

the sarcoplasmic reticulum takes it back up) activates the contractile machinery of the myofibrils, and a twitch of the muscle fiber results.

Neuromuscular Transmission

All vertebrate lower motor neurons make only excitatory connections with their skeletal muscle targets at synapse-like neuromuscular junctions (Fig. 14-2), where they release acetylcholine onto nicotinic receptors of postjunctional muscle fibers (as opposed to invertebrates, which have both excitatory and inhibitory lower motor neurons). Each adult skeletal muscle fiber has a single neuromuscular junction, but each one contains many release sites. The result is that a single action potential in a lower motor neuron causes substantial acetylcholine release and an excitatory postsynaptic potential (EPSP) in the postjunctional muscle fiber that is large enough to drive it past threshold. This in turn elicits a single muscle action potential and a twitch of the fiber. As the lower motor neuron's

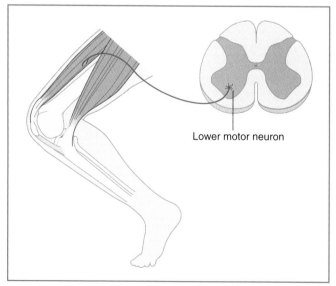

Figure 14-1. Lower motor neurons extend from the anterior horn of the spinal cord (or from cranial nerve motor nuclei) directly to skeletal muscle.

GENETICS & PHYSIOLOGY

Muscular Dystrophy

Duchenne's muscular dystrophy is a relatively common X-linked disorder caused by lack of dystrophin, a protein that links the actin filaments inside muscle fibers to a complex of membrane proteins and, through them, to the extracellular matrix. Muscle fibers, like nerve fibers, have a mechanical stability problem, and in the absence of dystrophin contraction can result in tears in the cell membrane, Ca^{++} entry, and cell death.

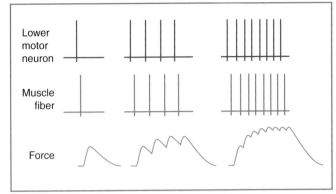

Figure 14-3. Each action potential in the axon of a lower motor neuron (top traces) results in an action potential in the muscle fiber it innervates (middle traces), slightly delayed because of the time taken by neuromuscular transmission. Each muscle fiber action potential causes a twitch (lower traces), and successive twitches summate.

PHARMACOLOGY

Paralyzing Prey

Curare, an alkaloid preparation long used by native South Americans as an arrow-tip poison, works by binding to nicotinic acetylcholine receptors and preventing skeletal muscle contraction. Synthetic versions are sometimes used in conjunction with anesthesia to prevent muscle contraction during surgery. (The curare has no effect on the CNS because alkaloids like this do not cross the blood-brain barrier.)

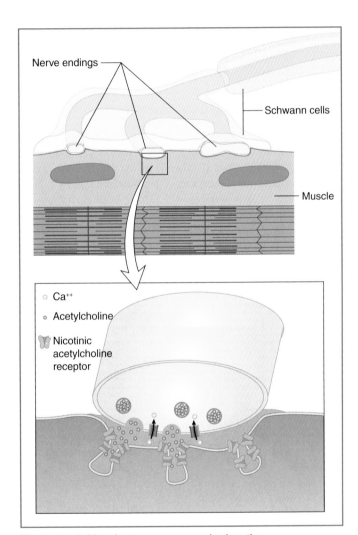

Figure 14-2. Vertebrate neuromuscular junction.

firing rate increases, so does the twitch frequency and the force generated by the muscle fiber (Fig. 14-3) because successive twitches can sum with each other in a process of temporal summation much like that seen in postsynaptic membranes. Thus, the only way to control the level of contraction of a skeletal muscle, at least on a moment-to-moment basis, is to control the firing rate of the lower motor neurons that

provide this input. Hence, the sum total of all the excitatory and inhibitory inputs to a given lower motor neuron at any given moment will determine the level of contraction of any muscle fibers it innervates.

Muscle Fiber Types

Skeletal muscle fibers come in three different functional types (Fig. 14-4). Some are slow-twitch fibers (often called type S) that, as the name implies, produce twitches with slow rise and fall times. The twitches are also small, so they cannot produce much force, but these fibers contain many mitochondria, use aerobic metabolism, and can maintain this low level of force for a long time without fatiguing. Some fast-twitch fibers produce large, brief twitches but contain few mitochondria and fatigue quickly (type FF, for *fast fatigable*). The third type is intermediate, producing fast but medium-sized twitches. They have some aerobic capacity and fatigue at an intermediate rate (type FR, for *fast fatigue-resistant*). Different species (and different individuals) have different proportions of these fiber types: birds that fly long distances, for example, have a high proportion of type S fibers, resulting in more "dark meat."

HISTOLOGY

Distinguishing Muscle Fiber Types

Muscles are mosaics of intermingled fiber types that can be distinguished from one another by means of stains for glycogen, glycolytic enzymes, oxidative enzymes, and other proteins. Different types of neuromuscular disorders cause distinctive changes in numbers, sizes, and appearances of different fiber types, so the use of such staining techniques on muscle biopsy specimens is an important diagnostic tool.

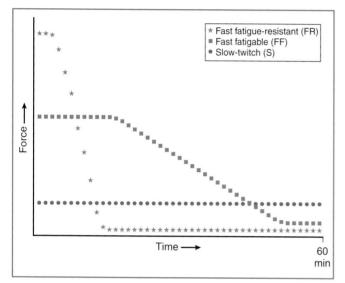

Figure 14-4. Size of the twitches produced by S, FR, and FF muscle fibers in response to successive stimuli every 10 seconds or so (too infrequently for there to be any summation).

TABLE 14-1. Spinal Cord Segments Innervating Major Muscles of Upper and Lower Extremities*

Muscle	Spinal Cord Segment
Deltoid	C5
Biceps	C6
Triceps	C7
Wrist flexors and extensors	C6, C7
Finger flexors and extensors	C7, C8
Quadriceps	L3, L4
Hamstrings	S1
Gastrocnemius	S1

*Only the segments with the largest number of motor neurons are indicated. Most pools of motor neurons extend over two to three segments, e.g., those for the triceps from C6 to C8 and those for the hamstrings from L5 to S2.

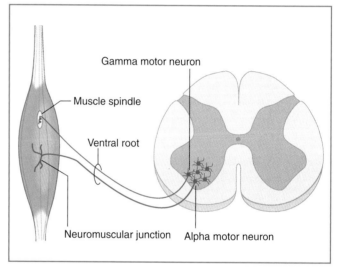

Figure 14-5. Pools of intermingled alpha and gamma motor neurons innervate individual skeletal muscles.

●●● LOWER MOTOR NEURONS

Spinal cord lower motor neurons (also called alpha motor neurons because of the Aα size of their axons) live in cigar-shaped clusters in the anterior horn. Each cluster contains the interspersed alpha and gamma motor neurons for one muscle, and extends through one to three spinal cord segments (Table 14-1), with gamma motor neurons for the same muscle interspersed among them (Fig. 14-5). There is a somatotopic arrangement of these clusters, with motor neurons for distal muscles lateral to those for proximal muscles, and motor neurons for flexors dorsal to those for extensors. The corresponding neurons for muscles innervated by cranial nerves form nuclei that extend longitudinally through a short length of the brainstem (Fig. 14-6 and Table 14-2).

Motor Units

Although each muscle fiber bears a single neuromuscular junction, each lower motor neuron has a number of terminal branches that collectively innervate multiple muscle fibers scattered through a large area of one muscle. The combination of a single lower motor neuron and all the muscle fibers it innervates is called a motor unit (Fig. 14-7) because this is the basic functional output unit of the motor control system. The sizes of motor units (i.e., the number of muscle fibers they contain) vary within a muscle, but the average size corresponds to the degree of precision with which a given muscle can be controlled. For example, the average size of the motor units in a large antigravity muscle is around 1000 fibers and that of the motor units in extraocular muscles is more like 10 fibers.

All muscle fibers in a given motor unit are of the same type, so there are three different types of motor unit: S, FR, and FF. In addition, the size of a lower motor neuron cell body is correlated with the kind of muscle fiber it innervates—the lower motor neurons of S units are the smallest and those of FF units the largest. This leads to a size principle governing the order in which motor units are recruited as a muscle

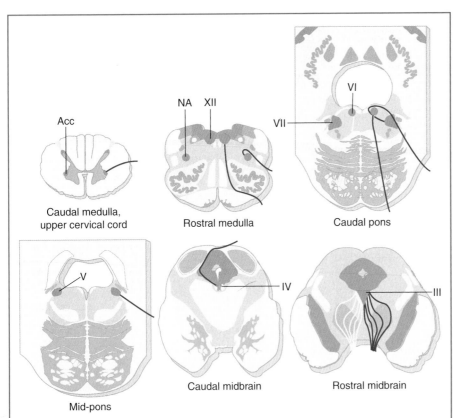

Figure 14-6. Locations of lower motor neurons with axons that travel through cranial nerves. Some of these axons take peculiar courses on their way out of the brainstem. Those for muscles of the larynx, pharynx, and face head for the fourth ventricle before turning around and exiting. This is especially prominent for the facial nerve, whose fibers travel through an internal genu in the floor of the ventricle. Trochlear fibers decussate at the pons-midbrain junction (actually a little caudal to the level shown), providing a rare example of lower motor neurons with axons that cross the midline before leaving the CNS. Acc, accessory nucleus; NA, nucleus ambiguus.

TABLE 14-2. Motor Neurons with Axons in Cranial Nerves

Muscle	Cell Bodies	Cranial Nerve
Inferior rectus	Rostral midbrain (oculomotor nucleus*)	III
Inferior oblique		
Medial rectus		
Superior rectus		
Levator palpebrae superioris		
Superior oblique	Caudal midbrain (trochlear nucleus)	IV
Mastication	Midpons (trigeminal motor nucleus)	V
Facial expression	Caudal pons (facial motor nucleus)	VII
Stapedius		
Larynx, pharynx	Rostral medulla (nucleus ambiguus)	X†
Tongue	Rostral medulla (hypoglossal nucleus)	XII
Sternocleido-mastoid	C1 to C5 (accessory nucleus)	XI
Trapezius		

*Also includes preganglionic parasympathetic neurons for the pupillary sphincter and ciliary muscle.
†Minor contribution via IX.

contracts more and more strongly (Fig. 14-8). A given amount of synaptic current will produce a larger voltage change in a small neuron than in a large neuron (because, all other things being equal, membrane resistance is inversely proportional to membrane area). So as synaptic drive to the pool of lower motor neurons for a muscle increases, S units are brought to threshold first. As they fire faster, FR units begin to reach threshold, followed by FF units. This corresponds to the way humans use muscles: small amounts of force can be produced for long periods (e.g., standing) and maximal force only briefly (e.g., jumping). It also makes it easier to have the force of a muscle contraction increase smoothly with increasing effort, because the increment provided by adding another unit is roughly proportional to the current force (e.g., increasing a weak contraction by 5% takes only a small amount of force, such as that provided by adding S units, whereas increasing a near-maximal contraction by 5% takes the greater force provided by adding FF units).

Inputs to Lower Motor Neurons

Each muscle receives its inputs from a single pool of lower motor neurons but is used in multiple kinds of movement. The same arm muscles, for example, are called into play in movements that range from automatic and stereotyped (e.g., reflexes) to those uniquely suited to the careful manipulation of a particular object. Corresponding to these multiple uses, each lower motor neuron receives thousands of inputs from multiple sources (see Fig. 2-25).

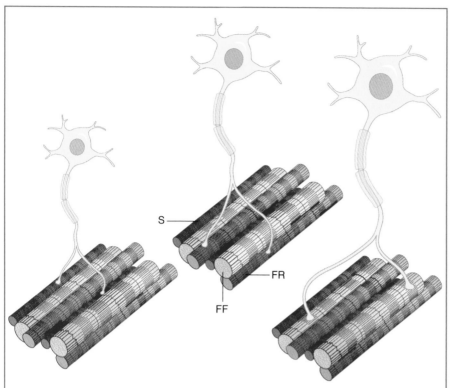

Figure 14-7. Basic organization of motor units.

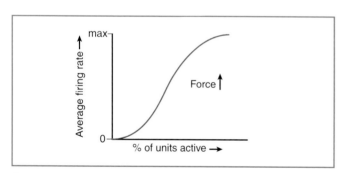

A

Figure 14-8. Orderly recruitment of motor units as the amount of force generated by a muscle increases. **A**, Within a given population of motor units, progressively more units become active and their firing rate increases. **B**, As units with slow-twitch fibers approach their maximum force production, units with fast fatigue-resistant fibers become active, followed by units with fast fatigable fibers.

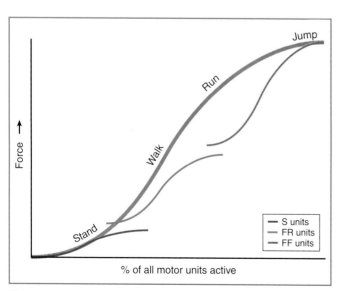

B

Reflexes

Reflexes are involuntary, more or less stereotyped, typically graded responses to particular sensory stimuli. Since they involve sensory inputs and motor outputs, every reflex using CNS circuitry must involve at a minimum a primary afferent neuron and a lower motor neuron. Most are more complex than this, but one—the stretch or deep tendon reflex (see Figs. 2-23 to 2-25) that is routinely tested in the neurologic examination—is actually that simple. Muscle spindle Ia afferents, stimulated by tapping a tendon and thereby briefly stretching the attached muscle, synapse directly on the motor neurons that innervate that muscle.

All other reflexes involve at least one interneuron. For example, the other major type of muscle afferent (i.e., Ib fibers from Golgi tendon organs) participates in reflexes that involve an inhibitory or excitatory interneuron. Hence, increasing the tension in a tendon, as in contracting a muscle against resistance, causes reflex inhibition or excitation of the motor neurons supplying that muscle. It was once thought that the inhibitory component might be a protective reflex designed to prevent excessive muscle contraction, but Golgi tendon organs and their reflexes actually play a more subtle role in fine motor control. For example, we have no trouble automatically adjusting the amount of force applied when grasping objects as diverse as rocks and raw eggs, and Golgi tendon organs provide the information about force required for these adjustments.

A third spinal reflex, which everyone has experienced, is the one that quickly and automatically withdraws a body part from something painful. This flexor or withdrawal reflex typically involves flexion of an entire limb, so multiple muscles and multiple spinal levels must participate (see Fig. 9-4).

Although reflexes are often thought of as fixed and invariable responses to a given stimulus, they are in fact modified on a moment-to-moment basis by the CNS to fit the circumstances. Stretch reflexes, for example, are automatically suppressed when they might get in the way (e.g., quadriceps stretch reflexes when someone sits down). Withdrawal reflexes of the lower extremity are suppressed or facilitated depending on which phase of the step cycle someone is in when a painful stimulus arrives.

Pattern Generators

The interneurons in the circuitry of most reflexes also provide one easy way to produce parts of more complex movements. Networks of these and other interneurons in the spinal cord or brainstem of vertebrates form the basic neural machinery for producing typically rhythmic movements such as walking, breathing, and chewing, as well as some nonrhythmic movements such as parts of facial expressions. The spinal cord of a lamprey, for example, can produce rhythmic bursts of ventral root action potentials appropriate for swimming movements, even when completely removed from the lamprey. Higher centers simply initiate or modify activity in these central pattern generators (or motor programs). In the case of walking, for example, descending pathways from the brainstem can initiate activity in the spinal pattern generator and control

its rate, causing gait to progress from walking to running to galloping. Depending on the species, however, descending pathways from the cortex to the brainstem or spinal cord are typically required to navigate around obstacles. Sensory inputs, while not necessary for the basic movements, are required to modify the movements to fit the environment (e.g., adjust to uneven surfaces).

The extent to which central pattern generators control rhythmic movements declines as species come to depend more and more on descending projections from the cortex. Quadriplegic cats can be induced to walk on a treadmill under appropriate experimental conditions, but this is much more difficult with humans. Finding better ways to facilitate this rhythmic activity may offer new treatment modalities for human spinal cord injury patients.

Upper Motor Neurons

Neurons that project either directly to lower motor neurons, or to the interneurons that influence lower motor neurons, are collectively referred to as upper motor neurons. Upper motor neurons have cell bodies in the brainstem and cerebral cortex, and they give rise to descending pathways that traverse the brainstem and spinal cord, as discussed later in this chapter.

Lower Motor Neuron Damage

The axons of lower motor neurons provide the only route through which the CNS can contact skeletal muscles (for this reason, they are sometimes called the final common pathway), so their destruction leads to a kind of weakness in which no contraction of a muscle is possible—not in voluntary movement or even in reflexes. As a result, the resting level of contraction of the muscle—its tone—is decreased or abolished, and the muscle is flaccid. In addition, chemical signaling normally occurring between the muscle and its lower motor neurons (see Chapter 20) is disrupted, and in response the muscle atrophies. Motor units begin to contract spontaneously, especially in early stages following damage (causing fasciculations apparent as rippling on the surface). Muscle fibers upregulate their production of acetylcholine receptors, become supersensitive, and contract in response to small amounts of stray acetylcholine (causing fibrillations, spontaneous contractions of individual muscle fibers that can be detected electrophysiologically).

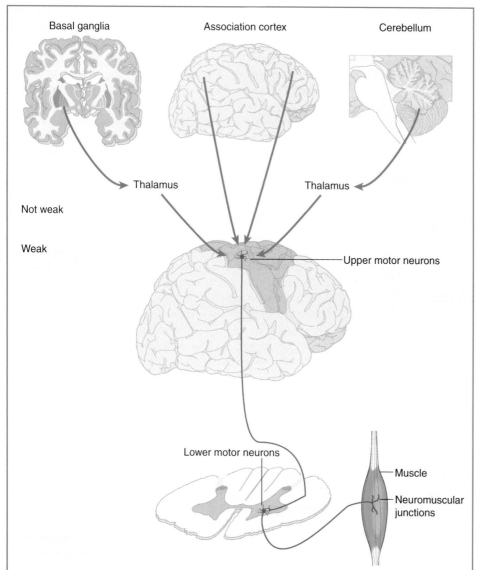

Figure 14-9. Areas of the nervous system prominently involved in the control of movement. Damage to any of these structures or areas can cause abnormalities of movement, but weakness is a prominent component of the syndrome only if structures in the lower part of the figure (or muscle itself) are damaged.

●●● UPPER MOTOR NEURONS

Voluntary movement requires more than just sending a message from primary motor cortex to pools of lower motor neurons. The process begins with a more or less conscious purpose for the movement, implying inputs from various (mostly frontal) areas of association cortex to motor cortex, followed by general planning of the movement and designing of its details. The planning and design are a collaborative function of the basal ganglia, cerebellum, and various cortical areas. Following initiation of a movement, the cerebellum plays a critical role in providing timing signals that ensure its accuracy. Processes that damage association cortex, the basal ganglia, or the cerebellum cause a variety of disorders, as described in Chapters 15, 16, and 19, in which movement is abnormal but weakness is not a prominent component (Fig. 14-9).

Descending Pathways

Upper motor neurons have their cell bodies in several places and axons that descend through different tracts (Fig. 14-10). The corticospinal tract is the most prominent in humans. Axons originating in several cortical areas (see Motor Cortex, below) descend through the posterior limb of the internal capsule, cerebral peduncle, basal pons, and medullary pyramids. At the spinomedullary junction, 85% to 90% of them cross the midline in the pyramidal decussation to form the lateral corticospinal tract, the principal tract mediating voluntary movement. (The minority of fibers that do not cross either continue into the ipsilateral lateral corticospinal tract or travel through the anterior funiculus as the less important anterior corticospinal tract.) Comparable upper motor neurons for cranial nerve motor nuclei have axons that travel through the corticobulbar tract (bulb is an old, seldom-used term for

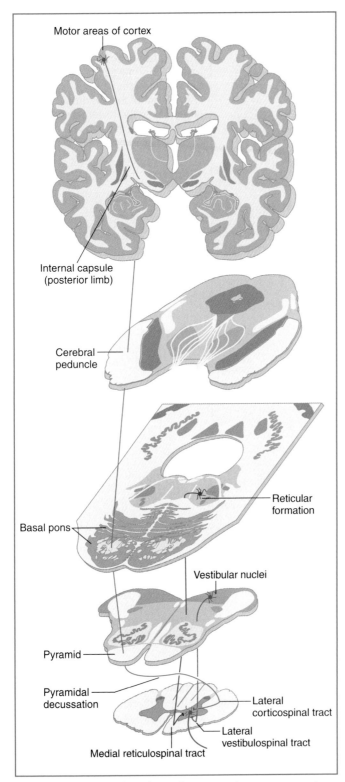

Figure 14-10. Major locations of upper motor neurons and their descending tracts in humans. There are actually multiple reticulospinal and vestibulospinal tracts; a major example of each is shown. There are also smaller projections (not shown) to motor neurons from sites such as the superior colliculus and red nucleus.

brainstem). Corticobulbar fibers accompany the corticospinal tract and peel off near the level of the nucleus they innervate (Fig. 14-11). Unlike the corticospinal tract, however, the corticobulbar fibers from each hemisphere are mostly distributed bilaterally. This corresponds nicely to the way in which the muscles innervated by cranial nerves are typically used: in chewing, swallowing, laughing, and other such activities we use muscles on both sides of the head simultaneously. The major exception is facial muscles below the level of the eye, which we use in a variety of asymmetric facial expressions. The lower motor neurons for these muscles receive a preponderance of crossed corticobulbar fibers and, as a result, damage to motor cortex, the internal capsule, or the cerebral peduncle on one side causes contralateral lower facial weakness. This is important clinically in diagnosing the basis of facial weakness, because damage to the facial nerve or facial motor nucleus causes weakness of the *entire* ipsilateral side of the face.

Reticulospinal tracts from the brainstem reticular formation are important alternatives to the corticospinal tract. The lateral vestibulospinal tract projects to all spinal levels and is involved in making postural adjustments in response to vestibular stimulation. The medial vestibulospinal tract projects to cervical levels and helps to keep your head stable as you move around. The tectospinal tract[1] projects from the superior colliculus to the cervical cord and plays a role in orienting to visual or auditory stimuli off in the periphery, but its importance in humans is probably limited. Finally, the rubrospinal tract (from the red nucleus) is an important alternative to the corticospinal tract in most mammals for the control of distal muscles. However, it too appears to be minor in humans.

Motor Cortex

Only about a third of the axons in the corticospinal tract originate in the primary motor cortex (or M1), a tapering strip in the precentral gyrus (Fig. 14-12). Another third or so come from premotor cortex, anterior to M1 on the lateral surface of the brain, and the supplementary motor area (SMA), anterior to M1 on the medial surface. Different parts of the body are represented systematically in each of these motor areas in one or more somatotopic maps; the map in M1 is largely parallel to that in somatosensory cortex (see Fig. 9-5), with the head represented near the lateral sulcus and the foot near the longitudinal fissure. The final third come from initially surprising places like somatosensory cortex and may not play much of a role in directing movement; somatosensory projections, for example, terminate in the posterior horn and are probably involved mostly in regulating the access of somatosensory information to ascending pathways. Corticospinal axons from motor areas, in contrast, affect lower motor neurons either directly or indirectly. Some synapse on interneurons (e.g., those in central pattern generators) that in turn affect lower motor neurons; others terminate directly on lower motor neurons themselves. The direct

[1]The superior and inferior colliculi together form the tectum ("roof") of the midbrain.

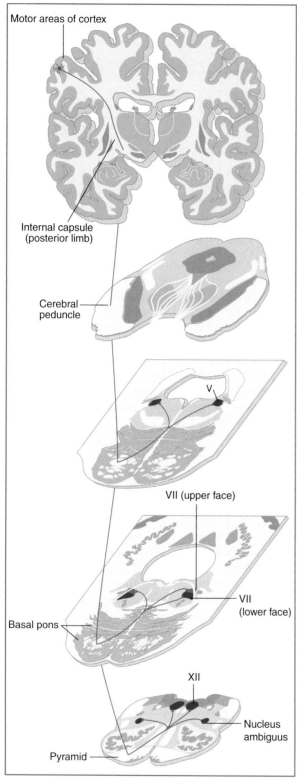

Figure 14-11. Corticobulbar tract. Corticobulbar inputs to all motor neurons except those for the lower face are shown as bilaterally symmetric, but there is actually considerable variability. Most individuals, for example, have more crossed than uncrossed projections to the trigeminal and hypoglossal nuclei, so after unilateral damage there is often mild, transient weakness of contralateral muscles of the jaw and tongue. There are no direct corticobulbar inputs to the oculomotor, trochlear, and abducens nuclei (see Chapter 17).

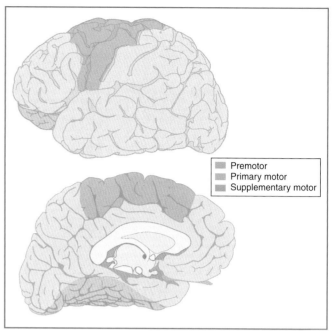

Figure 14-12. Principal neocortical areas containing upper motor neurons and relatively directly involved in the control of movement.

projections mostly reach lower motor neurons for muscles that can be controlled with precision and relative independence, such as the lower motor neurons for finger muscles in many primates, and are less common in other species. Axons descending from motor cortical areas also reach the reticular formation and vestibular nuclei, which do much of the background preparatory work that accompanies voluntary movement. Reaching out to smack a handball, for example, requires more than just contracting arm muscles because the arm movement (or virtually any other movement) changes the center of gravity, which in turn necessitates postural adjustments. These postural adjustments are effected through the reticulospinal and vestibulospinal tracts under orders from the corticospinal tract, and they actually begin before the arm movement.

CLINICAL MEDICINE

Manifestations of Somatotopic Maps

Seizures that begin in a localized part of the precentral gyrus may include muscle contractions that start in a restricted contralateral part of the body and then spread in a pattern that corresponds to the motor homunculus, e.g., start in the face and then move into the hand, arm, and finally the leg. They most commonly start in a hand or the face, because of the large cortical area devoted to these body parts. First described by the British neurologist John Hughlings Jackson in the mid-19th century, these are still known as jacksonian seizures.

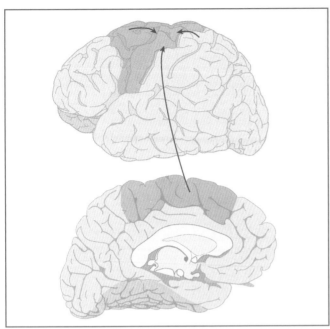

Figure 14-13. Major cortical inputs to primary motor cortex.

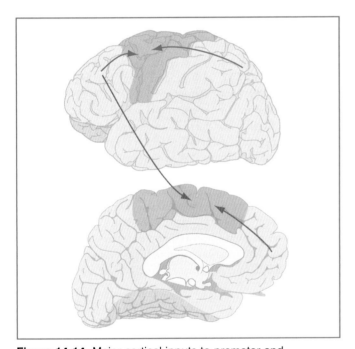

Figure 14-14. Major cortical inputs to premotor and supplementary motor cortex.

Although all three motor cortical areas project to the spinal cord (and brainstem), each has a different function. One indication of this is that each has a different pattern of connections. The major inputs to M1 come from the other two motor areas and from somatosensory cortex (Fig. 14-13), as though it were the last stop on the way down to lower motor neurons. The premotor and supplementary motor areas collect inputs from prefrontal cortex and then project to M1 (Fig. 14-14), as if they are somehow involved in formu-

TABLE 14-3. Effects of Upper Motor Neuron (UMN) and Lower Motor Neuron (LMN) Damage

Function Affected	UMN Damage	LMN Damage
Strength	Decreased	Decreased
Stretch reflexes	Increased	Decreased
Muscle tone	Increased	Decreased
Atrophy	Moderate	Severe
Other signs	Pathologic reflexes (e.g., Babinski sign) Clonus*	Fasciculations Fibrillations

*Rhythmic, alternating contraction of flexors and extensors at a joint in response to maintained stretch of a muscle. Typically elicited by dorsiflexing the foot.

lating the plan for movements. Premotor cortex also receives inputs from the parietal lobe and is thought to be important for movements related to sensory inputs (e.g., getting the hand to conform to the shape of an object being picked up). The lack of parietal input to the supplementary motor area is consistent with its being more involved in self-generated movements; activity in SMA increases even if movements are mentally rehearsed but not actually performed.

Upper Motor Neuron Damage

The effects of upper motor neuron damage depend on where the damage occurs. In the case of something like a middle cerebral artery occlusion that damages widespread cortical areas or the posterior limb of the internal capsule, the projections from cerebral cortex to the basal ganglia, the brainstem (reticular formation, etc.), and the spinal cord are all disrupted. Weakness results, typically more pronounced in the distal muscles whose lower motor neurons depend more on corticospinal input. However, the weakness is part of a syndrome very different from that following lower motor neuron damage (Table 14-3) because it is accompanied by spasticity and the unmasking of reflexes like the Babinski sign. Spasticity refers to a velocity-dependent increased resistance to stretch, typically worse in flexors of the upper extremity and extensors of the lower extremity (the antigravity muscles in primates like humans). This shows up as hyperactive stretch reflexes (hyperreflexia) and an increased resistance to passive stretch (usually described as increased muscle tone). If a spastic limb is forcibly flexed or extended, the increased resistance suddenly gives way in a clasp-knife response (like a penknife or clasp-knife snapping shut or open). The Babinski sign is dorsiflexion of the big toe and fanning of the others in response to something scratching the sole of the foot. It is one of several spinal cord and brainstem reflexes that are present at birth but are gradually suppressed as corticospinal and corticobulbar axons acquire myelin sheaths and become functional. These reflex connections persist, however, and upper motor neuron damage allows them to emerge again.

PATHOLOGY & CLINICAL MEDICINE

Damage to Both Upper and Lower Motor Neurons

Amyotrophic lateral sclerosis (ALS) is a devastating degenerative disease that selectively attacks both upper and lower motor neurons. Affected individuals have variable combinations of atrophy and fasciculations (from lower motor neuron loss), increased tone and reflexes (from upper motor neuron loss), and weakness (from both). The name comes from the combined muscle atrophy ("amyotrophic") and degeneration of the lateral corticospinal tract ("lateral sclerosis").

PHARMACOLOGY

Treatment of Spasticity

The sensitivity of stretch reflexes is controlled in part by spinal interneurons that make inhibitory synapses on the central terminals of stretch receptors, reducing the amount of glutamate they release onto motor neurons. Baclofen is a γ-aminobutyric acid (GABA) agonist that activates the metabotropic receptors at these synapses, effectively reducing the spasticity that accompanies disorders such as amyotrophic lateral sclerosis.

A much less common site of upper motor neuron damage is the medullary pyramids, and the difference in symptoms in such a case is instructive. Here the projections from cortex to basal ganglia and brainstem are spared, so some upper motor neurons and their connections are still functional (e.g., cortex → reticular formation → spinal cord). As a result, there is still a Babinski sign but less weakness and less spasticity. The most pronounced and lasting effect is on functions normally subserved by direct projections from motor cortex to lower motor neurons—precise movements, especially of the fingers.

Basal Ganglia

CONTENTS

The basal ganglia and cerebellum have major effects on movement production, produced not by projecting to lower motor neurons but rather by interacting with the cerebral cortex (Fig. 15-1; also see Fig. 16-1). As a result, damage to the basal ganglia or cerebellum results in distinctive movement disorders in which weakness is not a prominent component (see Fig. 14-9). Although connections with motor areas of the cerebral cortex underlie the best-known functions of the basal ganglia and cerebellum, both also interact with more widespread cortical areas and play a role in cognition and emotions.

●●● COMPONENTS OF THE BASAL GANGLIA

The basal ganglia comprise a series of interconnected nuclei in the cerebral hemisphere, diencephalon, and brainstem (Fig. 15-2). The principal components in the cerebral hemisphere are the striatum and globus pallidus. The striatum originates from a single mass of cells in the wall of the embryonic telencephalon and, as described in the next section, has similar connections throughout its extent. Later in development, however, the internal capsule grows through this mass, subdividing it into the caudate nucleus, putamen, and nucleus accumbens. The putamen is centrally located, underlying most of the insula. The caudate nucleus has an enlarged head that forms the lateral wall of the anterior horn of the lateral ventricle, continuing into a body that borders the body of ventricle, and curving into a slender tail in the inferior horn. A vestige of the common origin of the parts of the striatum is provided by nucleus accumbens, which is an anterior area of continuity between the putamen and the head of the caudate nucleus. Another sign of this common origin can be seen as

strands of gray matter that cross the internal capsule from the caudate nucleus to the putamen, often giving the striatum a striped appearance (hence its name). The globus pallidus has two subdivisions, an external segment adjacent to the putamen and an internal segment adjoining the internal capsule. Because the putamen and globus pallidus together form a wedge-shaped mass of gray matter, they are often referred to together as the lenticular nucleus (even though their connections are quite different). The list is completed by the diencephalic subthalamic nucleus and the substantia nigra, adjacent to the cerebral peduncle in the rostral midbrain.

Basal Ganglia Disorders

The best-known basal ganglia disorders are characterized by combinations of positive and negative signs—positive signs being involuntary muscle contractions in various patterns and negative signs being a paucity of muscle contraction. Parkinson's disease is the classic example. Positive signs include a resting tremor, especially pronounced in the hands, and a general increase in tone in all muscles, referred to as rigidity. Negative signs include slow movements (bradykinesia)

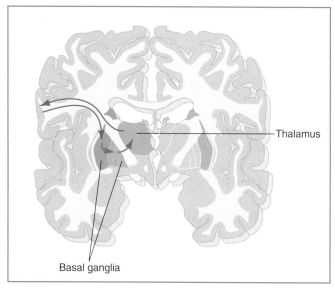

Figure 15-1. General pattern of connections of the basal ganglia. Throughout this chapter, connections are color-coded, with green indicating excitation and red indicating inhibition.

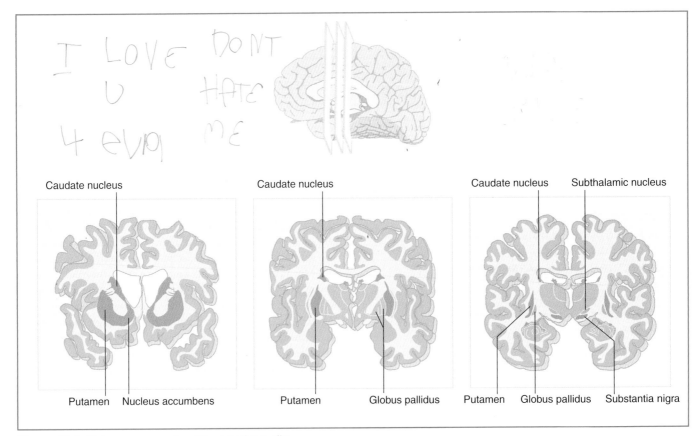

Figure 15-2. Major components of the basal ganglia.

and few movements (hypokinesia or akinesia). Stretch reflexes, however, are relatively normal, and the slow or limited movements, once begun, are of relatively normal strength. This is markedly different from the spasticity of upper motor neuron syndromes, in which the increased tone is concentrated in certain muscles, reflexes are increased, and the patient is weak. In addition, the increased tone of spasticity can be overcome in the clasp-knife response, which is not seen in Parkinson's; rather, rigidity often "gives" in little steps (cogwheeling) during movement of a rigid limb. Other basal ganglia disorders can be accompanied by different kinds of involuntary movements that fall into three general categories: rapid movements called chorea; slow, writhing movements called athetosis; and flailing movements of entire limbs, called ballism. In some disorders, tone is unchanged or decreased; in others, it is increased even more than in Parkinson's disease and can manifest itself as dystonia, in which body parts are twisted into fixed positions.

●●● CONNECTIONS OF THE BASAL GANGLIA

The basal ganglia have few projections downstream to the brainstem and spinal cord (i.e., they do not contain upper motor neurons). Instead, they affect movement and other functions by modifying the output from the cerebral cortex. The input portion of the basal ganglia is the striatum (caudate nucleus + putamen + nucleus accumbens), and the internal

segment of the globus pallidus (GPi) serves as the output portion. All axons leaving the striatum and the globus pallidus use γ-aminobutyric acid (GABA) as a neurotransmitter and make inhibitory synapses on their targets. Because neurons in GPi inhibit neurons in the thalamus, the net balance of excitatory and inhibitory inputs to each neuron in GPi determines the effect of the basal ganglia on cortical output (Fig. 15-3). This is the basis of a plausible framework for understanding the effects of the basal ganglia, as well as the positive and negative signs of basal ganglia disorders—diminished output from GPi disinhibits thalamic neurons and enhances thalamocortical outputs (i.e., results in positive signs), and increased output suppresses thalamocortical outputs (i.e., results in negative signs).

The major direct circuit through the basal ganglia (Fig. 15-4) involves a loop that starts in large areas of the cerebral cortex, projects to the striatum, and then projects to GPi. Output from GPi travels across or around the internal capsule and reaches the thalamus, which finally projects back to the cerebral cortex. Since all these connections are primarily uncrossed, any movement problem resulting from unilateral basal ganglia damage will appear in the contralateral side of the body. Corticostriatal projections are excitatory (glutamate), so increased input in this circuit causes inhibition of GPi neurons, thus facilitating excitatory thalamocortical transmission (glutamate again). Because there is a systematic mapping at each step of the way in this circuit, selectively increasing the

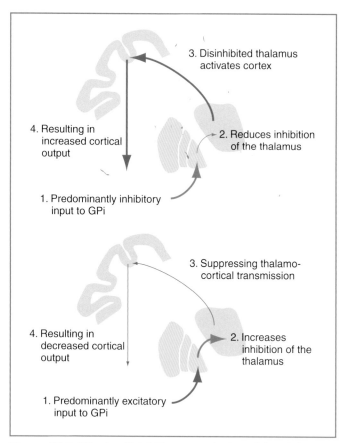

Figure 15-3. Effects of inhibition or excitation of the globus pallidus (internal segment) on cortical output.

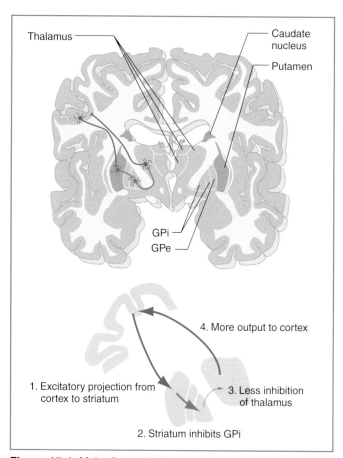

Figure 15-4. Main direct circuit through the basal ganglia. Although cortical projections are only shown reaching the putamen, the other parts of the striatum (caudate nucleus and nucleus accumbens) are connected up in similar circuits originating from different cortical areas (see also Fig. 15-8).

activity of particular striatal neurons can facilitate particular cortical outputs.

Subthalamic Nucleus

One major subset of striatal neurons provides the principal inhibitory input to GPi, and the subthalamic nucleus provides the principal excitatory input. A second major subset of striatal neurons projects to the external segment of the globus pallidus (GPe), which in turn projects to the subthalamic nucleus. The subthalamic nucleus sends excitatory (glutamate) projections to GPi, making it the key link in an indirect circuit through the basal ganglia (Fig. 15-5). The net effect of increased cortical input to this indirect circuit is disinhibition of the subthalamic nucleus. The resulting excitation of GPi in turn suppresses thalamocortical transmission (the opposite effect of activation of the direct circuit). Hence, selective excitation of particular sets of striatal neurons in the direct and indirect circuits could facilitate some cortical outputs and suppress others. Conversely, damaging the subthalamic nucleus might be expected to result in decreased inhibition of the thalamus by GPi and in the emergence of unwanted cortical outputs. Consistent with this, damage to the subthalamic nucleus causes hemiballismus, involuntary flailing movements of the contralateral limbs (Fig. 15-6).

Substantia Nigra

The substantia nigra is like two separate neural structures laminated together. The reticular part, adjacent to the cerebral peduncle, contains GABAergic neurons and is connected up almost exactly like a displaced piece of GPi—inputs from the striatum (direct circuit) and subthalamic nucleus, outputs to the thalamus. (It also has some outputs to the superior colliculus and, as described in Chapter 17, plays a role in eye movements.)

The compact part of the substantia nigra contains the pigmented neurons that got the substantia nigra ("black stuff") its name. These neurons project to the striatum, where they release dopamine and modulate the level of excitability of the striatal neurons in both the direct and indirect circuits. However, the two populations of striatal neurons have different postsynaptic receptors, and dopamine has opposite effects on them (a good example of the concept that the receptors determine the effect of a neurotransmitter). Dopamine binds to D_1 receptors of the striatal neurons in the direct circuit and depolarizes them (facilitating cortical outputs); in contrast, it binds to D_2 receptors of the striatal

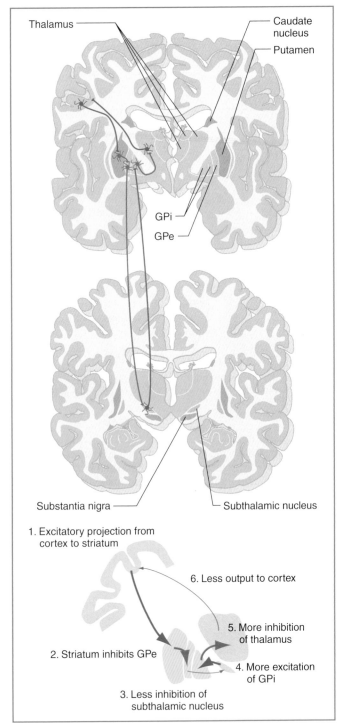

Figure 15-5. Indirect circuit through the basal ganglia. As in the case of the direct circuit, the caudate nucleus and nucleus accumbens participate in parallel circuits, each using its own part of the subthalamic nucleus.

neurons in the indirect circuit and hyperpolarizes them (also facilitating cortical outputs). Degeneration of these pigmented neurons causes Parkinson's disease, in which reduction of dopamine levels does just the reverse (Fig. 15-7)—it decreases activity in the direct pathway and increases activity in the indirect pathway, both of which result in increased inhibition of the thalamus by GPi.

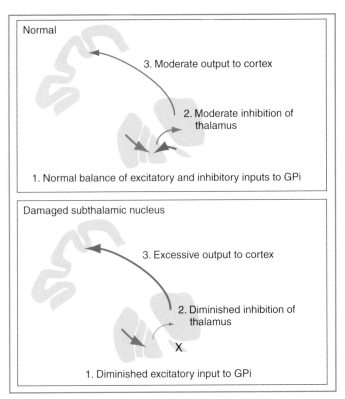

Figure 15-6. Effect of damage to the subthalamic nucleus.

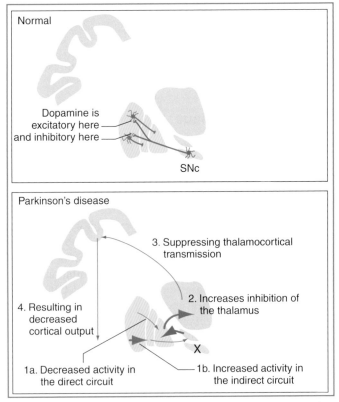

Figure 15-7. Role of the pigmented dopaminergic neurons in the compact part of the substantia nigra (SNc) in basal ganglia function (upper panel), and the effect of loss of these neurons (lower panel).

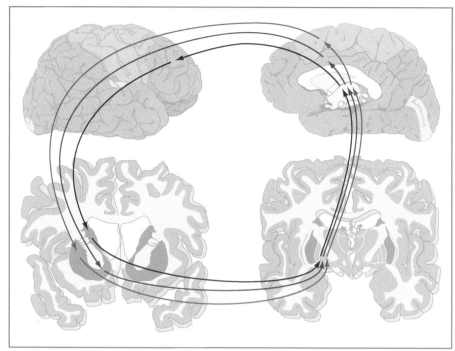

Figure 15-8. Parallel pathways through the basal ganglia. Only the direct circuit is shown, although all three parts of the striatum participate in parallel indirect circuits as well. In addition, to keep things simple, all three parts of the striatum are depicted as projecting to GPi. In fact, the caudate nucleus projects largely to the reticular part of the substantia nigra (posterior to the level of this section) and nucleus accumbens to the ventral pallidum (anterior to the level of this section).

PHARMACOLOGY

Replacing Lost Dopamine

Once it was discovered that Parkinson's disease is associated with loss of dopaminergic neurons, attempts were made to ameliorate the disease by replacing the lost dopamine. This cannot be done directly, because dopamine is a polar molecule that is mostly stopped by the blood-brain barrier. However, its precursor L-dopa (levodopa, dihydroxy-phenylalanine) does cross the barrier and is a mainstay in treating this disease.

CLINICAL MEDICINE

Surgical Treatment of Parkinson's Disease

A number of surgical approaches have been tried in an attempt to suppress some of the excess basal ganglia activity in Parkinson's disease (see Fig. 15-7), including electrolytic lesions in GPi and the subthalamic nucleus. To avoid irreversible damage, more recent techniques have used high-frequency stimulation through implanted electrodes, which paradoxically blocks activity in the stimulated structure. A currently favored target for deep brain stimulation is the subthalamic nucleus.

Parallel Pathways in the Basal Ganglia

There are several parallel subcircuits within the basal ganglia, all using the same generalized circuitry just described (Fig. 15-8). Each starts and ends with some cortical areas and uses its own distinctive portions of the striatum, globus pallidus, subthalamic nucleus, and thalamus. The first is primarily involved in the motor functions traditionally ascribed to the basal ganglia; it preferentially utilizes the putamen as its input portion of the basal ganglia. Somatosensory and motor areas of cortex project to the putamen, which in turn projects to the globus pallidus and then to the thalamus (ventral anterior and ventral lateral nuclei). The thalamic output then projects mainly to the supplementary motor area, which in turn projects to the motor cortex.

A second loop, this one involved in cognition, preferentially uses the caudate nucleus as its input portion of the basal ganglia. Association areas of the cerebral cortex project to the caudate nucleus, which in turn projects to the globus pallidus

(and the reticular part of the substantia nigra) and then to other parts of the thalamus (mostly the dorsomedial nucleus). From the thalamus, projections travel to prefrontal association areas. Bilateral damage restricted to the head of the caudate nucleus, although uncommon, causes not a movement disorder but rather changes in judgment similar to those that follow damage to prefrontal cortex.

There is even a limbic loop through the basal ganglia, again with a parallel organization. The hippocampus, amygdala, and limbic cortex project to nucleus accumbens and nearby ventral parts of the caudate and putamen (all collectively referred to as the ventral striatum). The ventral striatum then projects to a separate part of the globus pallidus just underneath the anterior commissure (the ventral pallidum), which in turn projects to parts of the thalamus (mostly other parts of the dorsomedial nucleus) connected to limbic cortex. These connections give nucleus accumbens a role in initiating behavior that is expected to be rewarding (see Chapter 18).

GENETICS

Huntington's Disease

Huntington's disease, which is inherited in autosomally dominant fashion, results from an expanded cytosine-adenosine-guanine (CAG) repeat on chromosome 4. The longer the repeat, the earlier is the onset of the disease and the worse its severity.

By virtue of these parallel pathways, the basal ganglia become involved in multiple cortical functions, and most basal ganglia disorders can produce nonmotor deficits that can be thought of as positive or negative signs affecting cognition or emotion. Many patients with Parkinson's disease, for example, also become demented or depressed. Huntington's disease is an inherited degenerative disease affecting the striatum. Patients with this disorder develop chorea and in later stages become demented, but often the first signs are changes in mood or personality.

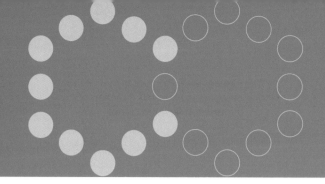

Cerebellum 16

The cerebellum, like the basal ganglia, affects movement but lacks connections with lower motor neurons. Instead, it acts through projections to upper motor neurons, both those in the cerebral cortex and those in the brainstem. The major cerebellar circuit in humans is reminiscent of the general pattern of connections used by the basal ganglia—a loop from cerebral cortex to the cerebellum and back to the cerebral cortex (Fig. 16-1). Cerebellar circuitry differs from that of the basal ganglia, however, in two major ways: unlike most other parts of the CNS, the cerebellum is wired so that one side affects the *ipsilateral* side of the body, and unlike the basal ganglia, the cerebellum makes extensive use of sensory inputs.

●●● BASIC ORGANIZATION OF THE CEREBELLUM

Cerebellar neurons live in two places—a cerebellar cortex extensively folded into transversely oriented folia and a series of three deep cerebellar nuclei on each side buried in the subcortical white matter (Fig. 16-2)—from medial to lateral, the fastigial, interposed, and dentate nuclei. Inputs arrive at the cerebellar cortex, which projects to the deep nuclei. The deep nuclei in turn provide the cerebellar output.

Cerebellar Cortex

Cerebellar cortex has a remarkably uniform, three-layered organization in all parts of the cerebellum (Fig. 16-3). Purkinje cells, one of the most striking types of neuron in the CNS, provide the only output from the cortex. Purkinje cell bodies form a single layer in the middle of the cortex and project their axons to the deep cerebellar nuclei, where they make inhibitory (GABA) synapses. Each also extends an elaborate,

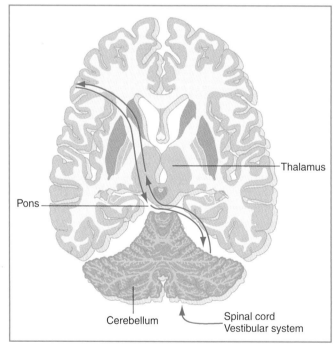

Figure 16-1. General pattern of connections of the cerebellum. Part of the basis for each side of the cerebellum being related to the ipsilateral side of the body is a crossing of the midline by traffic between the cerebellum and cerebrum. Projections from the cerebral cortex to the cerebellum cross on their way out of pontine nuclei (see also Figs. 16-9 and 16-10), and projections from the cerebellum back to the cerebrum cross on their way to the thalamus. Another part of the basis is uncrossed sensory inputs from the spinal cord and brainstem.

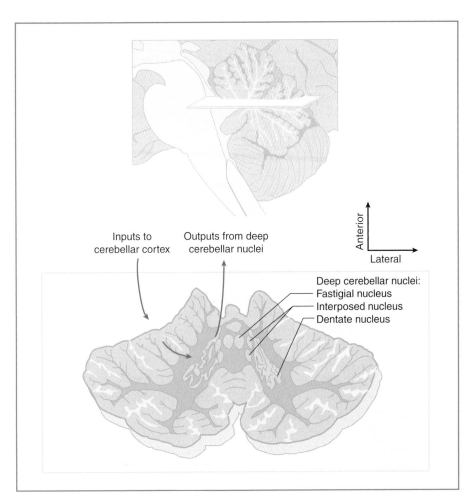

Figure 16-2. General layout of the cerebellum, with the direction of information flow indicated.

Inputs to cerebellar cortex

Outputs from deep cerebellar nuclei

Anterior

Lateral

Deep cerebellar nuclei:
Fastigial nucleus
Interposed nucleus
Dentate nucleus

extensive dendritic tree, flattened out in a plane perpendicular to the long axis of the folium, into the superficial molecular layer. Deep to the Purkinje cell layer is the granule cell layer, traversed by Purkinje cell axons and packed with an enormous number of tiny granule cells—about half of all the neurons in the entire CNS are granule cells! Each granule cell has a thin, unmyelinated axon that ascends to the molecular layer and bifurcates into a parallel fiber that extends 2 to 3 mm in each direction, parallel to the long axis of the folium and perpendicular to the dendritic trees of Purkinje cells in that folium. Along this course, each parallel fiber makes an excitatory synapse on hundreds of Purkinje cells, and each Purkinje cell dendritic tree is so extensive that it receives inputs from tens of thousands of parallel fibers.

Although there are several other neuronal types in cerebellar cortex, its basic circuitry can be described in terms of Purkinje cells, granule cells, and their inputs. Two types of afferent fiber reach the cerebellar cortex, one to Purkinje cells and one to granule cells. A single climbing fiber ascends to each Purkinje cell and divides into multiple branches that climb up its proximal dendrites (hence the name), along the way making thousands of excitatory synapses on these dendrites. Climbing fibers all arise in the contralateral inferior olivary nucleus (Fig. 16-4), a large nucleus in the rostral

medulla that underlies the olive (see Fig. 5-20). All other inputs to the cerebellar cortex[1] end on the dendrites of granule cells as mossy fibers (named for their microscopic appearance), where they make excitatory synapses. These two excitatory routes to Purkinje cells have markedly different effects, suggesting that they have different functions. The mossy fiber-granule cell-parallel fiber route leads to weak individual excitatory synapses, weak enough that many of them must be active at the same time to affect a Purkinje cell. The thousands of synapses made by a single climbing fiber, on the other hand, mean that a single action potential in a climbing fiber will have a powerful postsynaptic effect.

Just as the direct and indirect circuits perform fundamental operations of the basal ganglia, subserving particular functions by virtue of specific inputs to different parts of the striatum (see Fig. 15-8), this uniformly organized cortex performs the fundamental operations of the cerebellum. Specific inputs to different areas of cerebellar cortex, detailed later in this chapter, allow different parts of the cerebellum to subserve particular functions.

[1]This is not strictly true, because the cerebellar cortex, like other parts of the CNS, receives extensive modulatory inputs as well, most prominently serotonergic inputs from the brainstem reticular formation and noradrenergic inputs from the locus ceruleus.

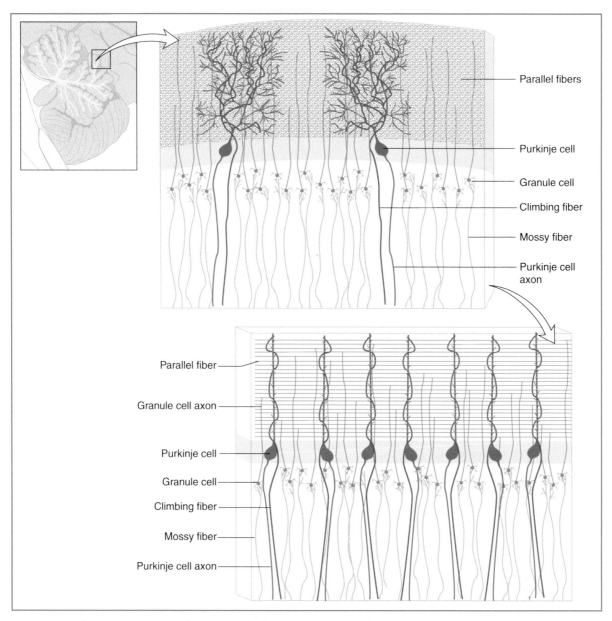

Figure 16-3. General structure of cerebellar cortex. Excitatory synapses are indicated in various shades of green, inhibitory Purkinje cells in red.

Cerebellar Peduncles

Mossy and climbing fibers enter the cerebellum, and the axons of cells in the deep nuclei exit, through a series of three cerebellar peduncles on each side (Fig. 16-5 and Table 16-1). The superior cerebellar peduncle is the major route taken by cerebellar efferents. It forms in the roof of the fourth ventricle, moves down into the brainstem, decussates in the caudal midbrain, and heads off to the thalamus. The middle cerebellar peduncle, the largest of the three, arises from pontine nuclei scattered through the contralateral half of the basal pons. This is the major route through which the cerebral cortex projects to the cerebellum: the principal input to the pontine nuclei is axons of cortical pyramidal cells that descend through the cerebral peduncle along with the corticospinal and corticobulbar tracts. The inferior cerebellar peduncle is the smallest of the three but the most complex. Most of its contents are climbing fibers from the contralateral inferior olivary nucleus, but it also contains spinocerebellar fibers ascending from ipsilateral spinal gray matter, comparable trigeminocerebellar fibers from the spinal trigeminal nucleus, and fibers traveling in both directions between the cerebellum and the vestibular system and reticular formation.

●●● SUBDIVISIONS OF THE CEREBELLUM

The transversely oriented fissures between the folia of cerebellar cortex make natural landmarks for dividing the

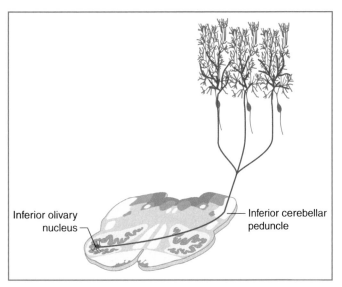

Figure 16-4. Origin of climbing fibers from the inferior olivary nucleus. The axon of each olivary neuron has several branches, each of which forms the single climbing fiber of one Purkinje cell.

TABLE 16-1. Contents of Cerebellar Peduncles

Peduncle	Source of Fibers
Superior	Deep cerebellar nuclei
Middle	Cerebral cortex (via pontine nuclei)
Inferior	Inferior olivary nucleus (climbing fibers)
	Spinal cord*
	Spinal trigeminal nucleus
	Vestibular nuclei and ganglion
	Reticular formation
	Fastigial nucleus
	Cerebellar cortex†

*One spinocerebellar tract (the anterior) enters through the superior cerebellar peduncle.
†Projections back to vestibular nuclei from restricted areas of cerebellar cortex.

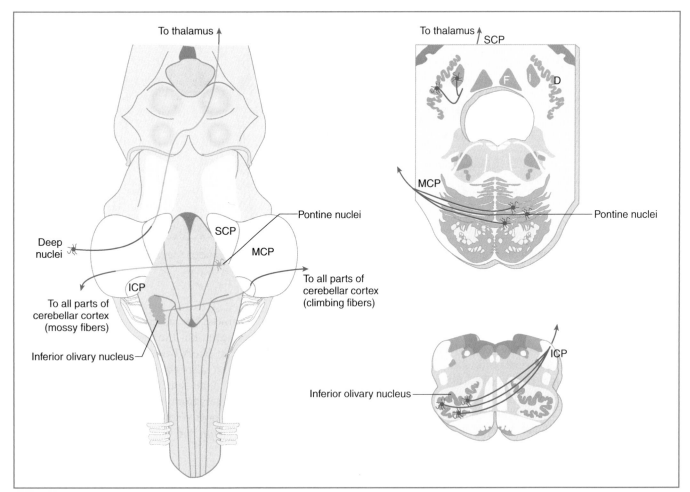

Figure 16-5. Major contents of the cerebellar peduncles. For simplicity, the inferior cerebellar peduncle is depicted as containing only climbing fibers, although in fact it contains much more (see also Table 16-1 and Fig. 16-10 for details). D, dentate nucleus; F, fastigial nucleus; I, interposed nucleus; ICP, inferior cerebellar peduncle; MCP, middle cerebellar peduncle; SCP, superior cerebellar peduncle.

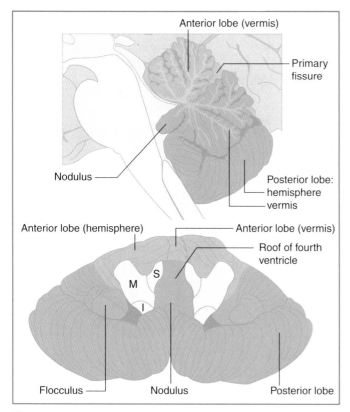

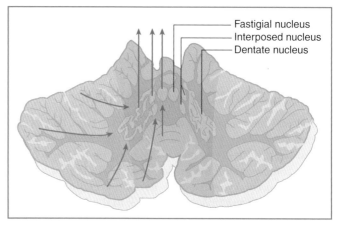

Figure 16-7. Longitudinal zones of the cerebellar anterior and posterior lobes, and their alignment with deep cerebellar nuclei.

Figure 16-6. Lobes of the cerebellum, as seen in a hemisected brain (*upper figure*) and in a view as though looking into the cerebellum from the floor of the fourth ventricle (*lower figure*). I, M, and S indicate the inferior, middle, and superior cerebellar peduncles.

cerebellum into lobes, just as landmarks like the central sulcus are used to divide each cerebral hemisphere into lobes. In terms of functional subdivisions, however, most of the cerebellum is organized into longitudinal strips that run perpendicular to the transverse fissures. The most obvious sign of this longitudinal subdivision is a narrow midline strip called the vermis, separated on each side by a shallow furrow from the much larger cerebellar hemispheres (Fig. 16-6).

Transverse Subdivision into Lobes

The most prominent cerebellar fissure is the primary fissure, which separates the anterior and posterior lobes (see Fig. 16-6). A less prominent fissure separates the posterior lobe from the small flocculonodular lobe. Each of these lobes is oriented transversely, extending from one hemisphere, through the vermis, and into the other hemisphere. For example, the nodulus is the vermal part of the flocculonodular lobe.

Longitudinal Subdivision into Functional Zones

In terms of functions and connections, however, it makes more sense to divide each half of the cerebellum into three longitudinal zones that cut across both the anterior and posterior lobe, each with a distinctive set of inputs and outputs (Table 16-2). The three longitudinal zones correspond to the three deep cerebellar nuclei (Fig. 16-7)—each half of the vermis projects to the ipsilateral fastigial nucleus, the medial part of the hemisphere (also called the intermediate or paravermal zone) projects to the interposed nucleus, and the

TABLE 16-2. Major Connections and Functions of Cerebellar Zones

	Lateral Hemisphere	Medial Hemisphere	Vermis	Flocculonodular Lobe
Deep nucleus	Dentate	Interposed	Fastigial	Fastigial, vestibular
Afferents*	Cerebral cortex	Cerebral cortex, spinal cord	Spinal cord, vestibular nuclei	Vestibular nuclei
Efferents	Thalamus to premotor cortex	Thalamus to motor cortex	Vestibular nuclei, reticular formation	Vestibular nuclei
Function	Planning movement	Correcting movement	Adjusting posture	Balance, slow eye movements

*Climbing fibers are not included, because they arrive in all zones from specific subsectors of the inferior olivary nucleus.

lateral part of the hemisphere projects to the dentate nucleus. The flocculonodular lobe is extensively interconnected with the vestibular system and is most usefully considered as a separate functional zone.

●●● LATERAL HEMISPHERES

The lateral hemispheres account for more than half of the human cerebellum, just as the dentate nucleus is the largest of the deep nuclei. The major inputs to each lateral hemisphere come (via pontine nuclei) from multiple contralateral areas of cerebral cortex, and its major outputs (via the dentate nucleus and thalamus) go back to the cerebral cortex. The particular cerebral cortical areas with which the lateral hemispheres interact provide some hints about their functions. Prominent inputs to the lateral hemispheres arise in premotor cortex, and numerous outputs project through VA/VL to primary motor and premotor cortex, suggesting that the lateral hemispheres somehow collaborate with the cerebral cortex in using sensory information to plan the details of movements. Consistent with this, many neurons in the dentate nucleus change their firing rates before a movement begins. The pathway from cerebral cortex to the cerebellum (Fig. 16-8) descends through the internal capsule, accompanies the corticospinal tract in the cerebral peduncle, and terminates in ipsilateral pontine nuclei. (There are actually so many corticopontine fibers in human brains that they account for more than 90% of the axons in each cerebral peduncle.) Pontine nuclei then give rise to pontocerebellar fibers that cross the midline and reach the cerebellar cortex through the middle cerebellar peduncle. The return route starts with Purkinje cells that project to the dentate nucleus. Dentatothalamic fibers leave in the superior cerebellar peduncle, decussate in the caudal midbrain, pass through or around the red nucleus, and terminate in the thalamus (mostly the ventral lateral and ventral anterior nuclei). Along the way, many dentatothalamic fibers give off collaterals to the red nucleus.

The lateral hemispheres are interconnected with broader areas of cortex than might be expected if their only responsibility were to help in the planning of movements; as discussed later in this chapter (see Fig. 16-12), they are now thought to collaborate in cognitive processes as well. Because of their extensive interconnections with neocortical areas, the lateral hemispheres are sometimes referred to as the neocerebellum or cerebrocerebellum.

Effects of Damage

Even the simplest movements require a precisely timed sequence of contractions and relaxations of multiple muscles. At the beginning of raising a glass to one's lips, for example, the biceps contracts and the triceps relaxes. As the glass approaches the lips, the hand is slowed and then stopped by decreasing the biceps contraction and contracting the triceps. Each lateral hemisphere plays an important role behind the scenes in planning the timing of each of these contractions and relaxations in ipsilateral muscles. As a result, damage

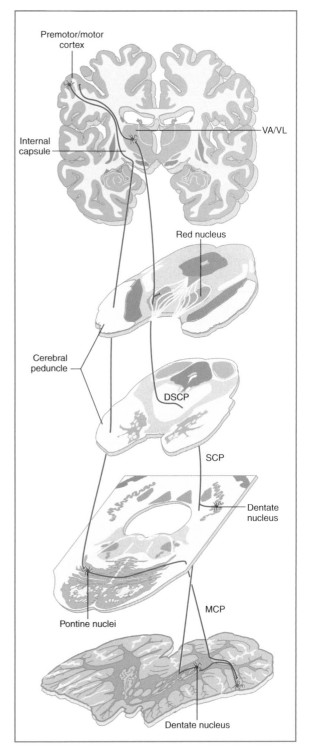

Figure 16-8. Pathway interconnecting the cerebral cortex and the lateral hemispheres of the cerebellum. The pathway crosses once on the way into the cerebellum and again on the way to the thalamus. As a result, one side of the cerebellum affects the contralateral cerebral hemisphere (and the ipsilateral side of the body). Only connections with motor cortical areas are shown although, as described in the text, neocortical association areas use the same pathway. DSCP, decussation of the superior cerebellar peduncles; MCP, middle cerebellar peduncle; SCP, superior cerebellar peduncle; VA/VL, ventral anterior and ventral lateral nuclei of the thalamus.

causes ipsilateral ataxia (uncoordinated movements), which is especially pronounced in the limbs.

MEDIAL HEMISPHERES

The medial part of each hemisphere also receives inputs from contralateral cerebral cortex (via pontine nuclei), but from more limited areas, in this case primarily the limb areas of primary motor cortex. These form multiple somatotopic maps, a major one in the anterior lobe, where the lower extremity is represented superior to the lower extremity, and another in the posterior lobe. Superimposed on these maps is an input from the spinal cord, via spinocerebellar tracts that convey information about the position of limbs and the activity of motor neurons. This makes the medial hemispheres eminently suited to compare intended movement (messages from motor cortex) with actual movement (messages from the spinal cord) and to issue correcting signals if needed. Consistent with this, most neurons in the interposed nucleus change their firing rates only after a movement has begun. The corrective feedback travels from the interposed nucleus back to the thalamus (mostly the ventral lateral nucleus), again through the superior cerebellar peduncle (Fig. 16-9). Along the way, some of these fibers give off collaterals to a particular small area of the red nucleus, which gives rise to the rubrospinal tract. This is one route through which the medial hemisphere can affect movement, but the human rubrospinal tract is very small and the major route is feedback to primary motor cortex.

Effects of Damage

Even the most carefully planned movement cannot account for unknown details, such as the weight of a glass and its contents. As a result, damage to the medial hemispheres also causes ataxia, not because the planning of movements is defective, but because a movement, once begun, cannot be corrected accurately. Overcorrections and undercorrections build on each other, and movements become ever more wobbly and inaccurate as a target is approached. This oscillation toward the end of a voluntary movement is referred to as intention tremor (as opposed to the resting tremor of Parkinson's disease, which diminishes or stops during movements).

VERMIS

The movement-related functions of the vermis of the anterior and posterior lobes center around the automatic postural adjustments made before and during limb movements, and this is reflected in its major connections with the parts of the brainstem that mediate these adjustments—the reticular formation and vestibular nuclei (Fig. 16-10). Inputs from cerebral cortex (via pontine nuclei) are relatively sparse, come largely from trunk areas of primary motor cortex, and are presumably involved in the coordination of voluntary trunk movements. To coordinate the timing of postural adjustments,

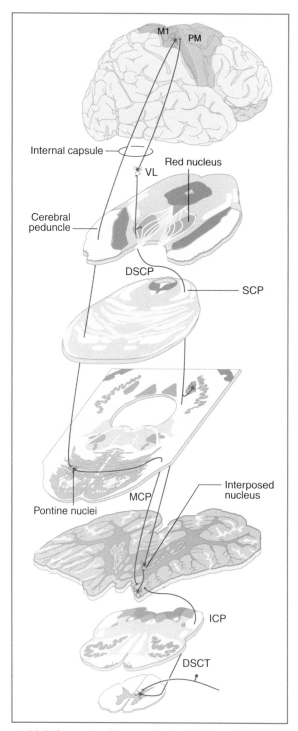

Figure 16-9. Inputs and outputs of the medial hemispheres of the cerebellum. As in the case of the lateral hemispheres, cerebral connections cross on the way in and the way out. Spinocerebellar inputs are mostly uncrossed, helping maintain the relationship between one half of the cerebellum and the ipsilateral side of the body. Several spinocerebellar tracts project to the medial hemispheres, but for simplicity only the dorsal spinocerebellar tract (named for its position in the spinal cord) is shown. DSCP, decussation of the superior cerebellar peduncles; DSCT, dorsal spinocerebellar tract; ICP, inferior cerebellar peduncle; M1, primary motor cortex; MCP, middle cerebellar peduncle; PM, premotor cortex; SCP, superior cerebellar peduncle; VL, ventral lateral nucleus of the thalamus.

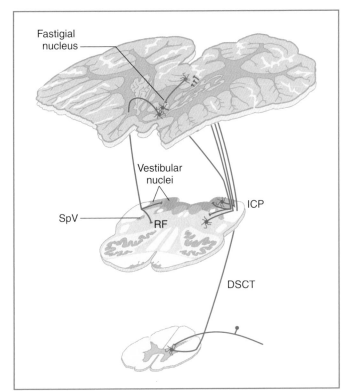

Figure 16-10. Inputs and outputs of the cerebellar vermis. Inputs are mostly uncrossed, but outputs are bilateral; those that cross loop over the top of the dentate nucleus inside the cerebellum, and both crossed and uncrossed traffic to and from the brainstem travels in the most medial part of the inferior cerebellar peduncle. Several spinocerebellar tracts project to the vermis, just as to the medial hemispheres, but for simplicity only the dorsal spinocerebellar tract (named for its position in the spinal cord) is shown. Not shown are comparable inputs representing the head, contributed by the spinal trigeminal nucleus. DSCT, dorsal spinocerebellar tract; ICP, inferior cerebellar peduncle; RF, reticular formation; SpV, spinal trigeminal nucleus.

Midline Cerebellar Damage

Thiamine deficiency, most commonly seen in the context of chronic alcoholism, causes focal degeneration in restricted areas of the brain. One site is the cerebellar cortex, especially its Purkinje cells, where (for unknown reasons) the vermis and medial hemispheres of the anterior lobe are selectively affected. The degeneration starts in the most anterior part of the anterior lobe and spreads posteriorly, leading to ataxia of the legs and trunk because of the orientation of the homunculus there.

Effects of Damage

Patients with midline cerebellar damage affecting the vermis have difficulty coordinating the movements of trunk muscles, which can make limb movements ataxic as a result. This is particularly obvious as a wide-based, staggering gait. In the unlikely event that damage is confined to the vermis, limb movements become relatively normal if the trunk is supported and postural adjustments become unnecessary.

●●● FLOCCULONODULAR LOBE

The flocculonodular lobe has particularly extensive interconnections with the vestibular system. Inputs arrive from the vestibular nuclei, and some vestibular nerve fibers even terminate directly in the nodulus (the only primary afferents to enter the cerebellum). Outputs reach the vestibular nuclei both through the fastigial nucleus and directly (the only Purkinje cell axons to leave the cerebellum). As might be expected from these connections, the flocculonodular lobe has an important role in the major vestibular functions of equilibrium and the control of eye movements designed to keep images stable on the retina (see Chapter 17).

Effects of Damage

Damage to the nodulus, like damage to other parts of the vermis, results in a wide-based, staggering gait. In this case, however, the unstable gait is accompanied by vertigo and nystagmus, symptoms similar to those following damage to the vestibular nuclei, nerve, or hair cells. This is one of the few instances in which damage to some part of the cerebellum causes changes in sensory experience. (Although the cerebellum receives large amounts of sensory information, it uses this information for the guidance of movement. Damage to the spinocerebellum, for example, causes ataxia but leaves the pathways to somatosensory cortex intact, so the patient has normal awareness of the ataxic movements.) As described

however, information about the current position of the trunk and the status of motor neurons is required. This is provided by spinocerebellar inputs ending in a pattern that continues the somatotopic maps begun in the medial hemispheres. Vermal outputs project (via the fastigial nucleus) bilaterally to the vestibular nuclei and reticular formation, consistent with the way in which trunk muscles on both sides of the body are used simultaneously. Because of their extensive use of inputs from the spinal cord, the medial hemispheres and the vermis of the anterior lobe are sometimes referred to collectively as the spinocerebellum.

The vermal maps of the trunk continue into the head, largely using information provided by the spinal trigeminal nucleus. As a result, the vermis also has a role in coordinating movement of the tongue, mouth, and eyes (see Chapter 17).

further in Chapter 17, damage to the flocculus causes deficits in the tracking eye movements used to keep the image of some moving object on the fovea.

●●● OTHER FUNCTIONS OF THE CEREBELLUM

The best-known functions of the cerebellum, like those of the basal ganglia, have to do with movement. However, just as in the case of the basal ganglia, it is now apparent that the cerebellum is involved in CNS functions beyond the roles traditionally ascribed to it in helping to coordinate movements.

Motor Learning

Movements change throughout life, partly because bodies change and reflexes and other relatively automatic movements need to be readjusted continually and partly because new motor skills are developed. The cerebellum, particularly through its connections with the inferior olivary nucleus and its climbing fibers, plays a critical role in various forms of motor learning. Examples include modification of the gain of the vestibulo-ocular reflex to compensate for the effects of wearing glasses; development of conditioned reflexes, such as automatically blinking in response to an innocuous sound that has been paired with something touching the cornea; and becoming more and more skillful at playing handball or a piano. In all of these cases, the powerful synaptic effects of climbing fibers in particular regions of the cerebellar cortex are thought to cause long-term decreases in the efficacy of any parallel fiber synapses that are simultaneously active in the same area (see Chapter 20).

Different parts of each inferior olivary nucleus project topographically to specific parts of the contralateral cerebellar cortex. This, together with the other input and output connections of cerebellar functional zones, provides the basis for multiple types of motor learning. The flocculus, for example, receives information about head movement from the vestibular nerve and nuclei, along with signals about response inaccuracy from a subset of climbing fibers. This allows the flocculus to play a key role in modification of the vestibulo-ocular reflex. The red nucleus, which is especially large in humans, probably also participates in motor learning. In most mammals, the bulk of the red nucleus gives rise to the crossed rubrospinal tract, an important alternative to the corticospinal tract. The rubrospinal tract of humans is tiny, however, and most cells of the red nucleus project instead to the ipsilateral inferior olivary nucleus (Fig. 16-11) via axons that travel through the middle of the reticular formation in the central tegmental tract. Converging inputs to the red nucleus from premotor cortex and deep cerebellar nuclei position it to play a role in the development of motor skills, although the details are not understood.

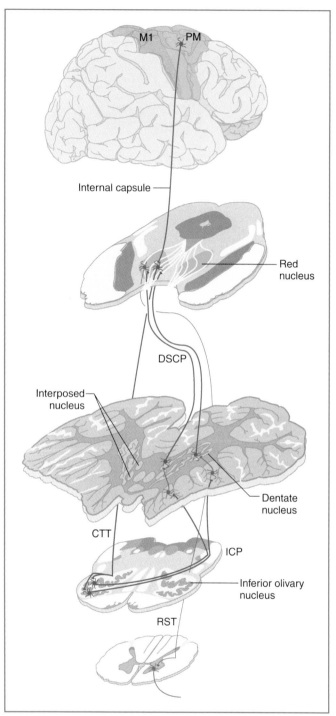

Figure 16-11. Interconnections of the cerebellum, red nucleus, and inferior olivary nucleus. The major set of connections form a loop from the inferior olivary nucleus, through the cerebellum, to the contralateral red nucleus, and back to the inferior olivary nucleus. There is also a small rubrospinal tract that projects to the contralateral cervical spinal cord. CTT, central tegmental tract; DSCP, decussation of the superior cerebellar peduncles; ICP, inferior cerebellar peduncle; M1, primary motor cortex; PM, premotor cortex; RST, rubrospinal tract.

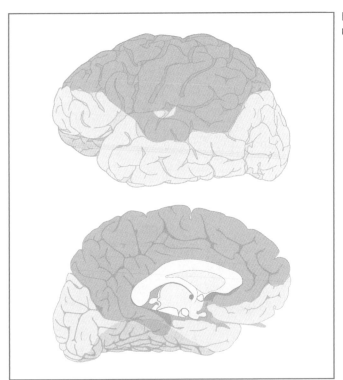

Figure 16-12. Areas of cerebral cortex that project to pontine nuclei, and through them to contralateral cerebellar cortex.

Cognition

The areas of cerebral cortex that project to pontine nuclei, and from there to the cerebellar cortex, extend into multimodal and limbic areas (Fig. 16-12) and are considerably more extensive than would be required for the planning and correction of movement. Similarly, each lateral hemisphere of the cerebellum projects through the dentate nucleus and thalamus not just to motor cortical areas but also to pre-frontal and somatosensory association areas. Consistent with these connections, functional imaging studies show increased blood flow in parts of the cerebellum during a variety of cognitive and sensory discrimination tasks whether or not movement is involved. Although the deficits are not as pronounced as those following damage to the cerebral cortex, damage to one cerebellar hemisphere causes impaired functioning of the contralateral cerebral hemisphere.

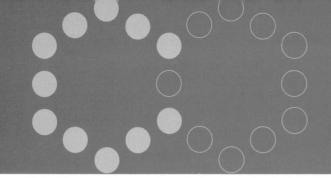

Control of Eye Movements 17

One consequence of the relatively slow transduction process used by photoreceptors is that rapidly changing levels of illumination, such as those that might be caused by details of an image moving quickly across the retina, cause receptor potentials that are smeared out in time and incapable of accurately encoding such details. Because of this, images need to remain stationary for a while on the retina in order to be seen clearly. Continuing with the eye-camera analogy, the eye behaves a lot like a camera with a shutter speed of about 100 ms, which would require support by a tripod for pictures not to be blurred. An additional problem for animals like humans results from having sharp, detailed vision in only a limited part of the retina (the fovea), requiring the fovea to be pointed accurately at objects of interest. Taken together, these two features necessitate two general categories of eye movement: those designed to get images onto the fovea (so we can start to see them clearly), and those designed to keep the images there (so we can continue to see them clearly). This is a nearly universal strategy used by animals with image-forming eyes, whether or not they have a fovea: periods of hundreds of milliseconds with images moving little on the retina, interrupted by fast, brief movements that change the direction of gaze.

There is a final complication for animals like humans that have two frontally directed eyes. Depth perception is made possible by keeping the eyes pointed in such a way that both foveae are directed at the same object of interest. If the system breaks down and the images on the two foveae do not correspond, diplopia (double vision) results. Two general kinds of movement are required to keep the eyes lined up this way

while we move or the world moves. First, as things move around at a given distance from us we need to move both eyes the same amount in the same direction; these are called conjugate movements. Second, as things move toward or away from us we need to use vergence movements to either converge or diverge our eyes.

All these movements require precisely controlled patterns of contraction of extraocular muscles, using mechanisms parallel to those described in the preceding three chapters—lower motor neurons, central pattern generators, and upper motor neurons, plus modulation by the basal ganglia and cerebellum.

●●● EXTRAOCULAR MUSCLES

Each eye is rotated in the orbit, like a ball in a socket, by the combined action of six extraocular muscles (Fig. 17-1). The medial, lateral, superior, and inferior rectus muscles originate from the back of the orbit and insert in the sclera of the anterior half of the eye. The superior oblique muscle also originates from the back of the orbit, but its tendon passes through a fibrous pulley (the trochlea) attached to the wall of the orbit before turning posteriorly and inserting in the sclera of the posterior half of the eye. Finally, the inferior oblique muscle originates from the floor of the orbit and passes diagonally backward to insert in the sclera of the posterior half of the eye.

The actions of the medial and lateral rectus are straightforward: the medial rectus rotates the eye toward the nose (adduction), and the lateral rectus rotates it away from the nose (abduction). The actions of the other four extraocular muscles are more complex because the direction in which each pulls is not usually in line with the optical axis of the eye (Fig. 17-2). The primary actions of the superior and inferior rectus are to rotate the eye upward and downward (elevation and depression, respectively), but each rotates the eye a little bit around other axes (Table 17-1). The superior and inferior obliques primarily rotate the top of the eye toward or away from the nose (intorsion and extorsion, respectively) although this can change depending on the direction in which the eye is pointed (Fig. 17-3).

Because of the multiple actions of the superior and inferior recti and the obliques, contractions and relaxations of all six extraocular muscles contribute to most eye movements. For example, even though the medial rectus is the principal adductor,

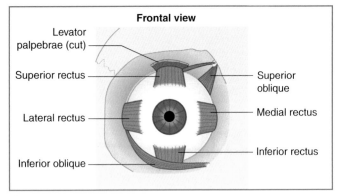

Frontal view

- Levator palpebrae (cut)
- Superior rectus
- Lateral rectus
- Inferior oblique
- Superior oblique
- Medial rectus
- Inferior rectus

A

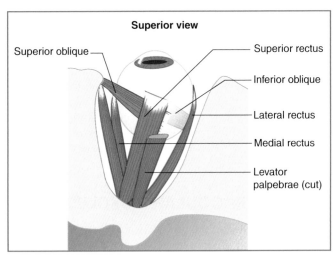

Superior view

- Superior oblique
- Superior rectus
- Inferior oblique
- Lateral rectus
- Medial rectus
- Levator palpebrae (cut)

B

Figure 17-1. Extraocular muscles of the right eye, seen from the front (**A**) and from above (**B**).

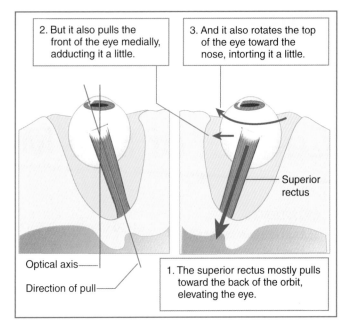

2. But it also pulls the front of the eye medially, adducting it a little.

3. And it also rotates the top of the eye toward the nose, intorting it a little.

Optical axis

Direction of pull

Superior rectus

1. The superior rectus mostly pulls toward the back of the orbit, elevating the eye.

Figure 17-2. The optical axis of the eye (the line from the center of the cornea to the fovea) points straight ahead during straight-ahead gaze, but the axis of the orbit points about 23 degrees laterally. The superior and inferior recti originate from the back of the orbit, and so their direction of pulling is not parallel to the optical axis. As a result, although the superior rectus primarily elevates the eye, it also has smaller adducting and intorting effects. (Similarly, although not indicated in the figure, the inferior rectus primarily depresses but also adducts and extorts a little.)

TABLE 17-1. Actions of Extraocular Muscles

Muscle	Major Action*	Other Action	Innervation
Lateral rectus	Abduction		CN VI
Medial rectus	Adduction		CN III
Inferior rectus	Depression	Adduction Extorsion	CN III
Superior rectus	Elevation	Adduction Intorsion	CN III
Inferior oblique	Extorsion	Abduction Elevation	CN III
Superior oblique	Intorsion	Abduction Depression	CN IV

*Major actions when the eye is pointed straight ahead. Some of the other actions can become more prominent, depending on the direction of gaze.

the superior and inferior recti also contribute; the lateral rectus and the obliques are antagonists in this movement, so their motor neurons are inhibited during adduction. To simplify the account in this chapter, however, the obliques will be largely omitted and the superior and inferior recti will be treated as though they contribute only to elevation and depression.

Lower Motor Neurons

The lower motor neurons for the six extraocular muscles are located in a series of three nuclei in the pons and midbrain (Fig. 17-4). The abducens nucleus (named for the action of the muscle) innervates the lateral rectus, the trochlear nucleus (named for the trochlea) innervates the superior oblique, and the oculomotor nucleus innervates the other four.

Looking to one side or the other requires simultaneous contraction of one lateral rectus and the contralateral medial rectus. This is coordinated by having not just lower motor neurons in the abducens nucleus but also a population of interneurons whose axons cross the midline and ascend through the medial longitudinal fasciculus (MLF) to contralateral

medial rectus motor neurons (Fig. 17-5). The same excitatory inputs that reach abducens motor neurons also reach these interneurons. As a result, damage to one abducens nucleus causes inability of *both* eyes to rotate toward the side of the damage. In contrast, damage to one MLF causes a selective inability to use the medial rectus on that side during conjugate gaze, even though the same muscle may still be able to contract during convergence.

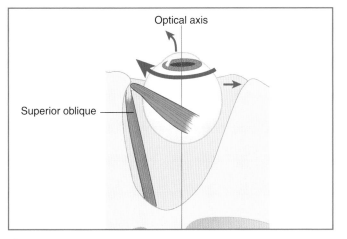

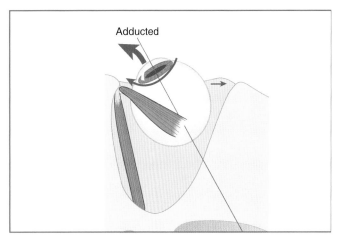

A

B

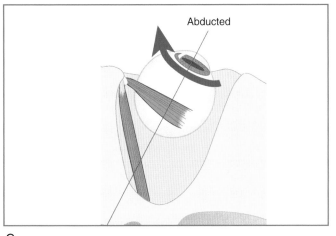

C

Figure 17-3. The pulling direction of the obliques is not aligned with either the optical axis or the orbital axis, and their actions change with the direction of gaze. The superior oblique inserts in the posterior half of the eye and pulls diagonally forward. **A,** As a result, during straight-ahead gaze, although it primarily intorts the eye, it also pulls the back of the eye a little bit medially and upward (i.e., abducts and depresses a little). **B,** During adduction, the direction of pull is more nearly in line with the optical axis, and the same muscle depresses more and intorts less. **C,** During abduction, the direction of pull can wind up perpendicular to the optical axis, and the action becomes purely intorsion. (Similarly, although not indicated in the figure, the inferior oblique primarily extorts when the eye is abducted, but it also elevates and abducts in other directions of gaze.)

PATHOLOGY

MS and the MLF

Multiple sclerosis (MS) is a demyelinating disease of the CNS with some favored white-matter targets. Among these is the medial longitudinal fasciculus (MLF), which may be affected early in the disease. The resulting selective weakness of the ipsilateral medial rectus is referred to as internuclear ophthalmoplegia, or INO. (Ophthalmoplegia means "paralysis of the eye," and internuclear refers to its being caused in this case by damage in between the abducens and oculomotor nuclei.)

CONJUGATE MOVEMENTS

For reasons described earlier, we need to make two different kinds of conjugate movements: fast movements (called saccades) that we use to get an image onto each fovea, and slow movements that we use to keep the image there. Typically, we can choose to make or not make these movements, implying that cortical areas can initiate or prevent them.

Fast Conjugate Movements

Saccades are extremely fast, almost step-like movements during which the eyes can rotate as much as 700 degrees per

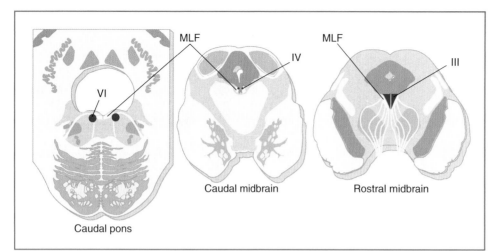

Figure 17-4. The brainstem nuclei containing the motor neurons for extraocular muscles. Trochlear and some oculomotor neurons are unusual in that they cross the midline before leaving the brainstem, but all the axons in CNs III, IV, and VI, once they leave the brainstem, travel to the ipsilateral eye.

MLF

MLF

VI

IV

III

Caudal pons

Caudal midbrain

Rostral midbrain

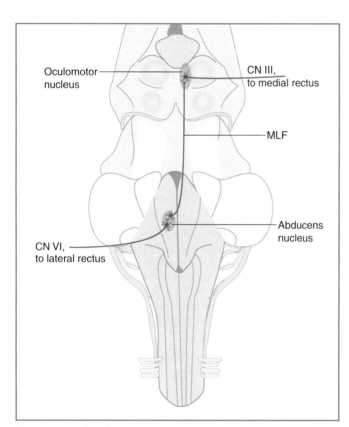

Oculomotor nucleus

CN III, to medial rectus

MLF

Abducens nucleus

CN VI, to lateral rectus

Figure 17-5. A subset of the axons in the MLF are those of abducens interneurons, projecting to medial rectus motor neurons.

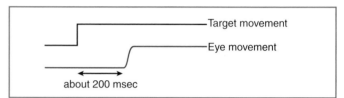

Target movement

Eye movement

about 200 msec

Figure 17-6. Saccade in response to abrupt movement of a target. Voluntary saccades are very fast movements but have a surprisingly long latency of around 200 ms.

ANATOMY & CLINICAL MEDICINE

The Midbrain and Vertical Gaze

Parts of the circuitry for upward saccades are located close to the dorsal surface of the midbrain, so one of the first signs of pressure in this area (e.g., from a pineal tumor) may be a relatively selective inability to look up.

second (Fig. 17-6). Getting an eye moving this quickly requires a very rapid burst of action potentials in the appropriate motor neurons, followed by a slower maintained rate suitable for keeping the eye in its new position. The required timing signals are set up by networks of neurons in the brainstem—basically, the central pattern generators for saccades. The motor neurons for all the muscles needed for vertical saccades are located in the midbrain, and the pattern generator is located

nearby in the reticular formation of the rostral midbrain. Each side of the midbrain projects to the oculomotor nuclei of both sides, so vertical saccades are not lost unless there is bilateral damage. For horizontal saccades, the interneurons and half of the motor neurons required for movement toward the ipsilateral side live in the pons, in the abducens nucleus (see Fig. 17-5), and the pattern generator is located nearby in the pontine reticular formation. The descriptive but unwieldy term paramedian pontine reticular formation, or PPRF, is often used for this area. Simultaneous inputs to both vertical and horizontal pattern generators can elicit saccades in any direction.

Saccades are used in multiple ways—to voluntarily change the direction of gaze, to jump from one part of a visual scene to another (including jumping from one group of words to another while reading), and to semiautomatically glance over at something moving in the periphery; they also are used as the fast phase of nystagmus (see Figs. 11-9 and 11-10).

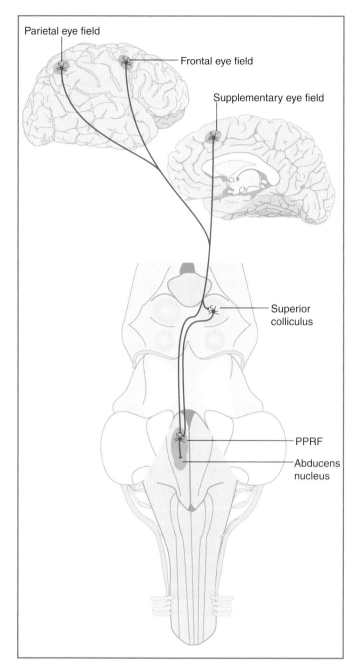

Parietal eye field

Frontal eye field

Supplementary eye field

Superior colliculus

PPRF

Abducens nucleus

Figure 17-7. Major inputs to the paramedian pontine reticular formation (PPRF) from cortical areas and the superior colliculus on the contralateral side.

PATHOLOGY & CLINICAL MEDICINE

Adversive Seizures

Seizures that originate in one frontal lobe may begin with forced turning of the head or eyes to the contralateral side, thereby earning the name *adversive seizures*.

muscle motor neurons in the cervical spinal cord, triggering gaze shifts directed upward, downward, or toward the contralateral side. At least three cortical areas also have a role in the initiation of saccades. The frontal eye field, located mostly in the walls of the precentral sulcus near the hand area in motor cortex, is involved in most voluntary eye movements. It initiates voluntary saccades and the saccades used in visually exploring a scene, in part by projecting directly to the saccade pattern generators and in part by projecting to the ipsilateral superior colliculus. Part of the supplementary motor area, sometimes referred to separately as the supplementary eye field, also projects to both the saccade pattern generators and the superior colliculus and probably is involved when sequences of saccades or combinations of saccades and body movements are required. Finally, the parietal eye field, in the banks of the intraparietal sulcus, projects to the superior colliculus and initiates automatic saccades to interesting things that appear in peripheral parts of the contralateral visual field.

Damage to the frontal or parietal eye field on one side causes a reduced ability to produce contralaterally directed saccades. This resolves quickly, however, usually in a matter of days, presumably because remaining intact cortical areas take over. Vertically directed saccades are not affected because both hemispheres participate in both upgaze and downgaze.

Slower Conjugate Movements

Once a saccade has pointed the foveae at something, different neural systems come into play to stabilize the image on the retina until gaze is shifted again by another saccade. Two general kinds of things can move an image off the fovea—movement of the fovea or movement of the object whose image is on the fovea—and separate but overlapping mechanisms are used to deal with these two possibilities. The vestibular system addresses most movements of the fovea, and the visual system addresses movement of objects in space.

Vestibulo-ocular Reflex

We have little awareness of how much or how quickly our heads move as we go about our daily activities, but unless there were eye movements in exactly the opposite direction, images would move across the retina and leave the fovea. The required compensatory eye movements are produced by the vestibulo-ocular reflex, or VOR (Fig. 17-8; also see Fig. 11-8). Because vestibular receptors are so fast and the reflex involves just a short, three-neuron circuit through the brainstem, the

Correspondingly, there are multiple inputs to the saccade pattern generators (Fig. 17-7). One prominent source is the superior colliculus of the rostral midbrain. Axons of some retinal ganglion cells bypass the lateral geniculate nucleus and project instead to the superior colliculus, forming a retinotopic map in its superficial layers. Many animals use this map as a major substrate of visual perception, but in primates the map is used primarily to direct head and eye movements toward objects in the periphery. Collicular neurons project to the saccade pattern generators and to neck

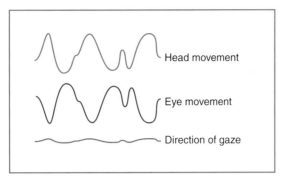

Figure 17-8. Compensation for head movement by the vestibulo-ocular reflex.

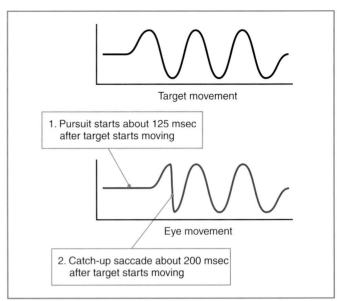

Figure 17-9. Smooth pursuit movements can "lock on" to smoothly, slowly moving targets but need about 125 ms to get started. The saccade system keeps track of how far the image of something interesting is from the fovea and can generate a saccade when needed to catch up.

PATHOLOGY & CLINICAL MEDICINE

Illusions of Movement

Because pursuit eye movements are relatively slow, fast head movements by patients with vestibular dysfunction cause images of the outside world to move across the retina. The brain interprets this as the world moving, and the patient experiences a disturbing illusion of movement called oscillopsia.

VOR has a latency of only 10–20 ms and can move the eyes at up to 300 degrees per second, making it able to counteract the high-frequency head movements that accompany walking and running around. The VOR is less effective in dealing with very slow or prolonged movements, because the vestibular system is sensitive to acceleration but not constant velocity. For low-frequency movements, the visual system takes over, using the mechanisms described in the next section.

The VOR, like other reflexes, can be modified to suit different circumstances. For example, we often shift gaze by turning our heads to look over at something. Unless the VOR were switched off during these head turns, the eyes would move in the opposite direction, preventing the gaze shift. VOR suppression, like changes in VOR gain (see Chapter 16), is accomplished by projections from the flocculus to the vestibular nuclei, enabling the eyes to remain stationary as the head turns.

Smooth Pursuit

If an object whose image is on the fovea begins to move, the visual system can detect this and initiate smooth pursuit eye movements to prevent the image from leaving the fovea. Because of the time required to get the movement information to visual cortex and develop the required feedback signals, however, smooth pursuit can only keep up with objects that move relatively slowly—no more than about 100 degrees per second. You can easily demonstrate the relative speeds of the VOR and smooth pursuit to yourself by staring at one of

your fingers while you move your head back and forth (VOR) or the finger back and forth (smooth pursuit), noting how fast each movement can get before the image of the finger becomes blurred. Because of this speed limitation, tracking objects in the real world typically involves a combination of saccades and smooth pursuit (Fig. 17-9). In addition, even though smooth pursuit is voluntary—a person can choose whether or not to track something—it cannot be done without an image moving across the fovea. You can demonstrate this to yourself, too: try to move your eyes back and forth slowly and smoothly with your eyes closed and you will feel them move instead in a series of saccades.

Smooth pursuit is like a reversed version of the VOR in that it is a smooth eye movement produced in the *absence* of vestibular stimulation, and in fact it probably evolved from the same circuitry used to cancel the VOR. This would explain the pathways involved in the generation of smooth pursuit (Fig. 17-10), which appear surprisingly intricate at first glance. Pursuit is initiated by the same cortical network that initiates saccades (with inputs from motion-sensitive areas of visual association cortex) and is implemented by the same flocculus-vestibular nuclei system that controls VOR cancellation. Signals from the cerebral cortex reach the flocculus via the pontine nuclei. Although there is some bilaterality in the pathway, projections from the cerebral cortex to the flocculus are mostly crossed, just like other corticocerebellar pathways. As a result, smooth pursuit in both directions is impaired after cortical damage, but the deficit is greater in the direction ipsilateral to the damage.

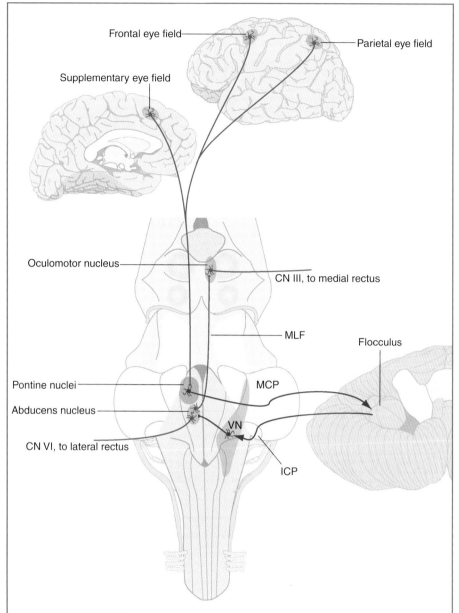

Figure 17-10. Pathways controlling horizontal smooth pursuit movements. Although there is more bilaterality in the pathway than indicated in the diagram, the projections from cerebral cortex to pontine nuclei are predominantly uncrossed. The result is that each cerebral hemisphere is more heavily involved in pursuit to the ipsilateral side than to the contralateral side. Similar projections through pontine nuclei, flocculi, and vestibular nuclei reach the oculomotor nuclei to control vertical smooth pursuit. ICP, inferior cerebellar peduncle; MCP, middle cerebellar peduncle; MLF, medial longitudinal fasciculus; VN, vestibular nuclei.

●●● VERGENCE MOVEMENTS

The vergence movements required to keep both foveae pointed at objects moving closer or farther away are accompanied by changes in the shape of the lens and changes in pupil diameter (see Fig. 12-18). The lower motor neurons and the preganglionic parasympathetic neurons required for this three-part response are located in the oculomotor nucleus, and the pattern generator for vergence and accommodation is located nearby in the midbrain reticular formation. Just as there are fast and slow conjugate movements, there are fast vergence movements for quickly switching gaze between objects at different distances and slower vergence movements for following objects moving in depth. The cortical areas involved in initiating these movements include the frontal eye fields

(which therefore seem to be involved in voluntary eye movements of all types) and more posterior parietal and occipital areas that analyze the blur and retinal disparity signals generated by objects moving in depth (Fig. 17-11).

●●● BASAL GANGLIA AND EYE MOVEMENTS

Most basal ganglia disorders (see Chapter 15) are characterized by various combinations of involuntary movements and movements of decreased velocity and amplitude. This extends to eye movements as well. Patients with Parkinson's disease, for example, make voluntary saccades and smooth pursuit movements that are smaller and slower than normal; patients with Huntington's disease often have involuntary

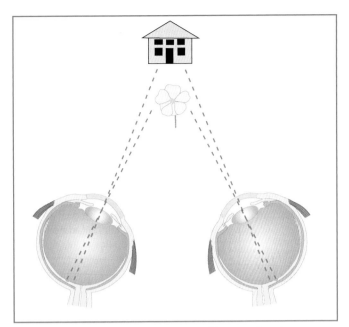

Figure 17-11. When looking at something nearby, the eyes converge and its image lands on both foveae. This causes images of objects farther away to fall into different parts of the two retinas. Visual areas of the cortex can use this kind of disparity information to help figure out how much convergence or divergence is needed when shifting gaze to objects at different distances.

saccades as they try to look at something. The basis for the involvement of the basal ganglia in eye movements is yet another loop parallel to those described in Chapter 15. In this case (Fig. 17-12), the loop starts with eye movement–related cortical areas that project to part of the caudate nucleus. This part of the caudate projects to the reticular part of the substantia nigra (rather than to the internal segment of the globus pallidus [GPi]), which in turn projects to the superior colliculus and, via the thalamus, to the frontal and supplementary eye fields. Increased inhibition of the superior colliculus by the reticular part of the substantia nigra in Parkinson's disease is thought to result in smaller and slower saccades, just as increased inhibition of the thalamus by GPi causes the hypokinesia and bradykinesia seen in other movements. Other patterns of imbalance in the excitatory and inhibitory inputs in this loop presumably explain the other eye movement abnormalities seen in basal ganglia disorders.

●●● CEREBELLUM AND EYE MOVEMENTS

Two parts of the cerebellum play a role in eye movements, the flocculonodular lobe and an additional part of the vermis dorsal to the nodulus, the latter sometimes referred to as the oculomotor vermis (Fig. 17-13). Some parts of this role are analogous to cerebellar participation in other movements and in motor learning, and other parts are unique.

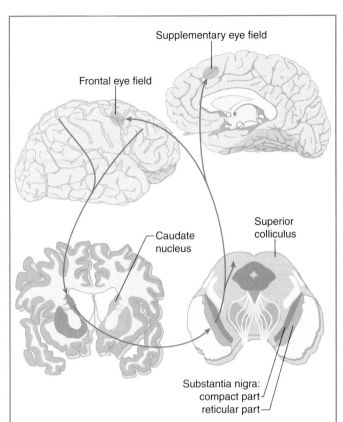

Figure 17-12. Connections through which the basal ganglia influence eye movements. This diagram shows only the direct pathway, comparable to the parallel loops in Fig. 15-8, but there is also an indirect pathway through which the subthalamic nucleus influences eye movements (see Fig. 15-5).

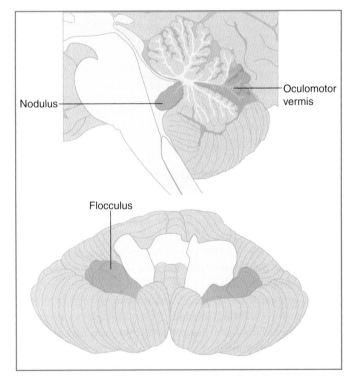

Figure 17-13. Parts of the cerebellum involved in eye movement control.

Eye movement–related areas of cerebral cortex project (via pontine nuclei) to the oculomotor vermis, which in turn projects via the fastigial nucleus to all the brainstem pattern generators for eye movements. Damage to this part of the vermis, or to the fastigial nucleus, or even to specific pontine nuclei, can cause saccades that undershoot or overshoot, or impaired smooth pursuit or vergence movements. The flocculonodular lobe also receives inputs from comparable areas of cerebral cortex (see Fig. 17-10), as well as extensive vestibular inputs, and projects back to the vestibular nuclei. Damage here, especially to the flocculus, causes impairment of smooth pursuit movements and loss of the ability to change the gain of the VOR. Combined damage to the flocculonodular lobe and the oculomotor vermis causes a loss of smooth pursuit movements, making these the only movements that depend on the cerebellum not just for their coordination but for their very production.

Homeostasis, Motivation, and Emotion

18

CONTENTS

Survival and reproduction are major goals of all creatures. Cells and the organisms in which they live battle entropy constantly, and cannot survive without a constant supply of energy to fuel their pumps and synthetic machinery. In addition, cells work well only in a restricted range of physiologic conditions, so homeostasis—keeping body temperature, blood pH, substrate concentrations, and a host of other variables within narrow limits—also is essential for survival. Homeostatic needs are largely addressed subconsciously by hormonal responses and by the autonomic nervous system (ANS), a network of afferent[1] and efferents that controls the activity of smooth muscle, cardiac muscle, and glands. For example, in a cold environment an animal can generate heat by hormonally induced changes in metabolism, or can retain heat by shifting blood flow to its interior. Environmental challenges also motivate behavioral responses, e.g., seeking out a warmer place or adding another layer of clothing. The hypothalamus plays a central role in this three-part response strategy, directing autonomic activity, regulating hormone secretion, and influencing behavior (Fig. 18-1).

Survival and reproduction require more than energy and homeostasis, however. For much of the world, it is eat or be eaten, so recognizing and remembering dangerous or favorable situations and behaviors also are vital. Similarly, successful reproduction is favored not just by autonomic and hormonal changes but also by particular patterns of behavior. The limbic system, including the hypothalamus, helps determine behavior by comparing risks and benefits in particular situations. It may be worth temporarily forgoing food even when hungry, for example, in a situation in which it would be socially unacceptable to eat, or it may not be a good idea for a cold animal to move to a warmer place where predators await.

●●● MAINTENANCE OF HOMEOSTASIS

The pathways and connections subserving visceral sensory and motor functions are in many ways parallel or analogous to those taking care of somatic functions. There are visceral primary afferents, the visceral equivalents of lower and upper motor neurons and central pattern generators, and visceral areas of cerebral cortex. There even are circuits through the basal ganglia and cerebellum that affect visceral functions and motivation.

[1] The original formulation of the autonomic nervous system included only visceral efferents. These days, most descriptions also include afferents from these same visceral structures.

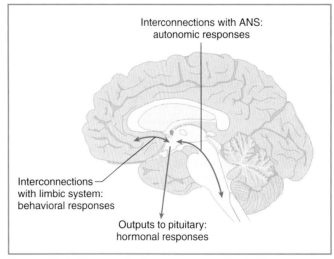

Figure 18-1. The hypothalamus as a nodal point in responses to homeostatic challenges.

Visceral Afferents

The senses of which we are consciously aware (described in Chapters 9 through 13) are based on primary afferents, many with large-diameter axons, tuned to a variety of adequate stimuli. Some of these are themselves sensory receptors, whereas others receive synaptic inputs from separate sensory receptor cells (see Fig. 4-2). Similarly, information about body chemistry, tension in the walls of hollow organs, and other visceral conditions of which we are typically at most only vaguely aware is conveyed to the CNS by an additional set of primary afferents. Most of these are long receptors with a peripheral sensory ending, a cell body in a dorsal root or cranial nerve ganglion, and a central process ending in the CNS, and most have small-diameter fibers in the Aδ or C category (see Fig. 2-22). A few receive inputs from short receptors in the periphery, and some visceral receptors are wholly contained within the CNS (e.g., neurons in the hypothalamus directly sensitive to temperature or blood-borne chemicals).

Some primary afferents from thoracic, abdominal, and pelvic viscera and blood vessels enter the spinal cord through the dorsal roots of the same spinal nerves that convey sympathetic and parasympathetic efferents (see the next section) and terminate in the posterior horn and intermediate gray matter (Fig. 18-2). Although most of these connections are part of the autonomic control circuits described later in this chapter, some branches of afferents conveying signals related to visceral damage terminate on the same anterolateral pathway neurons that receive inputs from nociceptors in the skin. This convergence of signals about cutaneous and visceral damage is part of the basis of referred pain, in which pathology affecting internal organs causes the experience of pain in other parts of the body. For example, cardiac ischemia can cause angina pectoris—pain felt not just in the chest but also in the left arm.

Other primary afferents from viscera and blood vessels of the thorax and abdomen, as well as those of the head, enter the brainstem primarily through the vagus and glossopharyngeal nerves, travel rostrally or caudally in the solitary tract, and terminate in the surrounding nucleus of the solitary tract (see Fig. 13-4). The nucleus of the solitary tract is the major integrating site for visceral sensory information, receiving these inputs as well as projections from spinal cord neurons conveying related data. It then distributes this information to visceral control centers in the brainstem and spinal cord and also through the ventral posteromedial (VPM) nucleus to visceral sensory cortex in the insula, adjacent to gustatory cortex (see Fig. 18-2). This is the point of entry into a cortical network including other parts of the insula and orbital cortex that underlies a general sense of discomfort or well-being and colors moods and emotions. Nearby areas of the insula, for example, receive inputs about pain, temperature, and pleasant, gentle stroking of the skin.

Visceral Efferents

The neurons that innervate smooth muscle, cardiac muscle, and glands, unlike the lower motor neurons that innervate

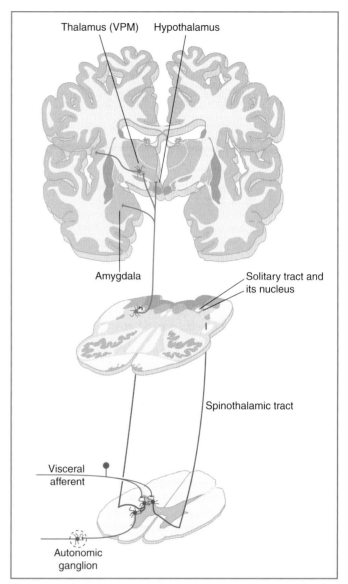

Figure 18-2. Distribution of visceral sensory information in the CNS. Visceral afferents enter the spinal cord and synapse on interneurons that form part of visceral reflex arcs and of pathways that reach brainstem sites such as the nucleus of the solitary tract. Some of the same afferents have branches that terminate on spinothalamic tract neurons, forming the substrate for referred pain. Similarly, visceral afferents enter the brainstem with CNs VII, IX, and X (not shown), traverse the solitary tract, and terminate in the nucleus of the solitary tract. The nucleus of the solitary tract in turn projects to an assortment of brainstem sites (not shown) as well as to the hypothalamus, amygdala, and, via the thalamus, to visceral sensory cortex in the insula.

skeletal muscle, live entirely outside the CNS in autonomic ganglia and fall into three groups. The enteric division of the autonomic nervous system is a network of sensory neurons, motor neurons, and interneurons located in the walls of the gastrointestinal tract. Although other parts of the ANS exert some control over the enteric network, it is capable of functioning largely on its own; as a result, processes such as

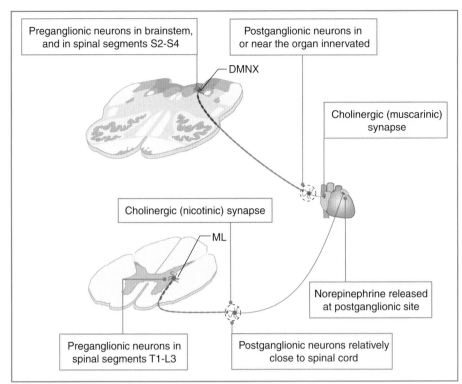

Figure 18-3. General layout of the sympathetic (lower part of figure) and parasympathetic (upper part of figure) divisions of the autonomic nervous system. Preganglionic sympathetic neurons are located in the intermediolateral cell column (IML) of the thoracic and upper lumbar spinal cord. Most preganglionic parasympathetic neurons are located in the dorsal motor nucleus of the vagus nerve (DMNX), in the medulla between the hypoglossal nucleus and the nucleus of the solitary tract; some, however, are located in other brainstem nuclei and in the sacral spinal cord. Not shown is the enteric division of the autonomic nervous system, an extensive collection of neurons in the walls of the gastrointestinal tract.

peristalsis, unlike coordinated contractions of other muscles, are able to proceed with no input from the CNS. The sympathetic and parasympathetic divisions of the ANS, in contrast, include preganglionic neurons with thinly myelinated axons that leave the CNS through spinal ventral roots or cranial nerves and synapse on neurons in peripheral autonomic ganglia (Fig. 18-3). The unmyelinated postganglionic axons of these autonomic ganglion cells then innervate visceral structures. (Although, strictly speaking, the term postganglionic should refer specifically to the axons of autonomic ganglion cells, these cells are commonly referred to as postganglionic neurons.)

Most autonomic neurons use multiple neurotransmitters in a variety of patterns, but the principal transmitter of both sympathetic and parasympathetic preganglionic neurons is acetylcholine, acting on nicotinic receptors. Postganglionic parasympathetic fibers also use acetylcholine (but acting on muscarinic receptors), whereas most postganglionic sympathetic fibers use norepinephrine (see Fig. 18-3).

Sympathetic System

Postganglionic sympathetic fibers extend to practically all parts of the body. Those for the head, neck and chest, as well as for blood vessels in skeletal muscle and for cutaneous targets such as sweat glands, originate from neurons in sympathetic chain ganglia (paravertebral ganglia) near the spinal cord (Fig. 18-4). Those for abdominal and pelvic viscera arise from prevertebral ganglia a little farther away from the spinal cord.

Preganglionic sympathetic neurons are all located in the spinal cord, forming a roughly topographically arranged column of cells in the lateral part of the intermediate gray matter (the intermediolateral cell column) extending from the first thoracic (T1) to the second or third lumbar (L2 or L3) segment (see Fig. 18-4). Upper thoracic segments control the sympathetic innervation of the head, neck, chest, and upper extremity, and lower thoracic and upper lumbar segments control that of abdominal and pelvic organs and the lower extremity. In thoracic segments, the intermediolateral cell column forms a pointed lateral extension (or lateral horn) of gray matter. Preganglionic sympathetic neurons have thinly myelinated axons that exit the spinal cord through the ventral roots of segments T1–L3, leave the corresponding spinal nerve through a white communicating ramus ("white" for the myelin), and enter the sympathetic chain on that side. Once there, the preganglionic fibers may synapse at that level, travel up or down the sympathetic chain to synapse with ganglion cells at other levels (Fig. 18-5), or pass through without synapsing and join splanchnic nerves on their way to prevertebral ganglia. (Some of the splanchnic nerve fibers end directly in the adrenal medulla, whose cells are neural crest derivatives that can be thought of as modified sympathetic ganglion cells specialized to release epinephrine and norepinephrine into the bloodstream.) Unmyelinated postganglionic fibers leave the sympathetic chain ganglia and join spinal nerves through gray communicating rami. Because the sympathetic chain extends the length of the spinal cord, all spinal nerves have gray rami; only T1–L3 have white rami (see Fig. 18-5).

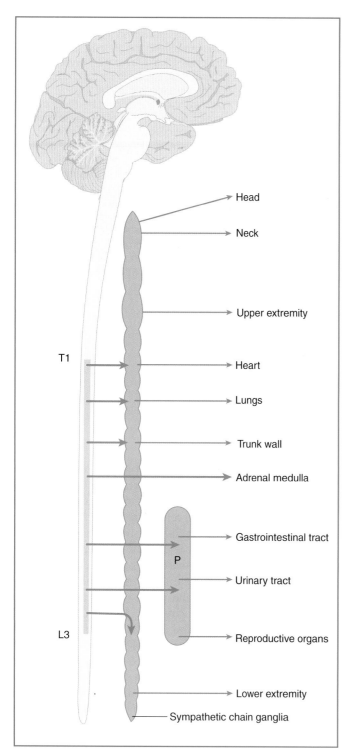

Figure 18-4. General pattern of distribution of sympathetic efferents. The actual pattern is not nearly so tidy as this diagram makes it appear, because preganglionic neurons for a given organ are distributed over several spinal cord segments, and their axons can ascend or descend multiple levels in the sympathetic chain before synapsing or leaving. P, prevertebral ganglia.

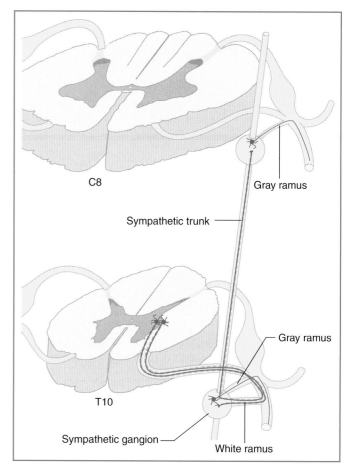

Figure 18-5. Distribution of sympathetic efferents through white and gray communicating rami.

Parasympathetic System

Postganglionic parasympathetic fibers also are unmyelinated but are short, originating from ganglia in or near the organs they innervate. Not only are they shorter than their sympathetic counterparts, but they also have a more restricted distribution, reaching the head, neck, and body cavities but not the limbs or the body surface.

Preganglionic parasympathetic neurons are found in both the spinal cord and brainstem (Fig. 18-6). Those in the lateral part of the intermediate gray matter of segments S2–S4 (where they do not form an obvious lateral horn) project to ganglia in or near the distal colon, bladder, and reproductive organs. Most of the rest are located in the dorsal motor nucleus of the vagus nerve, just medial to the sulcus limitans in the rostral medulla, and in nucleus ambiguus. Their thinly myelinated axons travel through the vagus to ganglia in the chest and most of the abdomen. Those for salivary and lacrimal glands are located in small clusters in the reticular formation near the pontomedullary junction, and their axons travel through the glossopharyngeal and facial nerves (Table 18-1). Finally, a clinically important group located in a subdivision of the oculomotor nucleus (the Edinger-Westphal nucleus) projects through the oculomotor nerve to the ciliary ganglion, which innervates the pupillary sphincter and ciliary muscle.

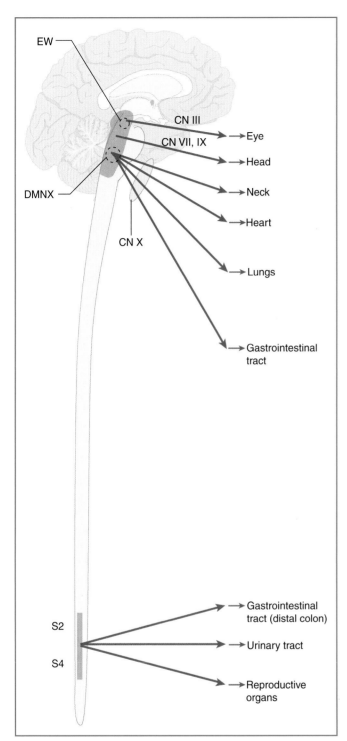

Figure 18-6. General pattern of distribution of parasympathetic efferents. Some of the vagal fibers shown as originating from the dorsal motor nucleus (especially those for the heart) actually arise in nucleus ambiguus. DMNX, dorsal motor nucleus of the vagus; EW, Edinger-Westphal nucleus (part of the oculomotor nucleus).

TABLE 18-1. Dominant Effects of Sympathetic and Parasympathetic Activation

Organ/Tissue	Sympathetic Effect	Parasympathetic Effect
Iris	Dilation of pupil	Constriction of pupil
Ciliary muscle		Contraction
Lacrimal gland		Increased secretion
Salivary glands	Decreased secretion	Increased secretion
Heart	Increased rate and output	Decreased rate and output
Bronchi	Dilation	Constriction
Gastrointestinal tract	Decreased peristalsis	Increased peristalsis
Digestive glands	Decreased secretion	Increased secretion
Arteries in viscera	Constriction	Dilation
Bladder detrusor	Relaxation	Contraction
Reproductive organs	Detumescence	Tumescence
Arteries in skin	Constriction	
Arteries in skeletal muscle	Dilation or constriction	
Sweat glands	Increased secretion*	
Adrenal medulla	Increased secretion	

*Via unusual postganglionic sympathetic fibers that are cholinergic.

Coordinated Autonomic Function

The sympathetic system has traditionally been considered to prepare the body for "fight or flight" activities, and the parasympathetic system to favor "rest and digest" activities. There is certainly some validity to this scheme in terms of the effects of global activation of each system (see Table 18-1)—for example, sympathetic activation diverts blood flow to skeletal muscles, increases heart rate, and causes systemic release of epinephrine and norepinephrine, whereas parasympathetic activation increases peristalsis and slows the heart—but it is an oversimplification. In normal daily activities, different parts of each system are activated selectively as appropriate, often in conjunction with skeletal muscle contraction or relaxation. Bladder control, as discussed later, is a good example, but there are many others in which blood flow is altered in particular parts of the body (e.g., sexual activity), specific nonvascular smooth muscles contract or relax (e.g., pupillary constriction), or patterns of skeletal muscle activity support homeostasis (e.g., breathing).

These patterns of coordinated autonomic/somatic activity are controlled through a pattern of connections largely parallel to those described in Chapters 14 to 17 for the control of skeletal muscles. A major difference is the central role of the hypothalamus in coordinating homeostatic responses and drive-related behaviors.

Autonomic Reflexes and Central Pattern Generators

Some responses involving autonomic efferents are relatively simple reflexes working in the background, based on visceral afferents, interneurons in places such as the nucleus of the solitary tract or the spinal intermediate gray matter, and sympathetic and parasympathetic efferents (see Fig. 18-2). Many others, however, demonstrate the integrated way in which the nervous system responds to environmental inputs, in that almost any kind of afferent may be involved, in combination with both somatic and autonomic efferents. Examples include pupillary constriction in response to light (see Fig. 12-17), salivation in response to tasty food or an appetizing aroma, and sympathetic responses to a painful stimulus or a frightening sound.

Complex response patterns that involve selected subsets of autonomic efferents or combinations of autonomic and somatic efferents are typically implemented by central pattern generators distributed through different levels of the brainstem. Neurons in the ventrolateral part of the medullary reticular formation, for example, receive inputs from the nucleus of the solitary tract and project to preganglionic sympathetic neurons in the spinal cord, coordinating the sympathetic responses to changes in blood pressure. Other groups of neurons in the reticular formation of the medulla and pons receive inputs from the nucleus of the solitary tract and modulate the depth and rate of respiration in response to changes in blood oxygenation.

Bladder Control and Micturition

The bladder is basically a muscular container that alternates between two states, a storage mode in which it accumulates and stores urine, briefly interrupted by periods of an elimination mode during which urination (micturition) occurs. We ordinarily have a high degree of voluntary control over when to switch from storage to elimination mode (i.e., are continent); the circuitry underlying the two modes and switching between them provides a good example of the coordinated, collaborative activity of the somatic and visceral systems.

Storage mode requires that the pressure inside the bladder —the intravesical pressure (Latin *vesica*, "bladder")—be lower than the outflow resistance. The principal mechanism for generating intravesical pressure is contraction of the detrusor, the smooth muscle in its wall, initiated by parasympathetic inputs from S2–S4 (Fig. 18-7). Several mechanisms contribute to outflow resistance, including smooth muscle in the neck of the bladder that forms an internal sphincter. The most important in terms of voluntary control of urination is the external urethral sphincter, a ring of skeletal muscle surrounding the proximal urethra. The external sphincter is composed of slow-twitch fibers (see Fig. 14-4), consistent with the requirement that it be tonically contracted for long periods of time, and is innervated by a cluster of lower motor neurons in the anterior horn of S2 (often referred to as Onuf's nucleus). During storage mode (Fig. 18-8), the external sphincter is contracted and the detrusor is relaxed, allowing the bladder

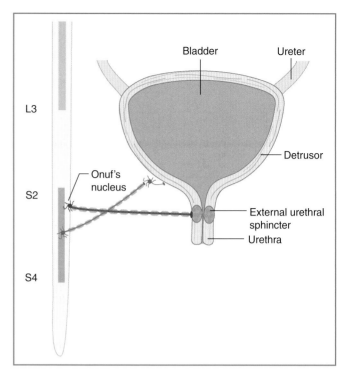

Figure 18-7. Efferent innervation of the bladder musculature. Sacral parasympathetics activate the detrusor muscle in the bladder wall, increasing the intravesical pressure. Motor neurons of Onuf's nucleus in the S2 anterior horn activate the external urethral sphincter, increasing outflow resistance.

to expand under low pressure. Detrusor relaxation is caused by sympathetic projections from lower thoracic and upper lumbar levels, which have a slight inhibitory effect on the detrusor but mostly act by inhibiting transmission through parasympathetic ganglia in and near the bladder.

A vesicovesical reflex is built into the spinal cord (Fig. 18-9), through which stretch receptors in the bladder wall stimulate parasympathetic output to the detrusor; this is the basis of involuntary micturition in infants. Switching to elimination mode voluntarily, however, is more complicated than this, because it involves reversing the components of storage mode, in a coordinated way, when it is socially acceptable to do so. This is accomplished through the pontine micturition center, essentially the central pattern generator for micturition, in the pontine reticular formation. The pontine micturition center monitors inputs from the spinal cord conveying information about bladder pressure, as well as hypothalamic and other

PHARMACOLOGY

Reining in an Overactive Detrusor

Some forms of urinary incontinence are caused by excessive activity of the detrusor muscle. One way to treat this is with cholinergic antagonists that act selectively at the type of muscarinic receptor that dominates in the bladder detrusor (M_3 receptors).

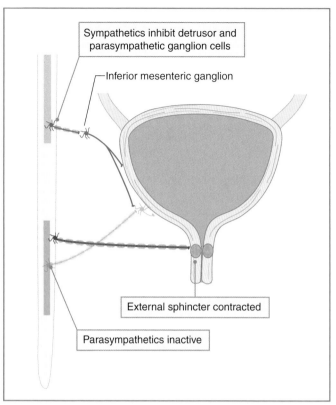

Figure 18-8. Maintenance of storage mode. Tonic activity of motor neurons in Onuf's nucleus contracts the external urethral sphincter, increasing outflow resistance. At the same time, sacral parasympathetic neurons are relatively inactive and sympathetic neurons of the inferior mesenteric ganglion (one of the prevertebral ganglia) inhibit both the detrusor and parasympathetic ganglion cells in the bladder wall.

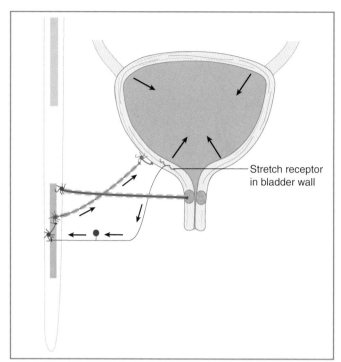

Figure 18-9. Vesicovesical reflex that mediates automatic emptying of the bladder in infants and in certain pathologic conditions. Contraction of the detrusor increases intravesical pressure and results in effective reflex emptying in infants, because the external sphincter is not tonically contracted. The reflex is less effective in adults, however, and is normally suppressed.

limbic inputs conveying information about the environment. When the time is right, it acts as a switch (Fig. 18-10), inhibiting the lower motor neurons in Onuf's nucleus and the sympathetic outflow to the bladder and at the same time activating the parasympathetic outflow to the bladder.

PATHOLOGY & CLINICAL MEDICINE

Bladder Function Disruption Due to Upper and Lower Motor Neuron Lesions

The neurons of the pontine micturition center are, in essence, the upper motor neurons for micturition. Damage between the pons and the thoracic spinal cord results in hyperactivity of the vesicovesical reflex, just as damage to other upper motor neurons results in hyperactive stretch reflexes. Because such damage also prevents relaxation of the external sphincter, intravesical pressure goes up, even while the bladder volume is low, until the sphincter is overcome; this sometimes is referred to as spastic bladder. In contrast, damage to the sacral spinal cord or cauda equina prevents detrusor contraction, resulting in a flaccid bladder that expands under low pressure until any remaining outflow resistance is overcome.

● ● ● HYPOTHALAMUS

The hypothalamus is the chief orchestrator of most activities related to homeostasis, reproduction, and dealing with stressful or dangerous situations. Although it is a relatively tiny structure—at about 4 g, much less than 1% of the CNS—the hypothalamus winds up being a nodal point in a remarkably large number of functional circuits, including those for feeding, fluid balance, temperature regulation, sleep-wake cycles, and sexual activity.

Corresponding to these multiple functions, the hypothalamus, like the thalamus, is subdivided into a series of anatomic zones (Fig. 18-11) containing arrays of nuclei with distinctive patterns of connections. The narrow periventricular zone, in the walls and floor of the third ventricle, is a continuation of the midbrain periaqueductal gray matter; in addition to being the home of some hypothalamic nuclei, the periventricular zone provides one route for axons to travel rostrally and caudally, interconnecting the hypothalamus and autonomic nuclei in the brainstem. The remainder of the hypothalamus on each side is subdivided into medial and lateral zones by the column of the fornix (see Fig. 20-9). The medial zone contains a series of nuclei. The lateral zone, in contrast, is a continuous area of scattered cells traversed by the medial forebrain bundle, a complex collection of fibers traveling in both directions between the cerebral hemisphere and the

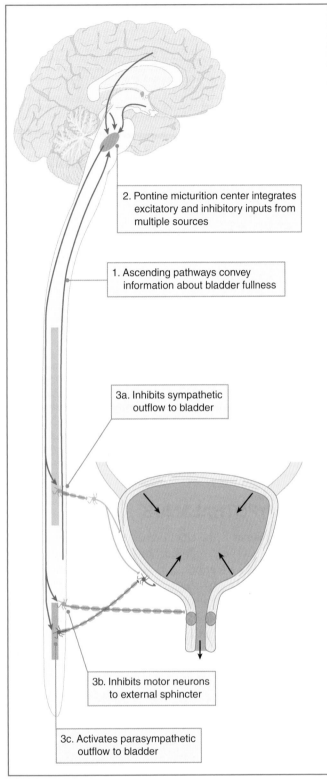

2. Pontine micturition center integrates excitatory and inhibitory inputs from multiple sources

1. Ascending pathways convey information about bladder fullness

3a. Inhibits sympathetic outflow to bladder

3b. Inhibits motor neurons to external sphincter

3c. Activates parasympathetic outflow to bladder

Figure 18-10. Normal adult micturition reflex. The pontine micturition center integrates information about bladder fullness with information from multiple sources about physiologic state, motivation, and social situation and acts like a switch. When switched on, descending pathways from the pontine micturition center cause coordinated contraction of the detrusor and relaxation of the external sphincter.

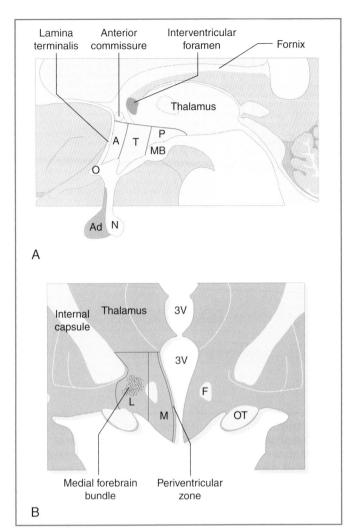

A

B

Figure 18-11. Longitudinal (**A**) and mediolateral (**B**) subdivisions of the hypothalamus. A, anterior zone; Ad, adenohypophysis (anterior pituitary); F, column of the fornix; L, lateral zone; M, medial zone; MB, mammillary body (part of the posterior hypothalamus); N, neurohypophysis (posterior pituitary); O, optic chiasm; OT, optic tract; P, posterior zone; T, tuberal zone; 3V, third ventricle.

brainstem and spinal cord. Some of these are afferents to or efferents from the hypothalamus; others, such as modulatory projections from the locus ceruleus and raphe nuclei to the cerebral cortex (see Figs. 5-22 and 5-23), are just passing through. The hypothalamus is also subdivided longitudinally into anterior, middle (or tuberal), and posterior zones. The anterior zone on each side contains preoptic nuclei adjacent to the lamina terminalis, a tiny suprachiasmatic nucleus above the optic chiasm, a supraoptic nucleus astride the optic tract, and a paraventricular nucleus higher up in the wall of the third ventricle. The tuberal zone is named for the tuber cinereum ("gray swelling"), the bulge on the inferior surface of the hypothalamus from which the infundibular stalk emerges. The posterior zone includes the mammillary bodies.

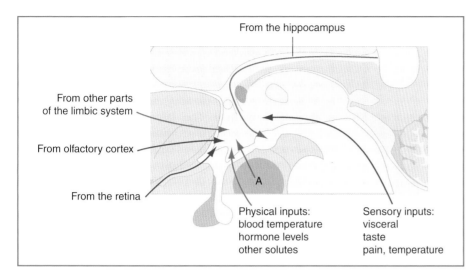

Figure 18-12. Inputs to the hypothalamus. Although numerous, these afferents fall into three general categories: sensory inputs, physical inputs, and inputs from other components of the limbic system. A, amygdala.

From the hippocampus

From other parts of the limbic system

From olfactory cortex

From the retina

Physical inputs:
blood temperature
hormone levels
other solutes

Sensory inputs:
visceral
taste
pain, temperature

Afferents to the Hypothalamus

The hypothalamus has two ways to keep track of internal conditions (Fig. 18-12). Visceral afferent information arrives from the nucleus of the solitary tract, either directly or after relays through other autonomic-related brainstem structures. In addition, a number of hypothalamic neurons are themselves sensory receptors that project to other parts of the hypothalamus. Some preoptic neurons are directly temperature-sensitive, and neurons in circumventricular organs in the walls of the third ventricle can sample the concentrations of hormones, glucose, and other solutes in blood passing by them (because these organs lack a blood-brain barrier). Other inputs with obvious relevance for feeding behavior and survival arrive from olfactory cortex, the gustatory part of the nucleus of the solitary tract, and anterolateral system fibers signaling tissue damage.

A last sensory input that might seem surprising comes from the retina, in the form of axons of intrinsically photosensitive ganglion cells that leave the optic chiasm and terminate directly in the suprachiasmatic nucleus. Although tiny, this nucleus is the master clock for most circadian ("about a day") rhythms in sleeping and waking, body temperature, hormone secretion, and other physiologic variables. It is not possible to build a biological clock that on its own would remain perfectly synchronized with our days over a lifetime. Instead, the suprachiasmatic clock has a period of about 25 hours, and external signals about day length entrain it to actual day length. The most important entraining signal is that provided by the retinal input, fluctuating with a 24-hour cycle.

The hypothalamus also receives substantial inputs from other parts of the limbic system, allowing it to play an important role in behavioral responses to various challenges (see Figs. 18-1 and 18-12). Some of these arrive from limbic cortex and from parts of the basal ganglia through the medial forebrain bundle. Major inputs from the amygdala reach the hypothalamus by passing under the lenticular nucleus, and also through the stria terminalis, a long bundle that curves

CLINICAL MEDICINE

Circadian Rhythms and Mental State

Patients with seasonal affective disorder (SAD) have depression that gets better and worse in a seasonal pattern. The incidence of SAD is higher in women and increases with proximity to the North or South Pole, suggesting that extreme changes in day length are involved in the etiology. Accordingly, the disorder is routinely treated by exposing the patient to bright light early in the morning when days are short.

around with the lateral ventricle in the groove between the thalamus and the caudate nucleus. Finally, the most anatomically prominent output from the hippocampus is the fornix, which also curves around with the lateral ventricle, ultimately reaching the mammillary body and other parts of the hypothalamus (see Fig. 20-9).

Efferents from the Hypothalamus

Hypothalamic outputs affect behavior and physiologic function by modulating activity in the cerebral cortex, influencing limbic structures and autonomic output, and controlling hormone production by the pituitary gland (Fig. 18-13; also see Fig. 18-1). Some groups of hypothalamic neurons project through the medial forebrain bundle to widespread cortical areas, providing diffuse modulatory inputs similar to those from the locus ceruleus and raphe nuclei (but using different neurotransmitters). These play an important role in the sleep-wake cycle (see Chapter 19) and presumably also in regulating levels of alertness. Multiple parts of the hypothalamus project back to the amygdala, and each mammillary body projects back to the ipsilateral hippocampus through a multistep pathway involving the anterior nucleus of the thalamus. Other hypothalamic nuclei project caudally through the medial forebrain bundle and the periventricular fiber system to central pattern generators (e.g., the pontine micturition center, respiratory

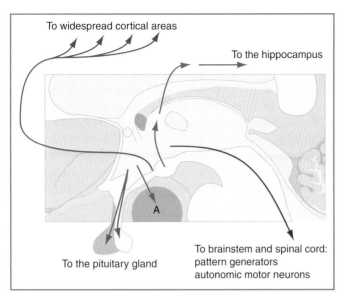

Figure 18-13. Outputs from the hypothalamus. A, amygdala.

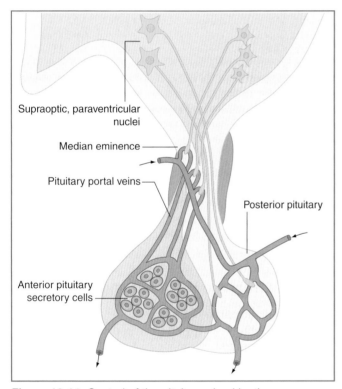

Figure 18-14. Control of the pituitary gland by the hypothalamus.

and cardiovascular centers) as well as directly to preganglionic autonomic neurons of the brainstem and spinal cord.

Hormone release from the two parts of the pituitary gland is controlled by two different mechanisms (Fig. 18-14). The posterior pituitary (or neurohypophysis) arises as a downward outgrowth from the diencephalon. Neurons in the supraoptic nucleus and some of the neurons in the paraventricular nucleus send their axons through the infundibular

stalk to terminations in the neurohypophysis. Action potentials traveling down these axons cause the release of oxytocin and vasopressin, in much the same way that neurotransmitters are released from other axon terminals. In this case, however, release occurs among a bed of capillaries with no blood-brain barrier, allowing the two hormones to reach the general circulation. The larger anterior pituitary (or adenohypophysis), in contrast, arises as an upward outgrowth from the roof of the mouth and contains non-neural secretory cells that produce one or two hormones from a long list (e.g., ACTH, growth hormone, thyrotropin, prolactin). Because the adenohypophysis is a non-neural structure, the capillaries have no barrier properties and hormones released there reach the general circulation. Hypothalamic neurons in the periventricular zone control secretion of adenohypophyseal hormones indirectly, through releasing hormones and release-inhibiting hormones liberated in the median eminence, the part of the tuber cinereum adjacent to the infundibular stalk. The median eminence is a circumventricular organ, allowing these hormones access to its capillaries, which then coalesce into pituitary portal veins that reach the adenohypophysis. The portal veins break up into a second capillary bed in the adenohypophysis, through which the releasing hormones and release-inhibiting hormones reach its secretory cells.

Regulation of Function by the Hypothalamus

A key concept in the way the hypothalamus regulates functions is the notion of set points. Different hypothalamic nuclei maintain records of the desired values of physiologic variables (set points, analogous to the setting of a thermostat). Afferents bring in information about the actual values of these variables and, if any differs too much from its set point, efferents prompt other parts of the CNS to take corrective actions (just as the furnace or air conditioner turns on when the room temperature differs too much from the thermostat setting).

Comparing the level of circulating thyrotropin to its desired level and releasing more or less thyrotropin-releasing hormone into the pituitary portal system is a simple example. Other functions regulated by the hypothalamus, however, are more complex, involving hormonal, autonomic, and somatic responses as well as changes in behavior. In these cases, the hypothalamus activates the appropriate pattern generators and, through the limbic system, affects behavior. A few examples follow. For each, only the autonomic and hormonal parts of the response pattern are discussed although, as described later, there are simultaneous changes in motivation and behavior.

Temperature Regulation

The principal thermostatic mechanism that leads to stability of body temperature is located in anterior parts of the hypothalamus, together with neurons that trigger heat-dissipation mechanisms; neurons that activate heat-generation and heat-conservation mechanisms are located in the

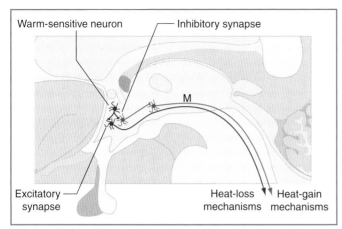

Figure 18-15. Automatic temperature regulation by the hypothalamus. Warm-sensitive preoptic neurons activate heat-loss mechanisms and inhibit heat-gain mechanisms, so as they fire faster, animals lose heat. As they slow down, heat-loss mechanisms become less active and heat-gain mechanisms are disinhibited. M, medial forebrain bundle.

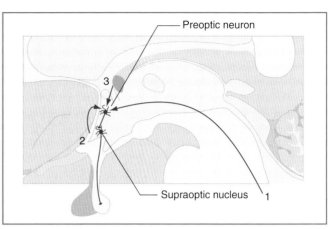

Figure 18-16. Regulation of water balance by the hypothalamus. Preoptic neurons integrate information about blood volume arriving from the nucleus of the solitary tract (1), about blood osmolality from the vascular organ of the lamina terminalis (2), and about kidney function by way of angiotensin II receptors in the subfornical organ (3). They use this information to regulate the rate of vasopressin release by neurons of the supraoptic (and paraventricular) nucleus.

MICROBIOLOGY & PHARMACOLOGY

Changing the Temperature Set Point

Infections of various kinds result in increased levels of prostaglandin E_2 that reach the temperature regulatory sites in the anterior hypothalamus, raising the set point and causing fever. Aspirin and acetaminophen reduce fever by inhibiting cyclooxygenase, a key enzyme in the synthesis of prostaglandin E_2.

posterior hypothalamus (Fig. 18-15). Neurons in the medial preoptic nucleus form an integrated view of the thermal condition of the body by being directly sensitive to increases in local temperature and also by receiving inputs about skin warming through the anterolateral pathway. As the body warms, they fire faster and cause cutaneous vasodilation and sweating (and panting in furry animals that cannot lose heat through their skin as effectively as humans can). Nearby cold-sensitive neurons project through the medial forebrain bundle to the posterior hypothalamus, which initiates cutaneous vasoconstriction, shivering, and piloerection (a vestige in humans that makes the fur of other animals a better insulator). If external temperature changes persist, additional hypothalamic connections alter the secretion of anterior pituitary hormones in ways that decrease or increase the metabolic production of heat.

Water Balance

The osmolality of tissue fluids also is maintained within narrow limits by a hypothalamic feedback mechanism similar to that used for temperature regulation (Fig. 18-16). As the amount of water in the body decreases, blood volume decreases and tissue osmolality increases; both changes are used to trigger water retention and acquisition. Glossopharyngeal

and vagal receptors in and near the heart convey information about blood volume to the nucleus of the solitary tract, which in turn relays it to the medial preoptic nucleus. Osmoreceptors in another circumventricular organ, the vascular organ of the lamina terminalis, also project to the medial preoptic nucleus. Finally, decreased perfusion pressure causes increased secretion of renin by the kidneys, activating the renin-angiotensin system and resulting in increased levels of circulating angiotensin II. Angiotensin II works at multiple levels to promote water retention and acquisition. In the brain, neurons in yet another circumventricular organ, the subfornical organ, detect increases in angiotensin II and project to—you guessed it—the medial preoptic nucleus. The medial preoptic nucleus integrates these multiple signals about water (and electrolyte) balance and projects to the supraoptic nucleus, regulating the rate of vasopressin release. Vasopressin (antidiuretic hormone) in turn decreases water excretion by the kidney.

Food Intake

Regulation of food intake and energy stores is more complicated, but feedback mechanisms analogous in many ways to those involved in temperature regulation and fluid balance nevertheless are at work. One way this shows up is in an apparent set point for body weight. Modest increases and decreases in food intake cause compensating changes in metabolic rate and no change in body weight. In most animals, a transient period of starvation is followed by a period of greater than normal eating once food becomes available again, but eating returns to pre-starvation levels once normal weight is reached.

For a long time, the hypothalamus was thought to contain feeding-related centers analogous to the regions that trigger heat loss and heat retention. Lesions in the medial tuberal part of the hypothalamus cause animals to eat excessively and gain weight, as though this part of the hypothalamus normally acts as a satiety center that tells animals when to stop eating. Conversely, lesions in the lateral tuberal part cause decreased eating and weight loss, as if this were normally a feeding center. It is now known that this is an oversimplification and that many different chemical signals participate in the regulation of feeding by acting at several levels of the CNS. However, one prominent site at which some of them act is the medial tuberal hypothalamus, which in turn affects the lateral tuberal region and other parts of the hypothalamus. For example, neurons in the medial tuberal region have receptors for ghrelin and leptin, two peptide hormones that enter the median eminence and have reciprocal effects on feeding. Oscillating levels of ghrelin are produced by the stomach throughout the day, reaching a peak just before eating and a minimum level between meals, stimulating animals to start eating. Leptin, in contrast, is produced by adipocytes in times of plenty and suppresses feeding. Abnormal ghrelin signaling, and especially leptin signaling, is now thought to underlie some cases of obesity. Superimposed on this process are short-term signals from the gastrointestinal tract about distention and chemical contents, mostly conveyed by the vagus nerve to the nucleus of the solitary tract, that tell an animal when to stop eating.

●●● LIMBIC SYSTEM

Stimuli and situations with implications for homeostasis and survival do more than cause autonomic and hormonal changes (see Fig. 18-1). They also cause drives and emotional reactions that motivate actions. If blood osmolality increases, for example, you not only secrete more vasopressin but also feel thirsty and look for something to drink. But you do not do that automatically; you weigh how thirsty you are against your current situation and make a decision about what to do. The limbic system is a collective term for the hypothalamus and other parts of the CNS that help you make the decision. Limbic structures serve as a bridge between the hypothalamus and multimodal association cortex, which collaborates with premotor and supplementary motor areas to design behavioral responses. All of this extends to the emotions associated with social interactions and other activities of daily living—anger, sadness, joy, fear, and so on—and their autonomic and behavioral concomitants.

It is apparent that there are two aspects to emotional states, a conscious feeling (implying cortical involvement) and an autonomic/hormonal output. An early attempt to define networks of neural connections that link the hypothalamus and multimodal association cortex was made by James Papez, who pointed out the interconnections between the hippocampus, hypothalamus, and cerebral cortex (Fig. 18-17) and hypothesized that the limbic lobe is important for the conscious awareness of feelings. He had the right idea, and the connections he pointed out are still known as the Papez circuit. However, it is now known that the amygdala and its connections with cerebral cortex and the

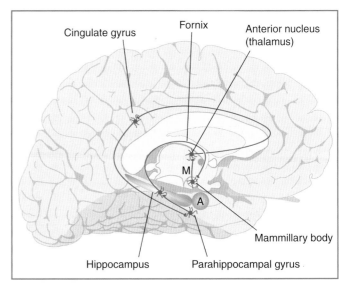

Figure 18-17. Papez circuit, originally proposed as an anatomic substrate for emotions because of the way it interconnects neocortex and the hypothalamus. It is now known that the amygdala (A), through connections discussed in the text (also see Fig. 18-18), is more centrally involved in emotional states. M, mammillothalamic tract.

hypothalamus and brainstem play a much more central role in emotional states and responses to them. Although the amygdala has widespread cortical connections (see below), those with a restricted part of the limbic lobe (the anterior part of the cingulate gyrus) and with orbital and nearby cortical areas are particularly important (Fig. 18-18). The hippocampus and the rest of the limbic lobe, in contrast, are more important for the formation of new memories of facts and events (see Chapter 20).

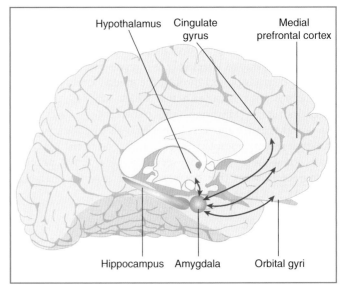

Figure 18-18. The general pattern of connections through which the amygdala interconnects the hypothalamus and limbic areas of cortex.

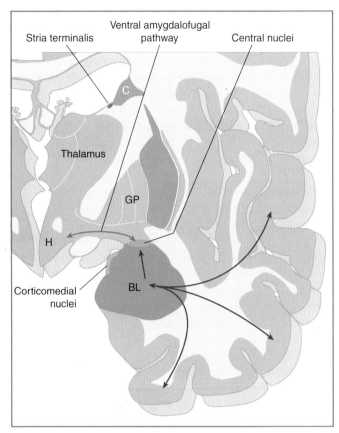

Figure 18-19. Major nuclear groups and connections of the amygdala. The corticomedial nuclei are interconnected with the olfactory system and are relatively small in humans. The central nuclei are extensively interconnected with the hypothalamus (H). Most of these fibers travel underneath the globus pallidus (GP) in a diffuse bundle sometimes called the ventral amygdalofugal pathway (not the best name, because it contains fibers going both from and to the amygdala); some travel through the stria terminalis, a tiny tract that leaves the amygdala posteriorly and curves around in the wall of the lateral ventricle, adjacent to the caudate nucleus (C). Finally, the basolateral nuclei (BL) are interconnected with cerebral cortex (see Figs. 18-20 and 18-21) and also project to the central nuclei, allowing the amygdala to serve as a bridge between the cerebral cortex and hypothalamus.

Connections of the Amygdala

The amygdala is a collection of a dozen or so nuclei located in the temporal lobe at the anterior end of the hippocampus, underlying the uncus. These nuclei can be sorted into corticomedial, basolateral, and central groups (Fig. 18-19). The corticomedial nuclei are an extension of the olfactory system and are particularly important for the processing of pheromonal information. The basolateral nuclei are extensively interconnected with the cerebral cortex, influencing conscious feelings, and project to the central nuclei. The central nuclei are interconnected with the hypothalamus and brainstem visceral nuclei, influencing the response patterns accompanying emotional states.

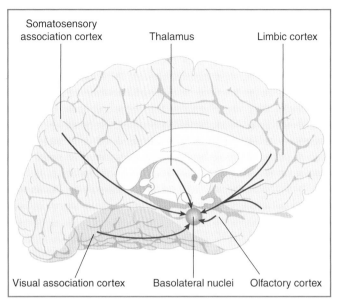

Figure 18-20. Major inputs to the basolateral nuclei of the amygdala. Not shown are additional inputs from gustatory cortex and auditory association cortex.

Cortical inputs to the basolateral nuclei (Fig. 18-20) arise in limbic areas, conveying information about mood, drives, and the rewarding or threatening aspects of objects and situations, and from sensory areas, conveying information about their nature. Somatosensory, auditory, and visual inputs come from association areas, although the gustatory and olfactory inputs are more direct. The outputs of the basolateral nuclei (Fig. 18-21) affect other parts of the CNS in ways that underscore feelings and emotional responses. They project back to limbic

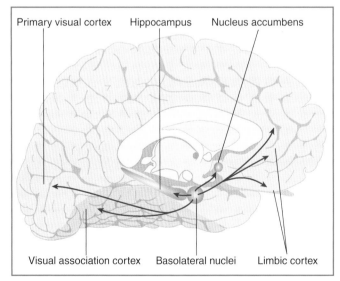

Figure 18-21. Major outputs from the basolateral nuclei of the amygdala. Projections back to sensory cortical areas are more extensive than inputs, reaching not just association areas, but also primary areas. To keep things simple, only those to visual areas are shown, but similar projections reach other sensory areas. Not shown are functionally important outputs to the central nuclei (see Fig. 18-19).

cortex, influencing behavior and emotions, and widely to cortical sensory areas, modulating their sensitivity as appropriate; for example, fearful faces and threatening sounds are detected more easily than neutral faces and sounds. They project to the nucleus accumbens and other parts of the ventral striatum, feeding into basal ganglia pathways that facilitate behaviors that are likely to be rewarding (see Fig. 15-8). Events with emotional significance are remembered better than inconsequential events, and correspondingly, the basolateral nuclei project to the hippocampus. Finally, the basolateral nuclei project to the central nuclei, which in turn project to the hypothalamus and to brainstem autonomic nuclei and central pattern generators.

Conditioned Fear

Brains are genetically programmed so that some things are intrinsically pleasant (e.g., sweet tastes) or unpleasant (e.g., pain). As animals go through life, they develop associations between intrinsically neutral stimuli or situations and pleasant or unpleasant outcomes. Such associations result in rapid emotional responses, as in the anticipation of a pleasant experience at the sight of an ice cream truck, anxiety at the sound of the voice of some individual, or fear after being touched on the shoulder while walking down a dark alley. The responses in many cases are initiated automatically and may be aborted once the details of the stimulus are apparent (e.g., discovering it was a friend who tapped you on the shoulder). The amygdala is intimately involved in the development of these associations, particularly those indicating possible danger. The best-studied example is conditioned fear, in which pairing a neutral sound with a subsequent painful stimulus eventually results in sympathetic responses (e.g., increased blood pressure and heart rate) to the sound alone (Fig. 18-22). The basolateral amygdala receives auditory inputs both directly and quickly from the medial geniculate nucleus, and indirectly and more slowly from auditory association cortex. The thalamic input serves as a kind of early warning system—if paired with a subsequent painful input, its synaptic strength increases (see Chapter 20) and it becomes able to trigger outputs to the central amygdala on its own. The cortical inputs have veto power, once the details of the stimulus become clearer.

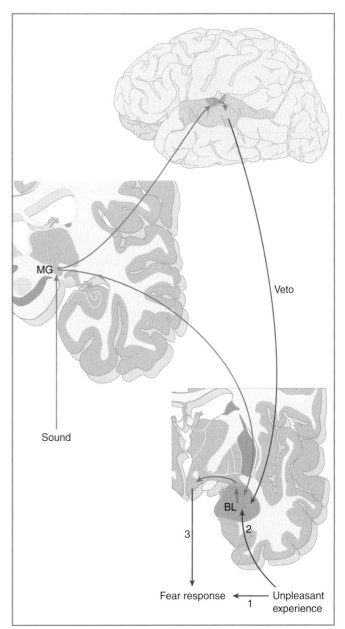

Figure 18-22. Conditioned fear and the amygdala. Intrinsically unpleasant experiences (e.g., pain) automatically trigger autonomic responses (1) and also alert the amygdala that something unpleasant has occurred (2). Information about sounds reaches the medial geniculate nucleus (MG), which in turn projects to both primary auditory cortex and the basolateral amygdala (BL). Association of pain with an innocuous sound causes changes in the strength of synapses in the basolateral amygdala, with the result that a previously innocuous sound can quickly trigger the same reaction as a painful stimulus (3). This kind of "early warning system" can be switched off if further analysis in auditory association cortex finds it to be unwarranted.

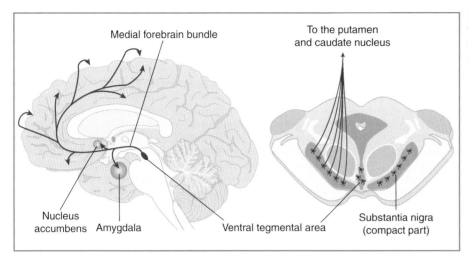

Figure 18-23. Dopaminergic projections from the ventral tegmental area to the amygdala, ventral striatum, and limbic and prefrontal cortex.

Limbic Connections of the Basal Ganglia and Cerebellum

Just as long loops interconnecting parts of the basal ganglia and cerebellum with motor areas of the cortex participate in the control of movement, similar loops interconnecting other parts of the basal ganglia and cerebellum with the limbic system participate in motivation and drive-related behaviors. Limbic cortex, the amygdala, and the hippocampus project to the ventral striatum, which projects directly to the hypothalamus as well as back to other parts of the limbic system through a typical basal ganglia loop (see Fig. 15-8). Neurons in the ventral tegmental area (VTA) of the rostral midbrain, near the compact part of the substantia nigra, provide modulatory dopaminergic inputs to the ventral striatum and prefrontal cortex (Fig. 18-23). One indication that the ventral striatum influences drive-related behavior is the observation that nearly anything expected to be pleasurable (food, sex, humor, drugs of abuse, and so on) is preceded by increased release of dopamine in the ventral striatum.

Similarly, there are loops from the cingulate and parahippocampal gyri to the cerebellum (via pontine nuclei) and back (via the thalamus), interconnections between the hypothalamus and cerebellum have been described, and emotional changes have been noted in patients with damage to the vermis.

Consciousness and Cognition   19

The distinctive cognitive abilities of humans, such as those used in language, problem-solving, and social interactions, develop on a background of consciousness—an awareness of one's self and surroundings, and an ability to focus attention. Consciousness results from collaborative activity of wide areas of the brainstem, diencephalon, and cerebral hemispheres, whereas the various different cognitive abilities depend on particular cortical areas and their connections, often with one hemisphere being more important than the other.

●●● CONSCIOUSNESS

Consciousness has both a content, reflecting the activity of particular cortical areas at any given point in time, and a level, reflecting the level of activity of an array of brainstem and diencephalic nuclei that give rise to diffuse modulatory projections to the thalamus and widespread areas of cortex (Fig. 19-1), using a variety of neurotransmitters with generally excitatory effects. Rostral parts of the locus ceruleus and raphe nuclei (see Figs. 5-22 and 5-23) provide norepinephrine and serotonin, respectively. Cholinergic neurons in the reticular formation of the rostral pons and caudal midbrain project to the thalamus, and a larger collection in the basal nucleus (of Meynert) project widely to the cerebral cortex. Finally, two clusters of hypothalamic neurons on each side also provide widespread projections to both thalamus and cortex. One set, in the posterior hypothalamus near the mammillary body (the tuberomammillary nucleus), uses histamine as a neurotransmitter. The second set, in the lateral tuberal hypothalamus, uses a recently discovered neuropeptide called orexin by some and hypocretin by others. The

brainstem components of this network are often referred to as the ascending reticular activating system because of the direction in which their axons travel and because these projections activate the forebrain and play a major role in maintaining consciousness.

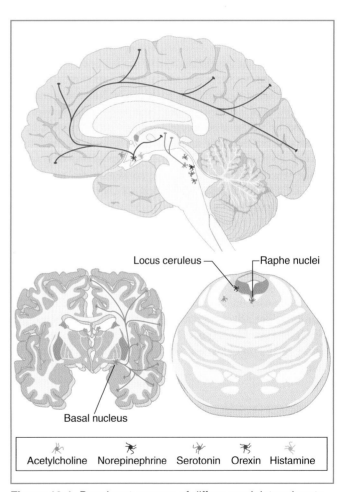

Locus ceruleus — — Raphe nuclei

Basal nucleus

| Acetylcholine | Norepinephrine | Serotonin | Orexin | Histamine |

Figure 19-1. Prominent sources of diffuse modulatory inputs to the cerebrum. Cholinergic neurons projecting to the cerebral cortex and thalamus are segregated in the basal nucleus and the pontine/midbrain reticular formation, respectively. All the others project widely throughout the cerebrum, as illustrated for the hypothalamic orexin neuron. (Other parts of the CNS also receive modulatory inputs; e.g., raphe nuclei in more caudal parts of the brainstem project to the brainstem, cerebellum, and spinal cord.)

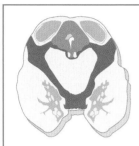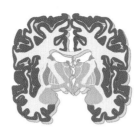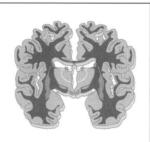

Figure 19-2. Examples of the kinds of lesions required to cause prolonged loss of consciousness: bilateral damage to the reticular formation of the midbrain or rostral pons (or the diencephalon, not shown) or extensive bilateral damage to cerebral cortex or white matter.

The level of consciousness varies throughout the day and night, from high levels of alertness, through distractedness and drowsiness, to the minimal levels present during sleep, depending on the patterns of activity in these modulatory nuclei.

Coma

The content of consciousness can be affected in predictable ways following damage to particular functional areas of cortex in either hemisphere, as described later in this chapter. However, consciousness itself also can be impaired or lost in certain pathologic conditions. In this case, bilateral damage is always required, affecting either large parts of the network of modulatory nuclei, the axons leaving the brainstem components of the network and traveling through the midbrain, or very large areas of cerebral cortex or subcortical white matter (Fig. 19-2). This is because consciousness results not from activity in any particular part of the CNS but rather from interactions among structures throughout the cerebrum; unlike certain cognitive abilities discussed later, neither cerebral hemisphere plays a critical role. Hence, even a massive stroke, if confined to one hemisphere, does not cause substantial long-term changes in level of consciousness (although it could cause major changes in the content of consciousness). In contrast, a relatively small lesion in the brainstem that affects ascending noradrenergic, serotonergic, and cholinergic fibers bilaterally results in coma, an extended period of unconsciousness from which someone cannot be aroused.

PHYSIOLOGY & CLINICAL MEDICINE

Breathing Patterns in Coma

Several pattern generators in the pons and medulla interact to produce normal, rhythmic breathing. As a result, characteristically altered breathing patterns accompany damage at particular sites in comatose patients. Cheyne-Stokes respiration—periods of hyperventilation alternating with apneic episodes—may indicate bilateral cerebral damage. Persistent hyperventilation may indicate midbrain damage that disrupts descending projections to the reparatory pattern generators, and intermittent cessation of breathing may indicate damage to the pattern generators themselves.

Coma does not persist indefinitely following brain damage. After a period of no more than a few weeks, almost all comatose patients either emerge from the coma, fail to survive, or enter a vegetative state in which some aspects of sleep-wake cycles and some brainstem functions resume but cortical functions remain absent.

Sleep and Wakefulness

All animals show rhythmic periods of increased and decreased activity. It is not always clear that the periods of inactivity are equivalent to what we think of as sleep, but in many instances this seems to be the case.

Sleep is a state of decreased but not abolished consciousness from which an individual can be aroused. Most of us sleep at night, in a quiet, comfortable place, and it was thought for a time that sleep is a passive process induced by withdrawal of sensory stimuli—the brain has nothing to work on, so it stops working for a while. This does not explain why we usually wake up 7 to 8 hours after we go to sleep whether sensory stimuli resume or not, and we now know that sleep is an actively induced state that involves carefully orchestrated changes in various components of the modulatory network. Specific parts of the brain turn the sleep state on and off at regular intervals.

Sleep Stages

Mammalian sleep has several stages, most easily defined by electroencephalographic criteria, and the stages have different physiologic and anatomic correlates. The electrical signals recorded as the electroencephalogram (EEG) are caused by synaptic current flowing into or out of the dendrites of cortical pyramidal cells, and normal, attentive wakefulness is accompanied by a low-voltage, desynchronized EEG that reflects different pyramidal cells doing different things at any point in time. Beginning with the onset of sleep, the EEG goes through four stages in which it gets progressively larger, slower and more synchronized, corresponding to falling more and more deeply asleep. In stage 4, the deepest of the four stages, the EEG is almost totally slow waves, so this stage is also referred to as slow-wave sleep. Then at intervals of 90 minutes or so, the EEG changes retrace themselves and some time is spent in a desynchronized EEG state that looks like an awake or lightly asleep condition; in fact, however, an individual in this state is often harder to awaken than someone in

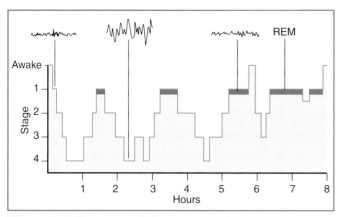

Figure 19-3. Sequence of sleep stage and electroencephalographic changes in a typical night's sleep of a young adult.

TABLE 19-1. Major Characteristics of Non-REM and REM Sleep

Feature	Non-REM Sleep	REM Sleep
EEG	Large, slow, synchronized (in deeper stages)	Small, fast, desynchronized
Dreams	Vague	Detailed, emotional
Muscle tone	Reduced	Almost abolished
Autonomic activity	↑ Parasympathetic	↑ Sympathetic

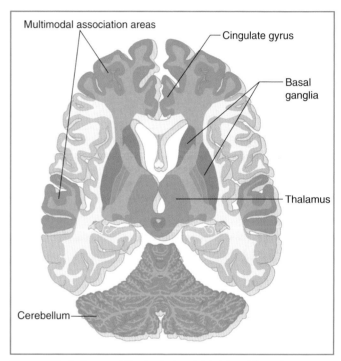

Figure 19-4. Areas of the brain in which blood flow decreases during deep stages of non-REM sleep, relative to wakefulness. (Based on Braun AR, Balkin TJ, Wesenten NJ, et al. Regional cerebral blood flow throughout the sleep-wake cycle: an $H_2^{15}O$ PET study. *Brain* 1997;120(pt 7):1173-1197.)

the depths of slow-wave sleep. This is a completely different sleep stage called REM sleep (rapid eye movement sleep), in which the eyes dart around beneath closed lids (as opposed to stages 1 to 4, which collectively are called non-REM sleep). We cycle through these sleep stages all night long, 4 to 6 cycles per night (Fig. 19-3). The non-REM episodes get shorter and the REM episodes get longer as the night progresses, so most non-REM sleep is experienced early in the night and most REM sleep closer to dawn.

Non-REM and REM sleep have strikingly different properties (Table 19-1). During non-REM sleep, heart rate, blood pressure, respiratory rate and the set point of the hypothalamic thermostat all decrease; gut motility increases. Blood flow to the brain decreases, particularly in the thalamus, basal ganglia, and multimodal and limbic areas of cortex (Fig. 19-4). Muscle tone decreases but is not abolished: we regularly roll around in bed during non-REM sleep, and slow-wave sleep is typically when sleepwalking occurs. People awakened from non-REM sleep often do not report dreams. If they do, the dreams have little detailed imagery. Slow-wave sleep, in general, sounds restful and restorative, although there is relatively little evidence that this is its function.

REM sleep is a much more peculiar state, with both tonic and phasic characteristics. Heart rate, blood pressure, and respiratory rate increase again and fluctuate irregularly. Muscle tone disappears almost completely owing to inhibition of both alpha and gamma motor neurons. The hypothalamic thermostat shuts off, and temperature regulation becomes "reptilian." Superimposed on this baseline are bursts of rapid eye movements and twitches of other muscles. Cerebral blood flow increases almost to waking levels, except in multimodal cortical association areas, where it stays depressed (Fig. 19-5). People awakened from REM sleep are very likely to report that they were dreaming, and that the dream had detailed visual imagery, a story, and emotional overtones. This fits nicely with the changes in blood flow: the seeming plausibility and the emotionality of events in dreams would be countered when awake by activity in multimodal areas.

We apparently need both slow-wave and REM sleep, and they seem to serve different needs. For example, someone selectively deprived of REM sleep will spend more time in REM sleep after the period of deprivation. In addition, the amount of time spent in REM sleep changes over our lifespan. Newborns spend half of their sleep time in REM, and for premature infants the figure may be 80% or more. Adults, in contrast, spend only 20% to 25% of their sleep time in REM and progressively less time in slow-wave sleep as they age.

Neurobiology of Sleep

Non-REM and REM sleep also have different anatomic substrates. In general terms, the modulatory activating network shown in Figure 19-1 is periodically inhibited by other parts of the CNS, resulting in non-REM sleep; during

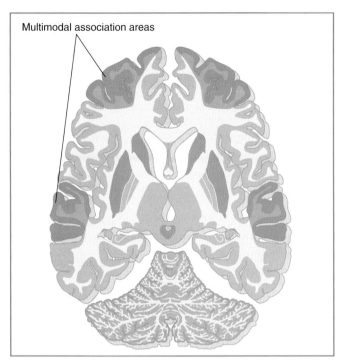

Figure 19-5. Areas of the brain in which blood flow remains diminished during REM sleep, relative to wakefulness. (Based on Braun AR, Balkin TJ, Wesenten NJ, et al. Regional cerebral blood flow throughout the sleep-wake cycle: an $H_2^{15}O$ PET study. *Brain* 1997;120(pt 7):1173-1197.)

non-REM sleep, neurons in the pontine reticular formation initiate periods of REM sleep.

Non-REM Sleep

The network of modulatory nuclei distributed through the hypothalamus and rostral brainstem have mostly excitatory interconnections with each other, maintaining the activity of all of them during wakefulness. The orexin neurons in the lateral hypothalamus may have a particularly important role in this, projecting to all other nuclei in the network (Fig. 19-6). Degeneration of these neurons causes narcolepsy, in which those affected have irresistible bouts of daytime sleepiness and pass directly into REM sleep. Non-REM sleep is initiated by patterned inhibition of the modulatory network by projections from the preoptic hypothalamus and parts of the medulla in and near the nucleus of the solitary tract (Fig. 19-7). Cholinergic neurons become virtually silent, all the other nuclei in the network slow down (Table 19-2), and consciousness is greatly diminished.

PHARMACOLOGY

Side Effects of Antihistamines

Antihistamines are used for symptomatic relief of allergic reactions caused by histamine release, but to the extent to which they block CNS histamine receptors they cause drowsiness as well. Diphenhydramine is used for this reason as a sleep aid.

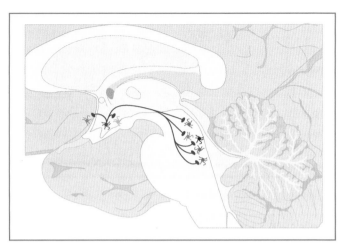

Figure 19-6. Orexin neurons in the lateral hypothalamus, in addition to their widespread projections to the cerebrum, make excitatory synapses on all the other components of the modulatory network that maintains wakefulness. (See also Fig. 19-1 for an explanation of the components of this network.)

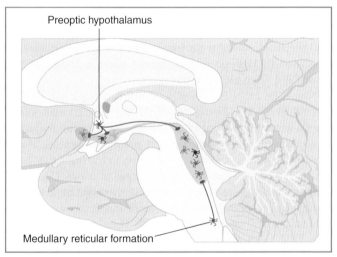

Figure 19-7. Inhibitory projections (red) from the preoptic hypothalamus and the medullary reticular formation periodically reduce the activity of neurons in the wakefulness-promoting network. (See also Fig. 19-1 for an explanation of the components of this network.) The way in which these two sets of inhibitory inputs are coordinated with each other in normal sleep-wake cycles is not understood.

TABLE 19-2. Changes in Firing Rates of Sleep-related Neurons During Non-REM and REM Sleep

Neurons	Awake State	Non-REM Sleep	REM Sleep
Preoptic hypothalamus	–	++	+
Raphe nuclei, locus ceruleus, orexin, histamine	++	+	–
Brainstem cholinergic	+	–	++

These features are broadly consistent with clinical observations. Patients with bilateral damage in the reticular formation of the midbrain or rostral pons, as noted above, are initially comatose because the brainstem components of the modulatory network are cut off from the cerebrum. (This state is different from non-REM sleep at least in part because the slowed input from neurons of the locus ceruleus and raphe nuclei [see Table 19-2] is missing.) They may subsequently enter a vegetative state, with some aspects of sleep-wake cycles maintained by hypothalamic parts of the network and independently by brainstem parts of the network; the continued lack of brainstem input prevents meaningful cortical activity. Remarkably, experimental animals with carefully controlled damage in the midpontine reticular formation, just a few millimeters caudal to where damage would cause coma, are constantly awake because inhibitory projections from the caudal brainstem are unable to reach the modulatory network.

REM Sleep

Unlike the distributed network that controls transitions between wakefulness and non-REM sleep, REM sleep is orchestrated by cholinergic neurons in the pontine reticular formation (Fig. 19-8) that periodically become active during non-REM sleep. These project directly or indirectly to the thalamus and basal nucleus, increasing the level of cortical activity (see Figs. 19-3 and 19-5 and Table 19-2); to the paramedian pontine reticular formation (PPRF) and other eye movement control centers, causing the rapid eye movements characteristic of this sleep stage; and indirectly to reticulospinal neurons in the rostral medulla that inhibit lower motor neurons and cause loss of muscle tone. Most narcoleptic patients have episodes of cataplexy, in which

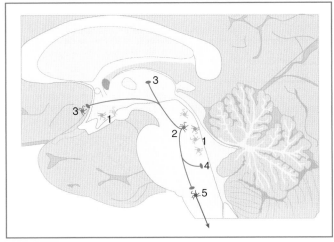

Figure 19-8. Circuitry underlying REM sleep. Although most components of the wakefulness-promoting network remain inactive during sleep (1), a set of cholinergic neurons in the pontine reticular formation becomes active (2). These in turn activate the thalamus and basal nucleus (3), causing a waking-like EEG, as well as saccade pattern generators (4), causing rapid eye movements, and inhibitory reticulospinal neurons (5), causing loss of muscle tone.

emotional situations elicit a sudden loss of muscle tone, caused by inappropriate triggering of the latter part of the REM circuitry.

The nature of the "clock" for the 90-minute periodicity of REM sleep is unknown, but periodic firing of orexin, raphe, and locus ceruleus neurons help terminate each episode by inhibiting the cholinergic neurons that initiated it.

Sleep Periodicity

Each species sleeps during a characteristic part of the day for a characteristic period of time. Humans, for example, sleep at night for about 8 hours, whereas other animals sleep for longer or shorter periods at different times of the day or night. The quantity of sleep is regulated homeostatically, so that too little sleep one night is typically followed by drowsiness the next day and easy falling asleep the next night for a longer than usual time. Regulation of the quantity of sleep is based in part on the accumulation of some substances in the CNS during wakefulness and their dissipation during sleep. Prominent among these is adenosine, which is released at greater rates by neuronal activity during wakefulness. Adenosine levels continue to rise throughout the day (or during the night in nocturnal animals), eventually causing drowsiness by inhibiting cholinergic neurons of the basal nucleus and other wakefulness-promoting neurons.

Superimposed on this increasing tendency to sleep as periods of activity progress is a circadian rhythm of sleep and wakefulness. Hence, whether sleep-deprived or not we get sleepy at night and are more alert during the day. This is based on direct and indirect projections from the suprachiasmatic nucleus to sleep and wake centers in the anterior and posterior hypothalamus.

●●● HIGHER CORTICAL FUNCTION

Many species respond in relatively rigid, predictable ways to stimuli of various sorts. Primates and some other mammals, in contrast, have a much broader and more flexible behavioral repertoire. Humans in particular have a seemingly limitless array of response patterns. This flexibility in responding is directly related to expanded amounts of association cortex (Fig. 19-9), which are interposed between sensory and motor cortices and provide the substrate for modifying responses to fit different situations.

Although the networks of interconnections between cortical areas are far-flung and complex, a simplified version of the connections underlying possible responses to seeing something (Fig. 19-10) exemplifies the general pattern. Primary visual cortex does some initial sorting of different aspects of the stimulus, then projects to multiple areas of unimodal visual association cortex. Dorsal association areas (often referred to as the "where" pathway) analyze the location and movement of the stimulus further, and ventral areas (the "what" pathway) analyze its shape, color, and identity. These unimodal areas then project to several multimodal association areas, where the visual appearance of the object is integrated with other properties such as its sound or tactile qualities. Particular multimodal areas subserve distinctive aspects of cognition related to the object, such as directing attention to it, naming and discussing it, assessing its significance in light of homeostatic needs and prior experiences,

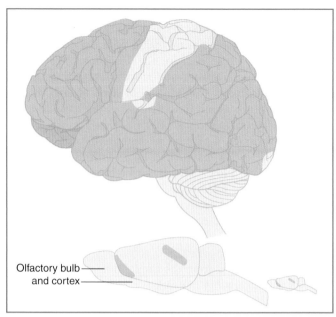

Figure 19-9. Relative amounts of association cortex in the brain of a human and of a typical rodent. The absolute differences are substantially greater, as indicated by the drawing of the rodent brain (lower right) to the same scale as that of the human brain.

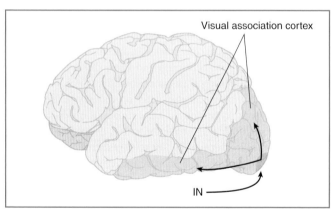

A

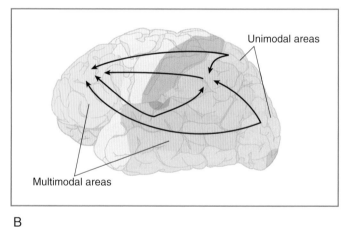

B

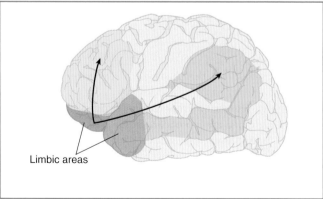

C

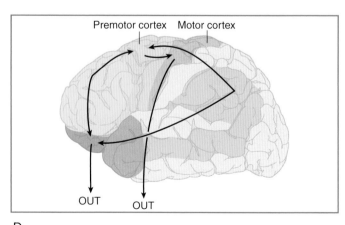

D

Figure 19-10. Simplified overview of information flow through cortical areas of different types. **A,** Information (in this case visual) arrives at a primary sensory area, is dissected into multiple components, and is distributed to unimodal association areas. **B,** Unimodal areas of multiple types project to multimodal areas. **C,** Memories and emotions are factored in through limbic inputs. **D,** Projections from multimodal areas to motor and limbic areas initiate some combination of behavioral and autonomic responses.

and deciding on a course of action. In a very general sense, posterior multimodal areas are more important for identifying and directing attention to things, and anterior areas for devising responses. However, multimodal areas are extensively interconnected with each other, and in effect they act collaboratively to sort things out and then initiate some combination of autonomic and behavioral responses through the limbic system and motor areas of cortex.

The primary visual cortices of the two hemispheres have asymmetric properties in the sense that each receives inputs from the contralateral half of the visual field of each eye (see Fig. 12-12). Asymmetries continue into association and limbic cortices, but in a broader, functional sense. In the unimodal visual association cortex of the occipitotemporal gyrus, for example, more cells in the left hemisphere are involved in encoding the shapes of letters and more cells in the right hemisphere are involved in encoding facial features. The hemisphere that is more important for language (the left, in a large majority of people) is commonly referred to as the dominant hemisphere. However, calling it the language-dominant hemisphere is probably more appropriate because, as described in various parts of this chapter, the "nondominant" hemisphere is in fact more important for a number of other functions. Under normal circumstances, we have little conscious awareness of these functional asymmetries because the corpus callosum and anterior commissure coordinate and unify the activities of the two hemispheres.

This broad framework provides a rationale for understanding the consequences of damage in different cortical areas. Lesions in unimodal areas cause loss of the ability to utilize some part of a single type of sensory information. Lesions in multimodal areas cause defects in particular cognitive abilities, no matter which sensory modality is utilized. Finally, lesions in limbic areas cause abnormal responses in emotional or drive-related situations, as well as memory deficits.

Unimodal Areas

Primary sensory and motor areas, as the principal routes through which sensory information reaches consciousness and voluntary movements are initiated, are the portals between the outside world and the rest of the cerebral cortex. As a result, damage to one of these areas typically causes a general deficit in the function it deals with—loss of vision in all or part of the contralateral visual fields after damage to primary visual cortex, for example, or contralateral weakness after damage to primary motor cortex.

Each primary sensory area projects to nearby unimodal association cortex (Fig. 19-11). Each of these in turn includes multiple subareas specialized for different aspects of the analysis of stimuli in that modality. Visual association cortex is the best understood, but other sensory systems have generally analogous sets of connections. Primary auditory and somatosensory cortexes even have their own equivalents of "what" and "where" pathways devoted to the identification

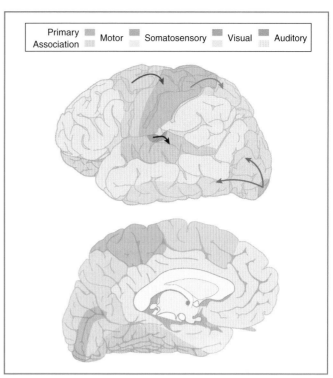

Primary Association | Motor | Somatosensory | Visual | Auditory

Figure 19-11. Unimodal association areas. Although not shown in the figure, primary gustatory/visceral cortex in the insula has an adjacent association area; the insula also contains additional auditory and somatosensory association areas.

and localization of auditory and somatosensory stimuli. Because of this fractionation of function in unimodal association areas, partial damage can cause selective losses of only certain functional aspects of a sensory system, resulting in disorders such as sensory-specific agnosias. Agnosia means "lack of knowledge," and refers to an inability to recognize classes of objects. In the sensory-specific agnosias caused by damage to unimodal association cortex, basic sensation is intact but the ability to recognize objects using that sensory modality is impaired. For example, damage to the face-processing area of visual association cortex (in the occipitotemporal gyrus) causes prosopagnosia, in which someone is unable to recognize previously familiar faces despite being able to see the facial features. The deficit is restricted to visual identification and is fairly selective for faces: familiar individuals can still be recognized by their voices or by watching them walk. Similarly, damage in somatosensory association cortex can cause tactile agnosia, in which the sense of touch is intact but the ability to recognize objects by palpation is impaired, and damage in auditory association cortex can cause auditory agnosia, in which sounds can be heard and described but not recognized.

Likewise, motor association cortex (premotor cortex and the supplementary motor area) is a mosaic of six or more areas, each specialized for some aspect of motor planning. Damage here causes minimal weakness but impairments in more complex aspects of movement, such as coordinating

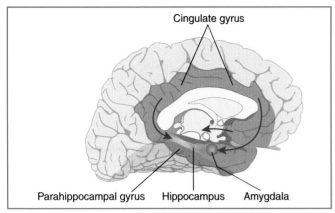

Figure 19-12. Limbic cortex as a series of unimodal areas that initiate responses through the hippocampus, amygdala, and hypothalamus, rather than through motor areas of cortex.

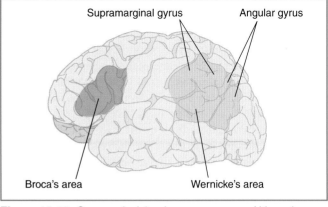

Figure 19-13. Core perisylvian language areas. Although traditional descriptions focus on Broca's and Wernicke's areas, additional areas such as the supramarginal and angular gyri are also involved in normal language functions.

the two sides of the body, performing sequences of movements, or getting movements to match objects.

Finally, limbic cortex can be thought of as a group of unimodal association areas that provide an interface between multimodal areas and the hypothalamus, amygdala, and hippocampus (Fig. 19-12). Its connections with the hypothalamus and amygdala help coordinate behavioral, autonomic, and hormonal responses (see Chapter 18), whereas those with the hippocampus play a central role in memory for facts and events (see Chapter 20).

Multimodal Areas

We routinely combine multiple attributes of objects and situations as part of everyday cognitive functions, e.g., noting the color, softness, and perhaps the smell of a piece of fruit and combining these with memories of prior experiences to anticipate its flavor. This is the province of multimodal association areas, which serve as portals not to the outside world but rather to aspects of conscious experience such as language, selective attention, emotional reactions, strategizing, and forming and accessing memories.

Language
Language, a system for communicating by means of symbols linked with objects and concepts, involves a neural substrate that exemplifies several recurring themes in the connections and functions of multimodal association cortex.
1. Language is intrinsically multimodal, because the essence of a word is its symbolic meaning rather than the modality through which it is presented or received. Hence, weakness of laryngeal muscles would cause impaired speaking (dysarthria) but would have no effect on written language. Similarly, blindness would make it impossible to read (unless reading Braille) but would have no effect on the comprehension of spoken language. Loss of language functions (aphasia) requires damage to multimodal language areas or their connections.

2. Posterior language areas are more involved in the comprehension of language, and anterior areas are more involved in its production (Table 19-3). Hence, posterior lesions result in fluent aphasias, in which language production is plentiful but inaccurate because comprehension is impaired. In contrast, lesions that include anterior language areas result in nonfluent aphasias, in which language production is sparse but comprehension may be relatively intact.

3. Language is one of the most prominently and consistently lateralized cognitive functions. About 95% of right-handers have a language-dominant left hemisphere. Left-handed individuals are more likely to have a language-dominant right hemisphere or to have language functions shared between the two hemispheres, but even so about 70% have a language-dominant left hemisphere.

The core language areas (Fig. 19-13) border the left lateral sulcus and are referred to as the perisylvian language zone (because the lateral sulcus is also known as the fissure of Sylvius, or sylvian fissure). Prominent among them are Wernicke's area, in the posterior part of the superior temporal gyrus, and Broca's area, in the posterior part of the inferior frontal gyrus. The arcuate fasciculus (see Fig. 5-8) interconnects anterior and posterior parts of the perisylvian zone. In the traditional model of language functions, Wernicke's area associates words with objects and concepts and forwards this information through the arcuate fasciculus to Broca's area, where plans for the production of language are devised. This accounts for prominent aspects of the major aphasia syndromes (see Table 19-3). Damage centered on Wernicke's area causes Wernicke's aphasia, essentially agnosia for words. This is a fluent aphasia in which comprehension is severely impaired and many paraphasias (incorrect words or parts of words) are produced (presumably because the inaccuracies are not comprehended). Damage centered on Broca's area, in contrast, causes Broca's aphasia, a nonfluent aphasia in which comprehension is less affected, and small numbers of meaningful words are produced with great effort.

TABLE 19-3. Aphasia Syndromes and Typical Associated Lesions

Aphasia	Fluency	Comprehension	Repetition	Typical Damage
Wernicke's	+	↓	↓	
Conduction	+	+	↓	
Transcortical sensory	+	↓	+	
Broca's	↓	+	↓	
Transcortical motor	↓	+	+	
Global	↓	↓	↓	

↓, Prominently impaired; +, *relatively* unimpaired (though rarely normal).

Damage between the two areas causes conduction aphasia, a fluent aphasia (because Broca's area is intact) in which comprehension is relatively good (because Wernicke's area is intact) but language output is paraphasic (supposedly because communication through the arcuate fasciculus is disrupted). Finally, damage to the entire perisylvian zone (as in a large middle cerebral artery stroke—see Fig. 7-13) causes global aphasia, a nonfluent aphasia in which comprehension is impaired. In all of these cases, repetition of spoken words is defective.

The network of neural structures involved in language comprehension and production is actually much more extensive than indicated in this traditional model, however, and includes extrasylvian cortical areas, multisynaptic connections between different cortical areas, parts of the basal ganglia, and even interactions with parts of the cerebellum. As a result, damage restricted to Wernicke's or Broca's area or the arcuate fasciculus does not cause profound, lasting language deficits; full-blown syndromes always involve damage to adjoining cortical areas and underlying white matter. In addition, the partitioning into comprehension areas and production areas is more relative than absolute. For example, the comprehension of patients with Broca's aphasia breaks down as sentences become longer or more complex.

Perisylvian language areas do not work independently of the rest of the cortex. Wernicke's area and the adjoining angular and supramarginal gyri collect information from surrounding sensory areas; Broca's area collaborates with other frontal areas. As a result, extrasylvian damage can cause a variety of syndromes called transcortical aphasias (see Table 19-3). Because the perisylvian zone is intact in these syndromes, a hallmark of transcortical aphasias is that repetition is relatively preserved.

Although the language-dominant hemisphere takes care of the mapping of symbols and the rules of grammar, the other hemisphere plays its own major role in communication. Much of the meaning in speech is conveyed not by the words themselves but by the rhythm and intonation used to deliver them. (Think about how easy it is to change the meaning of any few words—e.g., "I am"—from a simple statement, to an angry affirmation, to a question, just by changing the way they are said.) These aspects of language, referred to as prosody, are dealt with by a right-hemisphere network that is largely a mirror image of the left perisylvian zone. Thus, damage to the right inferior frontal gyrus causes a diminished ability to convey emotion or emphasis by voice or gesture, and damage to the right superior temporal gyrus causes difficulty comprehending emotion or emphasis in the voices or gestures of others.

Praxis

Just as we learn to string together correct words in correct sequences, we also learn to use other complex sequences of muscle contractions effortlessly in voluntary movements such as gestures and using tools. This ability, called praxis (Greek, "to act," "to do"), depends on patterns stored in or accessed by the multimodal association cortex of the language-dominant parietal lobe. Damage there can cause bilateral apraxia, a condition in which strength, sensation, and coordination are preserved but a patient is nevertheless unable to perform some types of skilled, purposeful movements. Apraxia comes in several forms, some affecting the limbs and others the mouth, and some affecting the ability to make sequences of movements only under certain conditions. An apraxic patient may be unable to blow out an imaginary match, for example, but have no trouble with a real one, or be unable to use either a real or an imaginary screwdriver properly. Because parietal multimodal cortex is extensively interconnected with premotor cortex, frontal damage in the language-dominant hemisphere also can cause apraxia (Fig. 19-14).

Attention and Spatial Orientation

Much more information comes into the CNS through all its sensory channels than it is able to analyze, and a major task is to focus attention on important items and keep track of how the body is oriented relative to them. Each hemisphere monitors the contralateral side of the world and body, but the right hemisphere, particularly right parietal multimodal cortex, plays the dominant role in forming global views; for attentional purposes, it monitors the ipsilateral side as well (Fig. 19-15). As a result, following right hemisphere damage, the left hemisphere is unable to compensate and some level of contralateral neglect often results. In mild forms, this may show up only as extinction, in which only the stimulus on the right is perceived when there are simultaneous bilateral stimuli (e.g., touches on both hands, sounds in both ears). In more severe forms, the left half of the world and even of

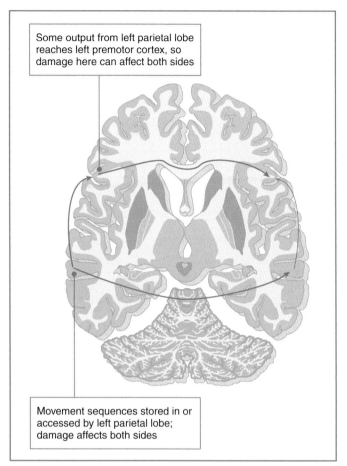

the body may essentially "disappear." Words on the left side of pages may be missed, food on the left side of a plate left uneaten, only the right side of the face shaved or right limbs dressed; ownership of the left limbs may even be denied. As in the case of apraxia, right parietal multimodal cortex is extensively interconnected with other multimodal areas, and forms of neglect have been reported following damage in the right frontal or temporal lobe.

The global view of the outside world formed by the right parietal lobe also is important for orienting to the world, for navigating through it, and for assembling the parts of a whole. Patients with damage here may have difficulty finding their way along familiar routes, putting puzzles together, or drawing geometric patterns.

Executive Functions

Making decisions about objects and situations perceived and attended to involves prefrontal cortex, and resourcefulness in doing so is consistent with the large expanse of this cortex in primates like humans. Collectively, these frontal problem-solving and decision-making functions, often referred to as executive functions, underlie the patterns of actions that we construe as the personality and character of others.

Figure 19-14. Left parietal dominance for skilled movements using either side of the body as the basis for some forms of apraxia.

In the figure:

Some output from left parietal lobe reaches left premotor cortex, so damage here can affect both sides

Movement sequences stored in or accessed by left parietal lobe; damage affects both sides

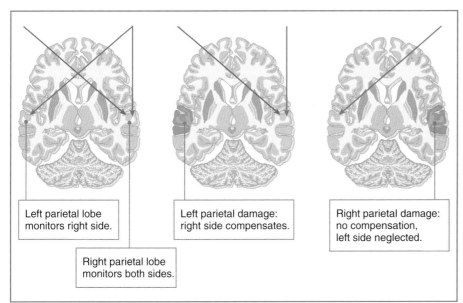

Figure 19-15. The probable basis of left-sided neglect following right hemisphere (usually parietal) damage.

Left parietal lobe monitors right side.

Right parietal lobe monitors both sides.

Left parietal damage: right side compensates.

Right parietal damage: no compensation, left side neglected.

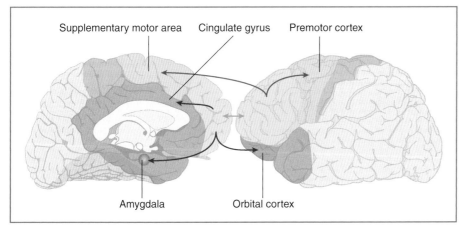

Supplementary motor area   Cingulate gyrus   Premotor cortex

Amygdala   Orbital cortex

Figure 19-16. Major connections of prefrontal cortex. Both dorsolateral and ventromedial areas receive inputs from numerous unimodal areas, from posterior multimodal areas (see also Fig. 19-10B), and from each other, but they have different emphases in their outputs. Dorsolateral areas focus on premotor and supplementary motor areas and the formulation of behavioral responses. Ventromedial areas focus on limbic cortex and the amygdala and motivational responses.

Prefrontal cortex, like other association areas, is a collection of multiple subareas. These fall into two broad categories (Fig. 19-16): the parts in the superior and middle frontal gyri on the lateral surface of the hemisphere (dorsolateral prefrontal cortex) and those on the medial surface, merging with the orbital gyri (ventromedial prefrontal cortex). Dorsolateral regions specialize in applying rules and strategies, e.g., deciding on a logical next move in a chess game. Ventromedial regions factor in motivational issues, such as the likelihood that a particular decision is socially acceptable or will lead to reward or loss. Prefrontal functions are not so strongly lateralized as those of other multimodal areas, and unilateral damage often has relatively limited effects.

Dorsolateral prefrontal cortex uses its widespread inputs from other association areas in part as the basis for working memory, the multiple bits of thought we can keep "in mind" at a given time and use for devising plans. A common example of the use of working memory is looking up a telephone number and remembering it long enough to key it in, but the same kind of memory is used constantly to keep

track of the flow of events around us. Patients with dorsolateral prefrontal damage have difficulty filtering out irrelevant aspects of a situation, changing strategies that are not working, initiating tasks, and shifting from one task to another.

The best-known case of ventromedial damage was that of Phineas Gage, who was the foreman of a railroad crew working near a small town in Vermont in the mid-1800s. A blasting accident propelled a 3-foot iron bar upward through his head, destroying most of his ventromedial prefrontal cortex bilaterally. Miraculously, he survived, but a marked personality change was noted after he recovered. Prior to the accident, he was industrious, responsible, and considerate. Afterward, he was impulsive, rude, and emotionally unpredictable.

Disconnection Syndromes

Because cognitive functions depend on networks of interconnected cortical areas (e.g., see Fig. 19-10), they can also be disrupted by white matter lesions that disconnect cortical

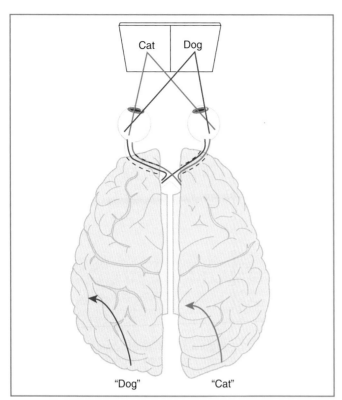

Figure 19-17. Severing the corpus callosum disconnects the language functions of the left hemisphere from functions of the right hemisphere. Because the left hand and the left visual fields are represented almost exclusively in the right hemisphere, such a patient would be unable to read words presented to the left ("Cat") and unable to name objects in the left hand (despite being able to use the object with that hand).

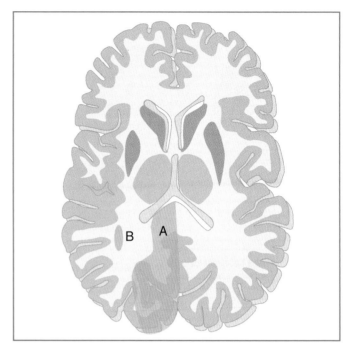

Figure 19-18. Lesions that could cause alexia without agraphia. Damage at site A would cause right homonymous hemianopia, so words in the right visual field obviously could not be read; in addition, information from the left visual field could not reach language areas because of damage to the splenium of the corpus callosum, so reading would be globally impaired. A much smaller lesion at site B would leave visual fields intact but could nevertheless selectively impair reading by preventing all visual information from reaching language areas.

areas from one another. The most extreme example of such a disconnection syndrome is caused by sectioning of the corpus callosum, a drastic surgery done in rare situations to prevent the spread of seizures from one hemisphere to the other. One aspect of the resulting disconnection would be a cutting off of the right hemisphere from language areas in the left hemisphere (Fig. 19-17). As a result, such a patient would be unable to name anything held in the left hand or read words flashed in the left visual hemifield; oddly enough, because the ears are represented bilaterally in auditory cortex (see Fig. 10-16), the same patient would be able to respond to words spoken in either ear.

One of the first disconnection syndromes described is pure word blindness, an acquired inability to read. Auditory comprehension is intact, because this is a form of visual agnosia selective for words. Writing is unaffected in this syndrome, so it is also called alexia without agraphia (literally, "loss of reading without loss of writing"). The first cause described for pure word blindness was a stroke in the territory of the left posterior cerebral artery territory (see Fig. 7-13), affecting left visual cortex and the posterior part of the corpus callosum (Fig. 19-18). Language areas in and near Wernicke's area and the angular gyrus that associate words with their

meanings were intact, since these areas are supplied by the middle cerebral artery. However, visual information was unable to reach these areas from the left hemisphere (damaged left occipital lobe) or from the right hemisphere (damaged corpus callosum). Smaller lesions causing this syndrome have since been described (see Fig. 19-18), underscoring that there are multiple locations at which visual information can be intercepted on its way to language areas.

Limbic Areas

The limbic lobe is the counterpart of premotor and supplementary motor cortex in mediating emotional expression and in the formation of some forms of memory.

The anterior cingulate gyrus and nearby areas are interposed between multiple association areas and the amygdala and hypothalamus (Fig. 19-19), positioning it to play an important role in the triggering and modulation of the expression and experience of emotion. Its connections with ventromedial prefrontal cortex and the amygdala also make anterior cingulate cortex part of the circuitry involved in comprehending the emotional significance of situations and events. Blood flow increases in this area, for example, not only during a painful experience but also when looking at a picture of someone else in uncomfortable

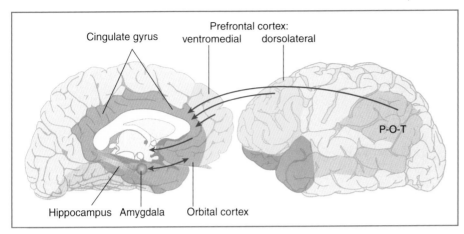

Figure 19-19. Major connections underlying the role of anterior limbic regions in comprehending and responding to the emotional significance of events. P-O-T, parietal-occipital-temporal multimodal association cortex.

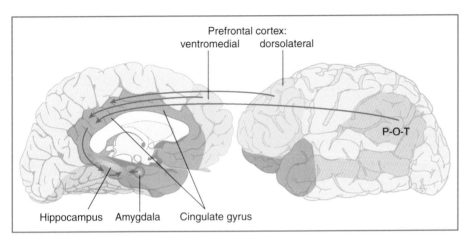

Figure 19-20. Major connections underlying the role of posterior limbic regions in collaborating with the hippocampus in memory formation. P-O-T, parietal-occipital-temporal multimodal association cortex.

PATHOLOGY & CLINICAL MEDICINE

Misidentification Syndromes

Some patients with prosopagnosia have autonomic responses to familiar faces (despite not recognizing them consciously), as though their face-processing circuits were still connected to the limbic system. An even more peculiar condition is the Capgras syndrome, in which someone recognizes friends and family but insists that they have been replaced by impostors. This is almost the reverse of prosopagnosia, as though the face-processing circuits have been disconnected from the limbic system and the brain devises an explanation for the lack of emotional responses to familiar faces.

circumstances. Conversely, disconnection of the anterior cingulate/ventromedial prefrontal/amygdala network from other association areas can cause a variety of peculiar syndromes in which objective recognition of people or objects or situations is relatively normal but realization of their emotional significance is lost.

Posterior cingulate cortex, together with its continuation as the parahippocampal gyrus, has particularly extensive inputs from both unimodal and multimodal association areas (Fig. 19-20) and, in turn, provides the major input to the hippocampus. This is a key part of the critical circuitry for forming new memories of facts and events, as described further in Chapter 20.

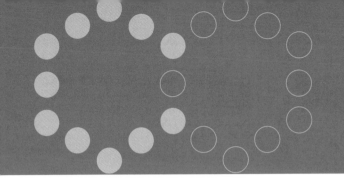

Formation, Maintenance, and Plasticity of Neuronal Connections

20

CONTENTS

MAJOR THEMES

DEVELOPMENT OF NEURONAL PATHWAYS AND CONNECTIONS
    Overproduction and Pruning
    Critical Periods

PLASTICITY OF NEURONAL CONNECTIONS IN ADULTS
    Learning and Memory
    Molecular Basis of Learning and Memory
    Repair of Damage in the Nervous System

The nervous system is not nearly so good at repairing itself as most other organs are, probably as a tradeoff that allows it to develop and maintain its amazing level of complexity. The repair mechanisms that do exist are largely variants of developmental mechanisms, and now there is hope that the same mechanisms can be coaxed to work better in adults following injury or disease.

●●● MAJOR THEMES

There is a progressive decrease in plasticity—the ability to alter connections in the nervous system—from fetal life to adulthood. Plasticity during development allows the nervous system to become tuned to the body and its environment but carries with it the hazard that an abnormal environment can cause permanently abnormal development. Stability of the adult brain, on the other hand, maintains its complexity (except when we purposely want to modify it, as in learning) but makes it vulnerable to damage.

Orderly development of connections, and to some extent the maintenance of connections once they have developed, involves chemical signaling in both directions between neurons and their targets.

In adults, the peripheral nervous system is much better at repairing itself than the CNS is, although we seem to be on the verge of being able to enhance CNS repair considerably.

●●● DEVELOPMENT OF NEURONAL PATHWAYS AND CONNECTIONS

Mammalian genomes are extensive and complicated, but not nearly enough to specify all the different neuronal types, arrangements, and connections in the nervous system. Hence, there must be developmental processes that allow all this complexity to unfold. The general idea that has emerged is that the arrangement of the nervous system is broadly specified genetically, then fine-tuned by interactions with other parts of the nervous system, other parts of the body, and the outside world.

Overproduction and Pruning

Overproduction and Death of Neurons

The nervous system develops as a series of modules, such as spinal cord segments, brainstem subdivisions, and parts of the cerebrum, each based on a set of neural progenitor cells in some part of the wall of the neural tube (e.g., see Fig. 6-10). Each module is subsequently modified as necessary to meet its particular functional requirements. This is perhaps most apparent in the spinal cord, where lumbar and especially cervical segments, which innervate limb muscles with many small motor units, contain many more lower motor neurons than do thoracic segments (Fig. 20-1). One way to do this might be to grow extra motor neurons at levels where they are needed. However, the initially surprising mechanism actually used is the production of substantially more neurons than needed, followed by death of the excess neurons. Presumably this ensures enough neurons for all the functions that need to be performed by any given module. Once a module is wired up in a preliminary fashion, unneeded neurons undergo programmed cell death, or apoptosis, a form of cellular suicide in which specific degradative enzymes

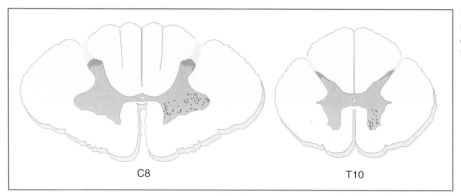

Figure 20-1. Relative numbers of motor neurons in a cross-section of the lower cervical (C8) and lower thoracic (T10) human spinal cord.

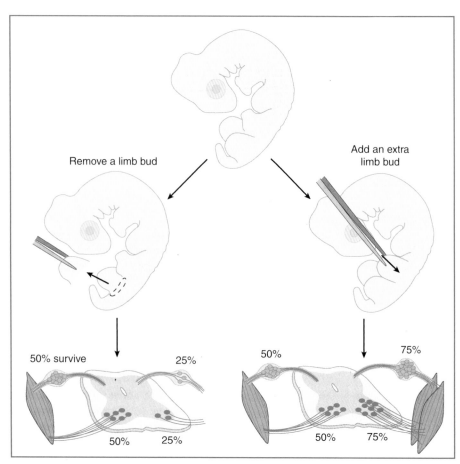

Figure 20-2. Removing or adding target tissue (in this case limb buds in a chick embryo) during development changes the degree of survival of motor neurons and dorsal root ganglion cells (and autonomic ganglion cells as well, although this is not indicated).

are synthesized and set loose. Overproduction of neurons followed by death of the surplus is not limited to motor neurons. At the level of the spinal cord, for example, segments with fewer motor neurons need fewer local interneurons and fewer upper motor neurons projecting to them. All over the nervous system, neurons are typically produced in two- to three-fold excess.

A major factor determining whether a neuron lives or dies is its degree of success in acquiring neurotrophic factors produced in limited quantities by postsynaptic targets and

other cells with which neurons interact.[1] This was first shown by increasing or decreasing the amount of peripheral target tissue in chick embryos, which results in saving or losing more motor neurons and dorsal root ganglion cells than normal (Fig. 20-2), but neurotrophic factors are generally active

[1]Hence, trophic, which means "nourishing," is something of a misnomer, because these factors, rather than providing metabolic support, actually prevent apoptosis.

throughout the nervous system, particularly during development. The most famous and first-described neurotrophic factor is nerve growth factor, which is critical for the survival of postganglionic sympathetic neurons and many dorsal root ganglion cells, but there are several others. Particular neuronal types are selective for specific neurotrophic factors or combinations of factors, which are transported retrogradely from postsynaptic neurons or tissues to the neuronal nucleus.

Overproduction and Pruning of Processes

Just as more neurons are produced than are needed, most of the neurons produce more branches than *they* need and then retract some. Innervation of muscle fibers is a particularly well-studied example. Each adult muscle fiber has a single neuromuscular junction, innervated by a single motor neuron (see Figs. 14-2 and 14-7), but this situation develops slowly as a result of an exchange of messages between muscle fibers and axonal endings. After the period of neuronal death, each of the remaining motor neurons innervates multiple muscle fibers, and each muscle fiber is innervated by multiple motor neurons (Fig. 20-3). The nerve terminals induce specializations such as acetylcholine receptor production and clustering of these receptors in the muscle membrane, and the muscle induces presynaptic active zones in the nerve terminals. The muscle fibers also produce neurotrophic factors, which act not just back in the neuronal cell body but also locally. The multiple nerve terminals compete for these factors until eventually all but one retracts. The "winner" takes over the neuromuscular junction, its active zones multiply, and the singly innervated adult junction results.

Similarly, cerebellar Purkinje cells (see Figs. 16-3 and 16-4) go through a period of innervation by multiple climbing fibers until one "wins." A period of overproduction of branches, competition, and pruning is widespread or universal in the CNS. For example, cortical pyramidal cells transiently produce axon branches that reach not only their expected targets but also inappropriate ones (Fig. 20-4); some in experimental animals are as bizarre as projections all the way from primary visual cortex to the spinal cord.

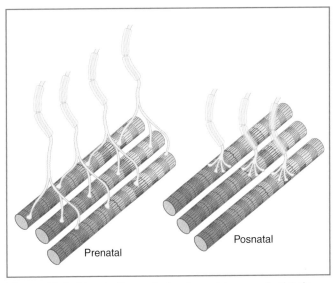

Figure 20-3. Muscle fibers start out receiving small, simple inputs from axons of multiple motor neurons, but by shortly after birth these have been pruned back until each fiber retains a single neuromuscular junction. The surviving junction becomes larger and more complex.

Critical Periods

This jockeying for synaptic territory is limited to a critical period, during which relatively permanent patterns of connections are set up. The best-studied example is the visual cortex, where ocular dominance columns (see Fig. 12-15) are only crudely formed at birth. As a result of postnatal binocular vision, terminals of lateral geniculate neurons conveying information from the right eye become dominant in some areas and those from the left eye in others. Once synapses have stabilized, the production of neurotrophic factors declines and change becomes more difficult. Thus, there is a critical period during which vision can influence the fine-tuning of visual cortex. If vision is abnormal during this critical period, then the final structure and function of visual

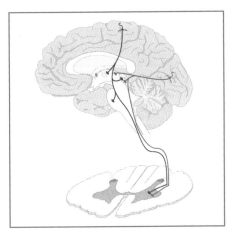

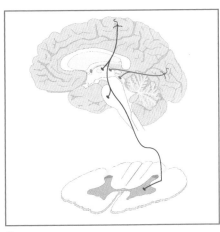

A   B

Figure 20-4. Pruning of branches of CNS axons during development. During the establishment of neuronal connections, pyramidal cells from different cortical areas make some synapses in functionally appropriate parts of the CNS and others in functionally inappropriate areas (**A**). In this case, a corticospinal neuron sends a branch to the superior colliculus, and a neuron in visual cortex sends a branch to the spinal cord. As neurons compete for trophic factors, the functionally inappropriate branches lose out and are retracted (**B**).

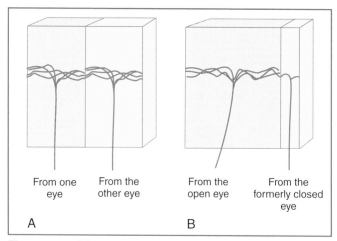

Figure 20-5. Effects of visual deprivation on the terminations of lateral geniculate axons in primary visual cortex. **A**, Geniculate axons convey information from only one eye, and they give rise to a profusion of synapses in one of the middle layers of primary visual cortex. Endings from one eye spread out over about 0.5 mm and alternate with endings from the other eye, forming the basis for ocular dominance columns (see Fig. 12-15). **B**, If one eye is covered during the critical period, its territory shrivels up irreversibly, inputs from the other eye expand to take over the vacated territory, and the vision in the temporarily deprived eye is degraded permanently.

cortex will be permanently abnormal. If, for example, input from one eye is blocked during the critical period, the normal eye will permanently dominate visual cortex and the covered eye will be functionally almost blind (Fig. 20-5). If the eyes are misaligned because of weakness of an extraocular muscle, binocular vision and depth perception will be permanently impaired. Other sensory systems (with the possible exception of the chemical senses) have analogous critical periods, all ending in the first few years of life. Similarly, inactivity of a muscle early in life causes permanent deficits in the inputs to its lower motor neurons.

There are critical periods for higher cortical functions as well. One famous demonstration was a comparison in the 1940s of the subsequent development of babies raised in a prison nursery (where they spent time with their mothers and other babies) and babies raised in a foundling home (where they were isolated most of the time). Starting at about 4 months of age, the babies raised in the foundling home became progressively more delayed developmentally—they were withdrawn, apathetic, inactive—and progressively more sickly. These differences were not reversible. Language development is another example. In a few unusual and unfortunate cases, children deprived of language exposure from birth had permanent deficits when exposed to language later, but more subtle deficits occur in all of us. At birth, infants can discriminate among all the speech sounds of all human languages, despite the fact that adults have difficulty discriminating differences not present in languages they learned when young. The change begins to occur during the first year of life and is determined by the language sounds infants hear

around them. Minimal exposure to sounds in other languages during this period permanently "rescues" the ability to discriminate among these sounds. This corresponds to the relative ease with which young children (compared to adults) can learn to speak a second language fluently and without an accent.

●●● PLASTICITY OF NEURONAL CONNECTIONS IN ADULTS

Once the nervous system has had time to wire itself up satisfactorily, critical periods end and change becomes more difficult. Modifications are still possible, however. For example, maps in areas like somatosensory and motor cortex (see Fig. 9-5), once thought to be fixed and immutable in adults, are now known to retain a significant degree of plasticity. This shows up as both practice effects and deprivation effects. Overuse of one finger compared to others (e.g., reading Braille for long periods of time) causes its area in somatotopic maps to expand at the expense of the areas devoted to the other fingers; disuse of a finger causes its area to contract. Both of these changes are reversible with changes in experience. In addition, long-term changes in synaptic connectivity continue throughout life as the basis for learning and memory.

Learning and Memory

A common first impulse is to consider learning and memory—the acquisition, storage, and ability to retrieve new information—as a unitary function. However, there are actually multiple systems in the brain subserving different kinds of memory (Fig. 20-6), broadly divisible into declarative and nondeclarative types. Declarative memories are those we have conscious access to and can *declare* to be true. They include memories of events (episodic memory), such as winning a recent handball game, and knowledge of facts (semantic memory), such as the temperature at which water freezes or the name of the mayor. Nondeclarative memories are also acquired through experience but are more automatic and come in a variety of forms. These include skills not just in moving but also in thinking (e.g., choosing and executing handball shots), habits (e.g., promptly opening a newspaper to a favorite section, changing patterns of speech depending on the surroundings), immediate emotional reactions to people or situations, and even modification of reflexes. Both declarative and nondeclarative memories are based on long-term changes in the strength of synapses (see Molecular

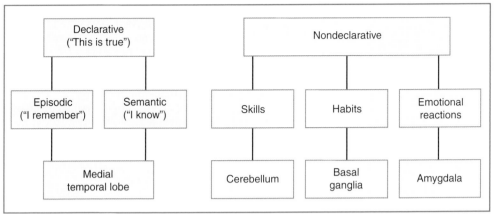

Figure 20-6. Major categories of memory. Although the locations of all the altered synapses that underlie each is not known with certainty, the indicated anatomic structures are prominently involved in the synaptic alterations.

Basis of Learning and Memory, below); the location of the modified synapses is related to the type of memory (see Fig. 20-6).

Declarative Memory

Declarative memories are acquired in stages, beginning as working memories maintained by activity of prefrontal cortex. Most things passing through working memory are simply discarded, but some are eventually consolidated in long-term memory. The hippocampus and nearby cortical areas play a central role in the consolidation of declarative memories.

The hippocampus itself is a cortical structure, but with a structure different from the six-layered neocortex shown in Figure 5-7. It consists of two interlocking strips of three-layered cortex, each C-shaped in cross-section, extending longitudinally through the medial temporal lobe in the floor of the lateral ventricle (Fig. 20-7). Major inputs to the hippocampus (Fig. 20-8) arrive from the anterior part of the parahippocampal gyrus (referred to as entorhinal cortex) and adjoining cortical areas, from the amygdala, and from cholinergic neurons in the septal nuclei, near the basal nucleus. Inputs to the parahippocampal gyrus from multiple association areas provide the information to be preserved as declarative memories. Inputs from the amygdala to the hippocampus influence *whether* something gets preserved as a declarative memory, providing a good example of the anatomic substrates of different memory types: the amygdala underlies nondeclarative memories manifested as emotional reactions to situations based on prior experiences, and the hippocampus underlies the consolidation of declarative memories of the details of those events. Finally, the modulatory cholinergic inputs are important for enhancing plastic changes in hippocampal synapses. The hippocampus then projects through the fornix (Fig. 20-9), one of the most distinctive fiber bundles in the CNS, to the mammillary bodies of the hypothalamus (see Fig. 18-17). It also projects directly back to the parahippocampal gyrus (Fig. 20-10) and from there to association areas. The links from association cortex to the hippocampus and back form much of the basis for maintaining memories during the process of consolidation; these connections, though less prominent anatomically than the fornix, may be more important functionally.

PHARMACOLOGY

Acetylcholine and Memory

Cholinergic projections from the septal nuclei to the hippocampus, acting through muscarinic receptors, are particularly important modulatory inputs to hippocampal neurons (see Fig. 20-11). Muscarinic antagonists, such as scopolamine, impair the acquisition of declarative memories; conversely, acetylcholinesterase blockers, such as physostigmine, enhance acquisition.

Bilateral damage to the hippocampus and parahippocampal gyrus causes severe anterograde amnesia, an inability to form declarative memories based on experiences subsequent to the damage. It also causes a variable degree of retrograde amnesia, a loss of memories formed prior to the damage. The retrograde amnesia is temporally graded, with memories less affected the older they are, consistent with the idea that long-term memories reside in networks of neocortical connections and not in the hippocampus itself; the degree to which they eventually become independent of the hippocampus is still disputed.

Molecular Basis of Learning and Memory

Synaptic connections are strengthened and weakened throughout the nervous system on time scales ranging from seconds to years (see Chapter 3). Some of these changes are part of such processes as focusing attention, regulating alertness, and adjusting muscle tone, but others are the physiologic basis of both declarative and nondeclarative memory.

On a moment-to-moment basis, the amount of transmitter released at a given synapse is influenced by factors such as Ca^{++} levels, the availability of synaptic vesicles, and the release of retrograde signals (see Figs. 3-12 and 3-13), but these changes are too brief to be important in learning. Longer-term changes involve increases and decreases in the numbers of receptor molecules in postsynaptic membranes. One well-studied example is long-term potentiation (LTP), which causes enhanced transmission lasting minutes to hours. LTP is based on Ca^{++} entry through *N*-methyl-D-aspartate

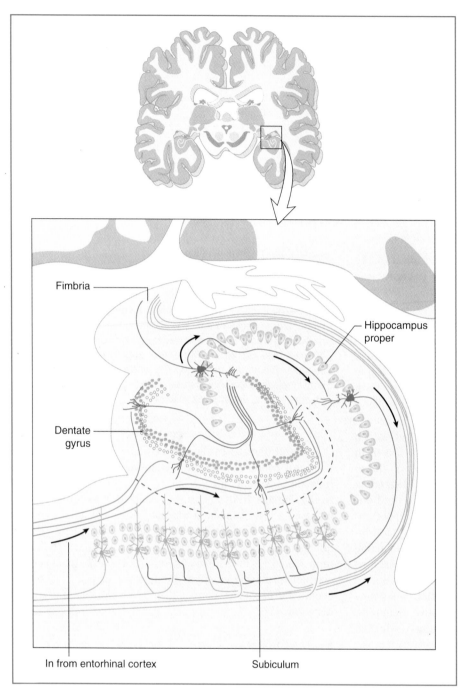

Fimbria

Hippocampus proper

Dentate gyrus

In from entorhinal cortex

Subiculum

Figure 20-7. Structure of the hippocampus. The hippocampus has three parts. One of the two interlocking C-shaped layers of cortex is the dentate gyrus; the other is the hippocampus proper. The transition zone from the hippocampus proper to the parahippocampal gyrus is the subiculum. Most inputs arrive in the dentate gyrus, most outputs arise from the subiculum.

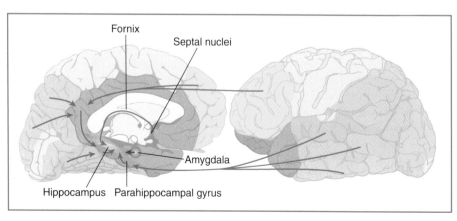

Fornix

Septal nuclei

Amygdala

Hippocampus   Parahippocampal gyrus

Figure 20-8. Inputs to the hippocampus.

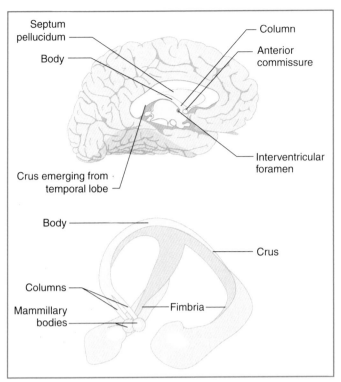

Figure 20-9. Course of the fornix. This long, curved fiber bundle starts out attached to the hippocampus as the fimbria ("fringe"), then leaves the posterior end of the hippocampus near the back (splenium) of the corpus callosum and continues as the crus ("arm") of the fornix. The two crura join to form the body, attached to the bottom of the septum pellucidum. The body then diverges at the level of the interventricular foramen into the two columns, which proceed to the mammillary bodies.

(NMDA) channels. Because NMDA channels open only in the presence of preexisting depolarization (see Fig. 3-10), this allows them to act as a molecular-level logic element, permitting Ca^{++} entry and synaptic strengthening only when two synaptic inputs are active simultaneously or when modulatory inputs signal a need for plasticity (Fig. 20-11). Conversely, other synaptic mechanisms can produce long-term depression (LTD), a weakening of synaptic strength that results from the removal of postsynaptic receptor molecules. LTP and

LTD also lead to very long-term changes based on alterations in the size or even existence of synapses; these stages involve communication with neuronal nuclei, alterations in gene expression, and the synthesis or removal of synaptic components (Fig. 20-12).

Repair of Damage in the Nervous System

If CNS or PNS neurons are destroyed by trauma or some disease process, the conventional wisdom until recently was that they cannot be replaced. With axons, it is a different story in the PNS, where axons can regrow. Until recently, it was thought that regrowth of CNS axons is never effective, but this view has also begun to change.

Wallerian Degeneration

If an axon in the PNS or CNS is severed, a characteristic series of responses ensues (Fig. 20-13). The process distal to the transection no longer receives shipments from the neuronal cell body, and synaptic transmission ceases. The distal process (along with its myelin, if present) slowly degenerates and is phagocytosed. This sequence of events is referred to as wallerian degeneration (the accompanying changes in water concentration make wallerian degeneration easy to see in T2-weighted MRIs). At the same time, the neuronal cell body swells, its nucleus moves to an eccentric position, and its chromatin uncoils. Nissl bodies seem to dwindle, because their rough endoplasmic reticulum disperses as the neuron tries to synthesize the components needed to rebuild itself (total RNA actually increases). This series of changes is called chromatolysis ("loss of color") because of the apparent loss of Nissl bodies. Presynaptic endings recognize that something is wrong and retract. All of these changes reverse themselves if the cell body manages to regenerate its axon and reach a target, or if it has enough undamaged axonal branches left. In many cases, diminished trophic interactions cause degenerative changes in neurons presynaptic and postsynaptic to the injured neuron, which themselves show degenerative changes—retrograde and anterograde transneuronal degeneration, respectively. (The atrophy of skeletal muscle fibers following lower motor neuron damage is an analogous form of anterograde transcellular degeneration.)

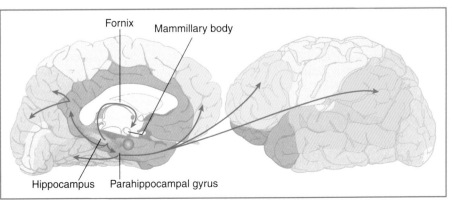

Figure 20-10. Outputs from the hippocampus.

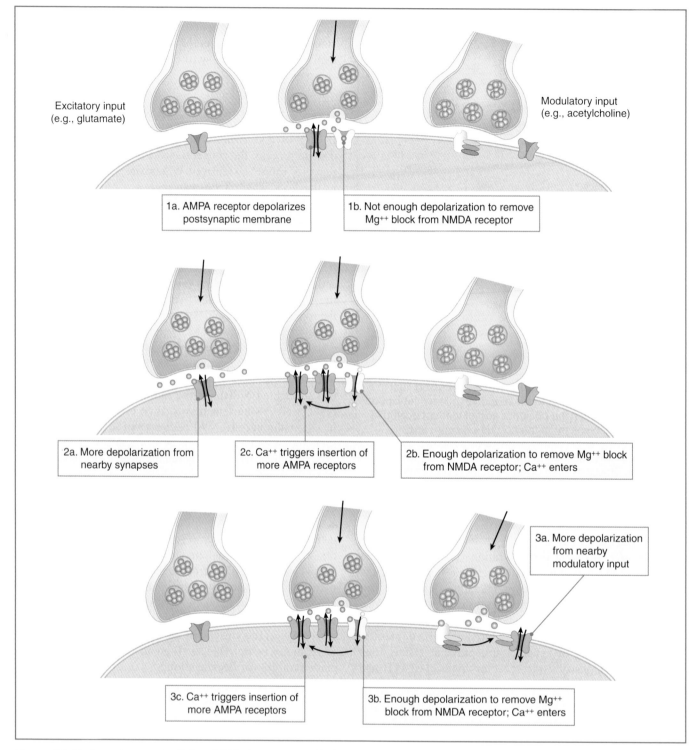

Figure 20-11. Long-term potentiation (LTP) at synapses with *N*-methyl-D-aspartate (NMDA) receptors. Single inputs (upper figure) activate only α-amino-3-hydroxy-5-methylisoxazole-4-propionic acid (AMPA) receptors. Added depolarization caused by activity of other excitatory synapses (middle figure) or modulatory inputs (lower figure) allows activation of NMDA receptors, inducing LTP. The potentiation can last hours, as long as extra AMPA receptors remain in the postsynaptic membrane.

Regeneration in the PNS

Following transection of a spinal or cranial nerve (other than the optic nerve, which is actually part of the CNS) or a peripheral nerve, macrophages move in to clean up the debris left behind by wallerian degeneration. As they do so, they also stimulate proliferation of Schwann cells, which in turn secrete trophic factors (e.g., nerve growth factor) that activate growth-related genetic programs and stimulate regrowth of processes proximal to the injury. The basal lamina remains behind after wallerian degeneration and provides guidance to

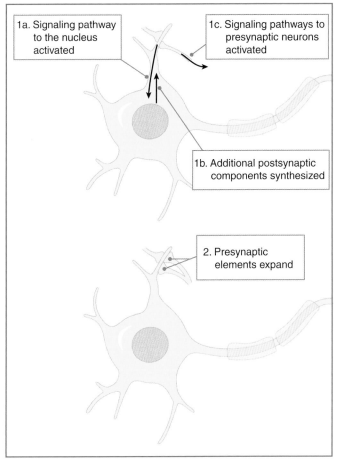

Figure 20-12. Very long-term changes in synaptic strength, caused by activation of genes (upper) and synthesis of additional synaptic components (lower).

regrowing processes. In fortunate cases, all of this combines to allow axons to regenerate back to their original targets, get remyelinated, and reestablish synaptic contacts. However, regrowing axons are not particularly selective about which endoneurial tube they grow down, so regeneration is seldom completely accurate. Crush injuries, in which basal laminae remain largely continuous through the injury site, have a better prognosis.

Regeneration in the CNS

After transection of a CNS pathway, microglia move in and slowly get rid of the degenerating distal processes. Astrocytes proliferate and form a glial scar that mechanically impedes regeneration. More importantly, growth-promoting factors are scarce in the adult brain, and growth-related genetic programs remain switched off. In addition, astrocytes and oligodendrocytes actually secrete growth-*inhibiting* factors—apparently the price we pay for stability when uninjured.

ANATOMY & CLINICAL MEDICINE

Miswiring in PNS Repair

Many of the signaling molecules present during development are absent or present in diminished amounts in adults, reducing the selectivity of regrowing peripheral nerve fibers. Axons of motor neurons may reinnervate the wrong muscle, leading to twitches in unintended muscles. After facial nerve damage, parasympathetic fibers formerly destined for ganglion cells in a salivary gland may instead wind up in the lacrimal gland, leading to tearing in response to food ("crocodile tears").

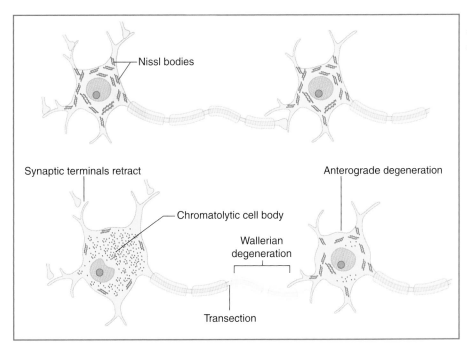

Figure 20-13. Wallerian degeneration, chromatolysis, and related retrograde and anterograde changes.

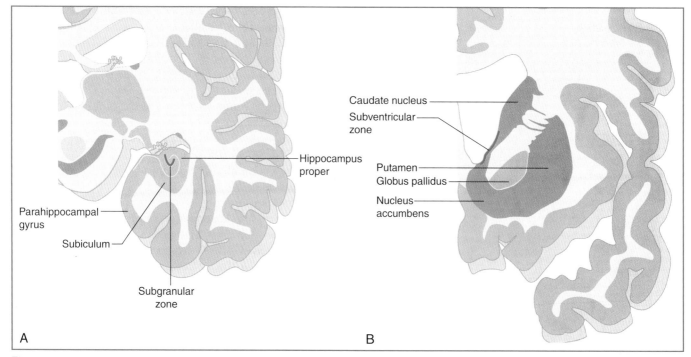

Figure 20-14. Zones where new neurons are produced in adult human brains. **A,** Stem cells at the edge of the granule cell layer of the hippocampal dentate gyrus (the subgranular zone) produce new dentate neurons throughout life. **B,** Stem cells between the head of the caudate nucleus and the ependymal lining of the lateral ventricle (the subventricular zone) produce new neurons that migrate to the olfactory bulb, at least in nonhuman primates and other mammals. The extent to which this occurs normally in humans is uncertain, but stem cells that can be coaxed experimentally to form new neurons are widely distributed in the lateral walls of human lateral ventricles.

Vertebrate CNS axons are not intrinsically incapable of regrowing; amphibians and some other nonmammalian species, for example, are able to reconstitute effective visual system connections following optic nerve transection. However, the inhospitable environment in which transected mammalian axons find themselves prevents all but some short-range sprouting by either injured axons or axons near denervated neurons. Over time, this sometimes results in some plastic changes. For example, following posterior column transection, some fibers of the spinal trigeminal tract may reach the nearby posterior column nuclei. This kind of regrowth, combined with unmasking of previously silent connections, can result in surprisingly large changes in cortical maps.

Hope for the Future

Several experimental strategies for promoting CNS regeneration have been tried in recent years, based on activating growth-related genetic programs and providing environments that foster growth of axons. The best of them point to promising treatment options in the future. An early approach took advantage of the hospitable environment provided by Schwann cells and used grafted segments of peripheral nerve as bridges across areas of injury. CNS axons can grow long distances through such grafts (showing that regrowth is possible), but once they emerge from the other end they are back in a hostile CNS environment and do not grow much farther. Alternative approaches try to mimic the conditions that are present early in development, utilizing trophic factors and blockade of growth-inhibiting factors. Others suppress inflammation and scar formation. Alone or combined, some of these techniques have allowed rodents to walk again after spinal cord transections.

Finally, in some cases it may be possible to replace neurons that have died. Implants of fetal dopaminergic neurons have produced improvements in some patients with Parkinson's disease, and fetal stem cells can be induced to form a variety of other neuronal types. More recently, the dogma that the adult CNS cannot produce new neurons has withered. Stem cells have been found in the walls of all the ventricles, and in two restricted parts of the brain it is now known that neurons are added or replaced throughout life (Fig. 20-14). Learning how to control stem cell proliferation and differentiation may be the wave of the future.

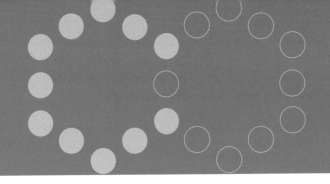

Case Studies

Case Study 1

A 66-year-old retired banker was brought by his wife to see his physician because of what she described as "personality changes" that had developed over the previous 3 months. Formerly active in his local community association and an avid golfer, he had taken to spending most of the day quietly watching television, rarely changing the channel. He frequently complained of a headache, but otherwise seldom spoke unless responding to someone else. When he did respond to someone, he was often tactless and rude. His wife also described increasingly odd behavior, explaining that 2 days previously she had asked him to take out the trash; he did so, then made multiple additional trips to put pieces of living room furniture out on the sidewalk.

In the physician's office, he was alert and cooperative but often made flippant comments. No sensory or motor abnormalities were noted. Asked to remember a series of three phrases, he kept repeating the first two words of the first phrase when asked about them 5 minutes later. Asked the meaning of "A rolling stone gathers no moss," he said, "Well, you know, it just rubs off."

1. **Where was there most likely to be damage in this man's CNS?**

2. **An MRI revealed a large, bilaterally symmetric tumor. Which cell type was most likely involved?**

3. **How do you account for the tumor being bilaterally symmetric?**

Case Study 2

A 7-year-old girl was evaluated for recurring attacks of weakness, each lasting 2 to 3 hours. Her parents said they usually occurred after she rode her bicycle for long distances or ran around a lot with other children but that recently she had had one after simply eating two bananas. Laboratory tests showed normal serum electrolytes, normal thyroid function, and normal nerve conduction velocities.

1. **What are the possible causes of weakness in this child?**

2. **Normal muscle fibers fire sustained trains of action potentials in response to moderate depolarization by current injection. The patient's muscle fibers, obtained by biopsy, depolarized more than normal in response to a comparable stimulus, fired a brief burst of action potentials, and then became electrically inexcitable. Why might a depolarizing, normally excitatory stimulus cause a muscle (or neuronal) membrane to become electrically inexcitable?**

3. **Why might exercise or eating bananas trigger such episodes?**

Case Study 3

Seizures are the manifestation of periods of uncontrolled, rapid, synchronized firing of groups of cortical neurons, sometimes in localized areas (partial seizures) and sometimes in widespread areas in both hemispheres (generalized seizures). Most medications used to reduce the frequency of seizures do one or more of the following:

   a. Bind to voltage-gated Na^+ channels and slow the rate at which they move from an inactivated state to the "resting" (deinactivated) state.

   b. Act at synapses that use GABA as a neurotransmitter, by enhancing the opening of GABA-gated ion channels, by blocking the reuptake of GABA from the synaptic cleft, or by blocking the enzymatic degradation of GABA.

   c. Block the type of voltage-gated Ca^{++} channel that is prominent in thalamic neurons.

1. **What might be the basis for the lowering of seizure frequency by each of these categories of drugs?**

Case Study 4

About a week after recovering from a moderately severe flu-like illness, a 26-year-old man reported feeling progressively more "dizzy." He went to bed early, and the next morning he was even more unstable and unable to stand or walk without support. His wife took him to a nearby urgent care facility, where it was noted that his strength was normal but stretch reflexes in his arms and legs were markedly diminished. When examined again 6 weeks later, he was able to walk but only with a wide-based, unsteady gait; he reported that in dark rooms, he was still unable to walk without support. His strength continued to be normal, but his reflexes were still nearly absent. He had a striking sensory disturbance in which he was unable to detect the direction in which an examiner deflected his fingers or toes unless he watched. A vibrating tuning fork applied to bony prominences throughout his body elicited no sensation, but when it was applied to his forehead he reported a "humming" sensation. He was able to discriminate warm, cool, and sharp objects normally. He had no trouble detecting touch anywhere on his body but was unable to sort objects by touch (e.g., pick out a particular kind of coin with his eyes closed).

1. Where in the nervous system could damage cause this pattern of sensory deficits?

2. Is there any place in the nervous system where damage could cause loss of reflexes and this pattern of sensory deficits?

3. How can you account for worsening of symptoms in dark rooms?

4. How do you account for the patient being able detect a vibrating tuning fork only when applied to his forehead?

Case Study 5

A 74-year-old woman had the sudden onset of weakness and numbness in her right arm and leg and difficulty seeing to the right. She was rushed to a local hospital, where she was found to be alert, cooperative, and able to answer questions appropriately. The right side of her mouth drooped, she was almost completely unable to move her right arm or leg, and she had a right Babinski sign. Her senses of touch and joint position in the right half of her body and face were severely impaired. She was vaguely aware of pinprick but unable to localize it. She was unable to see to the right of the midline with either eye.

1. Where is the most likely site of damage?

2. Which artery was most likely to have been involved?

Case Study 6

A. A newborn was found to have incomplete formation of the posterior skull. Most parts of both cerebral hemispheres were absent, replaced by masses of neural tissue that had herniated through the skull into a membrane-covered sac. The most likely cause of this malformation was defective—

a. Closure of the neural tube.

b. Differentiation of neural crest cells.

c. Formation of the pontine flexure.

d. Proliferation of neurons from stem cells.

e. Subdivision of a basically normal prosencephalon.

B. The Dandy-Walker malformation is characterized in part by congenital hydrocephalus involving the lateral, third, and fourth ventricles and agenesis of midline parts of the cerebellum. The most plausible cause of such a malformation is—

a. Delayed opening of the median and lateral apertures of the fourth ventricle.

b. Enlargement of the pineal gland, leading to compression of the cerebral aqueduct.

c. Excessive narrowing of the foramen magnum.

d. Occlusion of the central canal of the spinal cord.

e. Stenosis of the interventricular foramina.

Case Study 7

The 13-year-old shortstop of a Little League team was hit on the side of the head by a line drive. He did not lose consciousness and continued to play, but an hour later while sitting on the bench he fell over. He was helped to his feet and it was noted that his left arm and leg were weak and he was extremely lethargic and difficult to arouse. He was rushed to a hospital, where an urgent CT revealed a dense, convex mass over his right frontal and parietal lobes. As he was being wheeled out of the radiology suite, it was noted that he was even more difficult to arouse, that all four limbs were now weak, and that his right pupil was dilated and did not respond to light shone in either eye. An emergency neurosurgical procedure was performed.

1. **What was the dense mass most likely to be?**

2. **How can you account for his changes in consciousness?**

3. **How can you account for the weakness that developed in his right arm and leg?**

4. **How can you account for the changes in his right pupil?**

Case Study 8

A 34-year-old woman was eating dinner with her husband when her right foot started to twitch uncontrollably. Over a period of about 30 seconds, the twitching spread up her leg, then down her arm and into her hand, following which her head and eyes jerked forcibly to the right. After the twitching stopped, her right arm and leg were weak, slowly returning to normal in about an hour. The diagnosis was a focal seizure, and a CT scan at a local emergency room later that evening revealed the following:

- A golf ball–sized mass extended from the midline and indented the medial surface of her left frontal lobe near the top of the central sulcus. Before the injection of a contrast agent, the mass looked slightly lighter than the gray matter in either hemisphere.
- In a repeat CT scan after contrast injection, the mass looked completely white.
- Parts of the left frontal lobe adjacent to the mass looked darker than comparable areas in the right frontal lobe.

1. **How would you explain the initial CT appearance of the mass?**

2. **How would you explain the change in CT appearance after contrast injection?**

3. **How would you explain the CT appearance of parts of the CNS adjacent to the mass?**

4. **What might be the basis for the pattern of twitching in this seizure?**

Case Study 9

A worried 22-year-old woman arrived at her physician's office complaining of numbness and tingling in her legs and difficulty seeing with her left eye. She said the problem had started that morning and gotten progressively worse throughout the day. She was found to have impaired position sense and moderate weakness in her right leg although perception of pinprick there was normal. Position sense and strength were normal in her left leg, but she had difficulty perceiving pinprick there. Stroking the sole of her right foot caused dorsiflexion of the right big toe; when the sole of her left foot was stroked, she said it tickled and tried to withdraw the foot. Visual acuity of the right eye was 20/20. When she closed her right eye, she said everything looked fuzzy and dim, and visual acuity of that eye was 20/300. Both pupils were the same size; both constricted when light was shone into her right eye, and both dilated when the penlight was swung over to her left eye.

1. **What could account for the problems in her right leg?**

2. **What could account for the problems in her left leg?**

3. **What could account for her visual problems?**

4. **Is there any place in the nervous system where a single lesion could cause this collection of deficits?**

5. **How could shining a light into one eye cause both pupils to dilate?**

Case Study 10

A 39-year-old handball player began to notice difficulty hearing with his right ear about 16 months ago. The hearing problem slowly got worse, and a recent audiogram indicated a loss of about 65 dB measured by either air conduction or bone conduction. In addition, he has mild weakness of the entire right side of his face and diminished taste on the right anterior part of his tongue.

1. **What do the audiometric results indicate about possible causes of the hearing loss?**

2. **What does the pattern of facial weakness indicate about possible causes?**

3. **What does the gustatory loss indicate about possible causes?**

4. **What is the most likely cause of the patient's symptoms?**

Case Study 11

A 33-year-old woman began to have episodes about 3 years ago in which loud sounds caused her eyes to "twitch" and made the outside world appear to rotate, resulting in unsteadiness and loss of balance. Testing revealed that loud low-frequency sounds delivered to her right (but not left) ear caused a vertical-torsional nystagmus. During the fast phase, her eyes moved downward and rotated in a counterclockwise direction (as seen by others).

1. **What normally prevents sounds from stimulating vestibular parts of the labyrinth?**

2. **What might have led to vestibular responses to sound in this patient?**

Case Study 12

A 27-year-old woman complained to her physician that her periods had become increasingly irregular over the past year and had recently ceased entirely. Over the past month, she had developed an embarrassing discharge of milk from her breasts and a chronic headache. On the way into the doctor's office, she walked into the end of a low-lying tree branch on her right and suddenly realized that there had been several instances of not noticing something on one side or the other over the previous several weeks. In addition to ordering some blood tests, the physician examined her visual fields and found substantially diminished visual acuity in the upper temporal quadrant of the field of each eye, extending partway into the lower temporal quadrant.

1. **Where in the visual system could damage cause this pattern of loss?**

2. **What might be the significance of the loss being greater in upper parts of the fields than in lower parts?**

3. **What is the most likely cause of the loss of visual acuity?**

Case Study 13

A 22-year-old man fell asleep on his way home from work. His car drifted off the road and hit a tree, and he struck his head against the windshield. CT scanning revealed a frontal skull fracture and subdural hemorrhage. Following surgical treatment, the man complained that food seemed to have lost its taste and that only very spicy food seemed at all appetizing. In formal tests, he was able to identify swabs soaked in saline, sugar water, vinegar, and a quinine solution if they were applied directly to his tongue. He was unable to identify banana, cinnamon, or coffee when these were held under his nose, but he recoiled in response to smelling salts (ammonium carbonate).

1. **Why might a patient like this, with apparently normal taste buds, complain of loss of taste?**

2. **Why might head trauma cause a selective loss of olfaction?**

3. **What might account for the remaining ability to detect smelling salts?**

Case Study 14

A 52-year-old woman was evaluated for progressive weakness of her arms and legs. Three months earlier, she had noticed what she described as increasing "clumsiness" of her right hand (she is right-handed). Shortly after that, her hand started to feel stiff and weak. The stiffness and weakness spread over a period of weeks into her legs and her other hand, and she began to notice spontaneous twitches of her finger muscles. When examined, she had moderate weakness in the distal muscles of her arms and legs; marked atrophy of her hand muscles; fasciculations in her hands, calves, and tongue; increased tone in all four extremities; hyperactive stretch reflexes; and bilateral Babinski signs. Although she was distressed about her condition, her mental status and sensory examinations were normal.

1. **What is the significance of weakness accompanied by atrophy and fasciculations?**

2. **What is the significance of weakness accompanied by increased muscle tone and stretch reflexes?**

3. **Can this pattern of weakness be explained by damage at one site in the nervous system?**

Case Study 15

A 64-year-old man noticed the gradual onset of a tremor in his right hand; while sitting quietly in a chair, his thumb would rub against his fingers about four times per second. The tremor went away when he reached for something. Over the same time period (about 2 months), his right arm and hand felt progressively stiffer and clumsier, and he had trouble getting them to move. Once he began to use them, however, his strength seemed about the same on both sides. His physician noted increased tone in all the muscles of his right arm and no differences between the stretch reflexes of his two arms.

1. **In which part of this patient's nervous system would a degenerative process most likely be found?**

2. **In which parts of his basal ganglia was there likely to be increased activity?**

3. **In which parts of his basal ganglia was there likely to be decreased activity?**

Case Study 16

A 71-year-old hypertensive woman awoke one morning unable to move her right arm and leg. Her daughter, who lived next door, took her to the hospital, where she improved somewhat over the next several days. By the end of the week, her right leg was still so weak that she was unable to walk; she had increased knee-jerk and ankle-jerk reflexes on the right and a right Babinski sign. Her right arm had mostly recovered its strength, and her face was normal except for a slight drooping of the right side of her mouth. Her mental status was normal, as was sensation of all types. As the strength in her right arm improved, however, she noted that it had become extremely uncoordinated. She had marked ataxia, for example, when extending her right index finger from her nose to an examiner's finger and back, whether or not her eyes were open.

1. **What might account for the remaining weakness in the patient's leg?**

2. **What might account for the ataxia in the patient's arm?**

3. **Can this pattern of deficits be explained by damage at one site in the nervous system?**

Case Study 17

Following a cardiac catheterization, a 64-year-old woman awoke and found herself unable to open her left eye. She raised the eyelid with her left hand and noticed she had double vision. She started to reach for a mirror to look at her face and noticed that her right arm felt numb and clumsy.

Alarmed, she rang for a nurse, who in turn called a neurologist. The neurologist noted that the patient's left eye was deviated laterally and moved little when she tried to look up or down; when she tried to look to the right, her left eye got no farther than midposition. Her left pupil was dilated and did not respond to light shone in either eye. Perception of touch, pinprick, temperature, and joint position were slightly diminished in her right arm and leg and the right side of her face. When she tried to reach for something with her right hand, it oscillated widely whether or not her eyes were open. Similarly, if she tried to run her right foot up and down her left shin, it fell off the shin almost immediately.

1. **What might account for the deficits in the patient's left eye?**

2. **What might account for the sensory changes in her right arm and leg?**

3. **What might account for the coordination problems in her right arm and leg?**

4. **Can all these deficits be explained by damage at one location in the nervous system?**

Case Study 18

A 71-year-old man was talking to a friend at a cocktail party when he suddenly began to feel confused and disoriented. Thinking he had overindulged, he excused himself, got his wife to drive them both home, and went to bed. When he awoke the next morning, he realized there was something wrong with his vision. As he sat up, the ceiling of his bedroom seemed to disappear, and as he looked around the room, everything seemed colorless. When his wife came in to ask how he was, he recognized her voice, but was startled to find that he did not recognize her face. Formal testing confirmed all of this. Visual acuity was markedly diminished in the upper half of the visual field of each eye. He continued to complain that everything "looked gray," and he was unable to sort colored cards or name their colors. He was able to recognize friends and family members if he heard their voices or watched them walk around but not if he simply looked at their faces. Even though he could not recognize their faces, he often had a vague feeling of familiarity that was lacking when he looked at the faces of hospital staff members.

1. **Can this pattern of visual field loss be accounted for by damage at one location in the nervous system?**

2. **How can you account for the loss of color vision?**

3. **How can you account for the inability to recognize faces?**

4. What might be the basis of the patient's lingering feelings of familiarity when looking at the faces of people he knew?

5. What was the most likely arterial basis for this patient's apparent stroke?

Case Study 19

A woman heard a noise while driving down a highway with her 73-year-old husband on their way to a week's vacation. She looked at her husband and saw him slumped over, awake but looking confused and making grunting sounds. She drove straight to the nearest hospital, about a half-hour away, where it was quickly determined that he had suffered a massive stroke and was globally aphasic, completely paralyzed on the right side of his body and lower face and unable to see with his left eye. Thrombolytic agents were administered, and he improved rapidly. By the next day, he had made a substantial recovery, but some deficits were still evident. He was virtually silent unless someone asked him a question, and then he responded with just a few labored words. When asked what still bothered him, for example, he pointed to his right arm with his left hand and said "Arm...bad." This apparently referred to the fact that, although his right leg and lower face had largely recovered, his right hand and arm were still weak and numb. He seemed to understand everything that was said to him, and he was able to repeat complete sentences with little effort (in striking contrast to his difficulty with answering questions).

1. Where was there most likely to be residual damage that might account for his remaining language deficits?

2. How might the damage referred to in the previous question be related to weakness and numbness of the right arm?

3. What is the most likely arterial basis for this patient's remaining deficits?

Case Study 20

A 23-year-old woman was injured in combat by a bullet that severed her spinal cord at a midthoracic level. Before and for weeks after the surgeries that repaired the damage as well as possible, her legs were limp and stretch reflexes were absent. Her bladder was catheterized, because without this the bladder distended to a much greater than normal size, until small amounts of urine dribbled out. Beginning at about 5 weeks after the injury, stretch reflexes began to return and bilateral Babinski signs appeared. By about 10 weeks, this had progressed to severe spasticity. Over the same time period, her bladder detrusor began contracting forcefully at lower than normal volumes; despite this, the bladder failed to empty completely, so catheterization was continued.

1. How can you account for the initial flaccid state of the leg muscles?

2. What might account for the progressive changes in function of the leg muscles?

3. How can you account for the initial state of the bladder?

4. What might account for the progressive changes in bladder function?

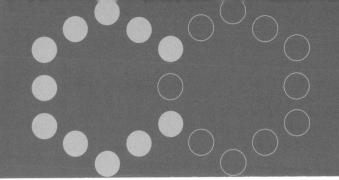

Case Study Answers

CASE STUDY 1

1. Prefrontal cortex is centrally involved in planning, short-term memory, initiative, and problem solving. Major disruption of these functions, as in this patient, typically reflects bilateral damage.
2. Astrocytomas are the most common primary brain neoplasms. Glioblastoma multiforme accounts for most of these.
3. Astrocytes are adapted to living and moving in the spaces between neurons. This enables astrocytoma cells to move along white matter tracts, in this case across the genu of the corpus callosum and into symmetric areas of prefrontal white matter. Because of their shape, these tumors are sometimes referred to as butterfly gliomas.

CASE STUDY 2

1. Weakness implies probable malfunction of upper motor neurons, lower motor neurons, neuromuscular junctions, or muscles themselves (see Fig. 14-9).
2. Voltage-gated Na^+ channels are the key substrate of action potentials (see Fig. 2-14), and blocking their activity makes muscle and neuronal membranes inexcitable. This patient's muscle membranes clearly contain a complement of such channels because they are able to fire bursts of action potentials. However, voltage-gated Na^+ channels inactivate after opening and are unavailable until the membrane repolarizes (see Fig. 2-14); hence, keeping Na^+ channels in the inactivated state makes a membrane inexcitable. Patients with some forms of periodic paralysis have a relatively small percentage of mutant Na^+ channels that inactivate abnormally slowly. After a burst of action potentials, they remain open, continue to depolarize the membrane, and prevent normal channels from deinactivating.
3. Increasing plasma K^+ concentration from the normal resting value of about 4 mmol/L to 6–7 mmol/L is sufficient to cause the sequence of events described in answer 2.2. Enough K^+ is released from skeletal muscle during exercise to reach this value, and K^+-rich foods such as bananas, fruit juices, and avocadoes can do the same thing.

CASE STUDY 3

1a. The duration of the absolute and relative refractory periods is largely determined by the rate at which voltage-gated Na^+ channels deinactivate (see Figs. 2-16 and 2-17). Slightly slowing this rate would reduce the maximum firing frequency of neurons but have no effect on their low-frequency behavior.
1b. GABA is the principal neurotransmitter mediating fast inhibitory transmission in the brain, so agents that enhance GABA transmission would generally reduce the excitability of neurons in the cortex (and elsewhere). This could be done by increasing the conductance of ligand-gated GABA receptors, or by making more GABA available.
1c. Some forms of epilepsy are characterized by rhythmic bursts of action potentials that arise from oscillatory interactions between the thalamus and the cortex. The thalamic contribution to the interaction is based on the slow waves produced by the opening of voltage-gated Ca^{++} channels (see Fig. 5-14), so blocking these channels helps break the cycle.

CASE STUDY 4

1. These are the sensory modalities conveyed by large-diameter peripheral nerve fibers (see Fig. 2-22), reaching consciousness through the posterior column–medial lemniscus pathway (see Fig. 9-5). Global damage anywhere along the way would cause a relatively selective deficit in perceiving vibration, joint position, and the finer aspects of touch.
2. Damage in the posterior column–medial lemniscus pathway would need to be in the upper cervical spinal cord or higher to affect both arms and legs. The branches of large-diameter fibers that form the afferent limb of stretch reflexes are given off locally, so such damage would leave reflexes unaffected. This leaves large-diameter sensory nerve fibers as the likely culprit. These fibers, and the ganglion cells from which they arise, are different enough antigenically from small-diameter fibers and their ganglion cells that autoimmune processes sometimes affect them selectively (as in this case).

3. The sense of equilibrium normally involves integration of position sense with vestibular and visual information. Loss of one of these three can be compensated for, but loss of two is debilitating. This is the basis of Romberg's sign (see Integration Box 11-4).

4. Vibration of bony prominences in the head (but not the body) can reach the cochlea by bone conduction and be detected as sound ("humming").

CASE STUDY 5

1. Right homonymous hemianopia indicates damage on the left, behind the optic chiasm (see Fig. 12-11). This, combined with right somatosensory and upper motor neuron problems, places the damage in the left hemisphere. If this were an extensive cortical stroke, language areas between somatosensory and visual cortex would have been affected. Thalamic damage could account for the somatosensory and visual deficits, but not the weakness. The only place where critical components of all three systems are compacted together is posterior parts of the internal capsule (see Fig. 5-18 and Table 5-2).

2. Deep cerebral structures like the internal capsule are supplied by small perforating branches from within and near the circle of Willis (see Figs. 7-12 and 7-14). A particularly large branch arising from the internal carotid artery, called the anterior choroidal artery, supplies most of the posterior limb and retrolenticular parts of the internal capsule, as well as sending branches to the optic tract and lateral geniculate nucleus.

CASE STUDY 6

A. The correct answer is a. Posterior defects of the skull or vertebral column characteristically accompany defective neural tube closure (a). Neural crest cells (b) develop into the PNS, but do not induce formation of the posterior skull or vertebral column. The pontine flexure (c) leads to formation of the fourth ventricle. Neuronal proliferation (d) mostly occurs after neural tube closure and induction of the skull and vertebral column. Defective subdivision of the prosencephalon (e) leads to abnormalities in the holoprosencephaly spectrum, typically accompanied by facial abnormalities but an intact skull.

B. The correct answer is a. Hydrocephalus involving all the ventricles points to a problem either at the apertures of the fourth ventricle (a) or outside the ventricles. Aqueductal stenosis (b) causes hydrocephalus of the third and lateral ventricles. Blockage of the interventricular foramina (e) causes hydrocephalus of only the lateral ventricles. Occlusion of the foramen magnum (c) or central canal (d) does not block the primary path of circulation of CSF

(see Fig. 7-11) and does not result in hydrocephalus. Increased pressure in the fourth ventricle during development could reasonably be expected to disrupt formation of the vermis, the part of the cerebellum nearest the roof of this ventricle.

CASE STUDY 7

1. Head trauma can cause either subdural or epidural bleeding. Because it is harder to separate the dura from the skull than to separate the arachnoid from the dura, epidural hemorrhages are usually relatively short and convex, and subdural hemorrhages relatively long and crescent-shaped (compare Figs. 8-6 and 8-7).

2. Acutely expanding intracranial masses can cause pressure on the midbrain, affecting ascending modulatory pathways and causing depressed consciousness (see Fig. 19-2A).

3. Expanding supratentorial masses can cause the uncus on that side to herniate medially and downward through the tentorial notch, compressing the opposite cerebral peduncle against the other edge of the tentorium cerebelli. The result is weakness and Babinski's sign on the same side as the expanding mass.

4. A herniating uncus also typically pinches the oculomotor nerve between itself and the midbrain, causing an ipsilateral dilated pupil.

CASE STUDY 8

1. The degree of lightness in CT studies is a reflection of x-ray density. This was a meningioma growing from the falx cerebri. Although meningiomas are highly vascular tumors, the CNS also has an extremely dense blood supply, so vascularity is not the basis of the tumor's x-ray density. Instead, it is a reflection of a tendency by meningiomas to accumulate calcium deposits.

2. Some tumors have a functional blood-brain barrier and do not change their appearance much following injection of contrast agents. Meningiomas, however, are derived from arachnoid cells and are outside the CNS. They have no blood-brain barrier and so are x-ray dense after contrast injection.

3. Brain tissue irritated by pressure from the tumor can become edematous, and the increased water concentration makes it less x-ray dense than other areas of the brain.

4. This pattern of spread corresponds to the arrangement of body parts in motor (and somatosensory) cortex (see Fig. 9-5). It was first described by the British neurologist John Hughlings Jackson, and these are still referred to as jacksonian seizures.

CASE STUDY 9

1. A selective deficit in position sense in the right leg is likely to indicate damage to the right fasciculus gracilis in the thoracic or upper lumbar spinal cord, or partial damage to the posterior column–medial lemniscus pathway at some level rostral to this. Weakness of the right leg, coupled with a Babinski sign, indicates damage to the corticospinal system. This could be damage on the right side of the thoracic or upper lumbar spinal cord (lateral corticospinal tract), partial damage at higher spinal levels on the right, or partial damage on the left above the pyramidal decussation.

2. A selective deficit in pain and temperature perception indicates damage to the anterolateral pathway on the right side of the thoracic or upper lumbar spinal cord, or partial damage at some higher CNS level.

3. A visual deficit confined to one eye indicates damage anterior to the optic chiasm (e.g., retina, optic nerve).

4. The problems in this patient's legs can most easily be explained by damage on the right side of the thoracic or upper lumbar spinal cord. (Damage higher in the spinal cord would affect more than the legs. Damage in the brainstem or higher would affect only the contralateral side of the body.) However, spinal cord damage would obviously not cause visual deficits, so multiple lesions must be involved in this case. This is a classic presentation of multiple sclerosis, in this case involving demyelinating plaques in the spinal cord and optic nerve.

5. Shining light in the normal eye causes both a direct and a consensual reflex, and both pupils constrict (see Fig. 12-17). Moving the light to the impaired eye decreases the afferent input to the pupillary light reflex, causing both pupils to constrict less (i.e., dilate). Moving a light back and forth between the eyes like this is called a swinging flashlight test, and pupillary dilation in response indicates an afferent pupillary defect.

CASE STUDY 10

1. If the hearing loss were greater when measured by air conduction than by bone conduction, this would indicate a problem in the outer or middle ear. Hearing loss that is similar whether measured by air conduction or by bone conduction indicates probable damage to the cochlea or the eighth nerve.

2. Weakness of one side of the face indicates lower motor neuron damage (i.e., damage to the ipsilateral facial nerve or facial motor nucleus). A supranuclear lesion (e.g., in the cerebral peduncle, internal capsule, or motor cortex) would cause weakness of the contralateral lower face, sparing the forehead (see Fig. 14-11).

3. Taste buds on the anterior two thirds of the tongue are supplied by the facial nerve. Central branches of these fibers terminate in the nucleus of the solitary tract, but damage here or at more rostral levels of the gustatory pathway would be unlikely to selectively affect the anterior part of the tongue.

4. Although it would be possible for damage at the pontomedullary junction, spreading into the caudal pons, to cause this set of findings, this would also be likely to affect the spinothalamic tract, medial lemniscus, or other brainstem structures. The findings are more consistent with a PNS lesion, in this case a vestibular schwannoma that has begun to compress the facial nerve.

CASE STUDY 11

1. Because scala tympani ends blindly at the round window membrane, perilymphatic pressure changes caused by vibrations of the stapes footplate can deflect the cochlear duct and stimulate the organ of Corti (see Fig. 10-10). These same pressure changes, however, are distributed equally in the perilymph surrounding the utricle, saccule, and semicircular ducts, so there is no net force to move them in any direction.

2. Any process that allows pressure gradients to develop around some part of the vestibular labyrinth would make that part responsive to sound-induced perilymphatic pressure pulses. Although there are several possible causes, perhaps the most common is erosion of the very thin layer of bone separating the superior semicircular canal from the middle cranial fossa. The result is comparable to having a second round window membrane, this one adjacent to the superior semicircular duct, leading to deformation of this duct in response to stapes footplate movements. The vertical-torsional nystagmus in this patient is that expected from stimulation of the right superior duct.

CASE STUDY 12

1. Damage in different parts of the fields of the two eyes (i.e., in a bitemporal or, much less commonly, a binasal pattern) almost always indicates damage to the optic chiasm (see Fig. 12-11). A bitemporal deficit (as in this case) results from damage more or less in the middle of the chiasm, whereas a binasal deficit would require lateral damage on both sides of the chiasm.

2. Ganglion cell axons maintain a roughly retinotopic arrangement through the optic nerve and chiasm, with axons from inferior parts of the retina traveling most inferiorly. Something pushing upward from below the optic chiasm would damage these fibers first and, because the eye's optics reverse things on the retina, affect upper parts of the visual fields more than lower parts.

3. The pituitary gland is situated directly below the optic chiasm (see Fig. 18-11), and prolactinomas are the most

common pituitary tumors. Oversecretion of prolactin causes amenorrhea and galactorrhea in women, and impotence and decreased libido in men.

CASE STUDY 13

1. Gustatory, olfactory, somatosensory, and other inputs are all integrated to yield a perception of flavor, and olfaction plays a dominant role (see Fig. 13-10). A majority of patients complaining of taste deficits actually have an olfactory deficit.
2. The thin axons of olfactory receptor cells can easily be sheared off as they pass through the cribriform plate (see Fig. 13-8).
3. Trigeminal endings in the lingual and olfactory epithelia detect spicy and pungent substances.

CASE STUDY 14

1. Fasciculations and marked atrophy are indicative of weakness caused by lower motor neuron damage, but *decreased* muscle tone and reflexes usually accompany this, so something does not fit.
2. Increased muscle tone and hyperactive reflexes (and Babinski's signs) are indicative of weakness caused by upper motor neuron damage, but this should not be accompanied by marked atrophy or fasciculations, so something does not fit here either.
3. The pattern of weakness suggests combined damage to upper and lower motor neurons, with the remaining lower motor neurons mediating the effects of upper motor neuron damage. The cell bodies of upper and lower motor neurons live in different parts of the CNS. Although it is conceivable that some process could affect both the cell bodies of lower motor neurons and the nearby synaptic terminals of upper motor neurons, this is instead the pattern seen in amyotrophic lateral sclerosis, an inexorable degenerative disease affecting both sets of neurons.

CASE STUDY 15

1. This is a representative initial presentation of Parkinson's disease, caused by degeneration of the dopaminergic neurons in the compact part of the substantia nigra. Parkinson's disease often starts asymmetrically and, because the major connections of the basal ganglia are mostly uncrossed (see Figs. 15-4 and 15-5), the degeneration is greater in the substantia nigra contralateral to the worse symptoms (in this case the left substantia nigra).

2. Increased activity is likely to occur in striatal neurons in the indirect pathway, leading to increased activity in the subthalamic nucleus and the internal segment of the globus pallidus (see Fig. 15-7).
3. Decreased activity is likely to occur in striatal neurons in the direct pathway and in the external segment of the globus pallidus (see Fig. 15-7).

CASE STUDY 16

1. Weakness of the right leg, coupled with increased reflexes and a Babinski sign, indicates damage to the corticospinal system (see Fig. 14-10). This could be damage on the right side of the thoracic or upper lumbar spinal cord (lateral corticospinal tract), partial damage at higher spinal levels on the right, or partial damage on the left above the pyramidal decussation (in the pyramid, basal pons, cerebral peduncle, internal capsule, or motor areas of the cortex).
2. This kind of right-arm ataxia indicates damage to the right cerebellar hemisphere or its inputs or outputs (see Figs. 16-8 and 16-9). Inputs descend from left motor cortical areas, through the internal capsule, cerebral peduncle, and basal pons to reach left pontine nuclei, which project to the cerebellum through the right middle cerebellar peduncle. Outputs leave through the right superior cerebellar peduncle, cross in the caudal midbrain, and reach the left thalamus, which projects to motor areas of the cortex through the internal capsule.
3. This seemingly odd combination of weakness and incoordination is referred to as ataxic hemiparesis. It is most commonly caused by a small infarct in the posterior limb of the internal capsule or the basal pons, where corticospinal and corticopontine fibers are in close proximity. A capsular infarct would need to be small enough to affect a subset of both corticospinal and corticopontine fibers, but spare the nearby somatosensory projections from VPL and VPM. A small pontine infarct could cause a similar syndrome by affecting corticospinal fibers for the leg, together with nearby pontine nuclei that transmit information used for arm coordination.

CASE STUDY 17

1. Weakness of the left superior, inferior, and medial recti, along with the pupillary sphincter, indicates damage to the left oculomotor nerve, either inside the rostral midbrain or outside the brainstem. Further testing would probably have revealed weakness of the left inferior oblique. (Damage to one oculomotor nucleus is much less common and, because the axons of superior rectus motor neurons cross before exiting [unlike those of almost all

other lower motor neurons], such damage would cause deficits in both eyes.)

2. Defective somatic sensation in all modalities on the right indicates damage on the left somewhere above the midpons, after trigeminal contributions have been added to somatosensory pathways (see Figs. 9-5 and 9-6).

3. Ataxia in the right arm and leg could be caused by damage in a variety of sites, prominently including the right half of the cerebellum or its input or output pathways. Most of these are on the right side of the CNS, but the superior cerebellar peduncles decussate in the caudal midbrain, so the output from the right half of the cerebellum travels through the left rostral midbrain (see Figs. 16-8 and 16-9). (Damage to the posterior column–medial lemniscus pathway can also cause ataxia, but this would diminish with eyes open.)

4. Bundles of oculomotor axons, the medial lemniscus and spinothalamic tract, and the crossed superior cerebellar peduncle are all adjacent to each other in the rostral midbrain, putting the damage in this patient in the left rostral midbrain.

CASE STUDY 18

1. Bilateral damage is required to account for loss of the upper left and right quadrants of both visual fields. This could be symmetric damage to the inferior parts of both retinas or optic nerves (unlikely but conceivable), to the lower part of the optic radiations (see Fig. 12-12) as they loop through the white matter of the temporal lobes, or to the lower parts of primary visual cortex (see Fig. 12-13).

2. Visual association areas in the inferior temporal and occipital lobes are involved in further analysis of form and color (see Fig. 12-16). Damage to posterior parts of the occipitotemporal gyrus can cause achromatopsia, or loss of color vision. Bilateral damage is usually required to cause complete loss, although unilateral damage can cause contralateral hemiachromatopsia.

3. Another consequence of this involvement in further analysis of form and color is that damage to the occipitotemporal gyrus can also cause deficits in identifying objects by shape, and this can be more or less selective for faces (prosopagnosia). Although right-hemisphere damage has occasionally been reported to cause prosopagnosia, most patients with this syndrome have bilateral damage.

4. The amygdala plays a key role in linking stimuli to emotional responses, and continued activation of the amygdala has been demonstrated in some patients who are no longer consciously aware of familiar or threatening objects.

5. The posterior cerebral artery supplies the inferior and medial surfaces of the temporal and occipital lobes (see Figs. 7-12 and 7-13).

CASE STUDY 19

1. Intact ability to repeat indicates damage outside the perisylvian language zone. Diminished fluency with mostly intact comprehension indicates anterior damage. This is transcortical motor aphasia (see Table 19-3).

2. Posterior continuation of the damage described in question 19.1 would cross the precentral and postcentral gyri in the region of the arm/hand representation.

3. This is a tough one. Occlusion of an artery leaving either the circle of Willis or the vertebrobasilar system causes damage that is typically worse in the territory fed by proximal parts of the artery (e.g., after middle cerebral artery occlusion, damage is worse in the perisylvian zone than farther away from the lateral sulcus). This is because other arteries can partially supply more peripheral parts of the territory through end-to-end anastomoses (see Fig. 7-13). The damage in 19.1 and 19.2, in contrast, seems to be near the area of overlap between middle cerebral and anterior cerebral arteries, in what is referred to as a watershed zone. Watershed infarcts can result from reduction in blood flow in multiple arteries at the same time, e.g., after cardiac arrest. This patient's left internal carotid artery was occluded, leading to reduced flow in the left ophthalmic, anterior cerebral, and middle cerebral arteries. The reduced flow in the anterior and middle cerebrals (either because of incomplete occlusion or coming from the circle of Willis) was able to save proximal parts of their territories from infarction, but the flow had run out before distal parts of the arteries were reached.

CASE STUDY 20

1. Following acute spinal cord injury, a state of spinal shock ensues, in which most functions of segments below the injury simply cease. Although the mechanism is not fully understood, a major part of it is the loss of the descending inputs that normally converge on somatic (and autonomic) motor neurons. Without these, the remaining inputs from sensory fibers and spinal interneurons are thought to be insufficient to depolarize motor neurons to threshold.

2. Multiple mechanisms contribute to plasticity after injury; not all of these are understood either. One factor is upregulation of neurotransmitter receptors in partially denervated neurons, with the result that they become hypersensitive to transmitters released by remaining inputs. Another is sprouting by the remaining inputs to occupy vacated synaptic sites. The net result of these and other mechanisms is that reflex inputs have abnormally powerful effects, and normally suppressed circuitry (such as that underlying Babinski sign) reemerges and is strengthened.

3. During spinal shock, autonomic motor neurons, like somatic motor neurons, are inactive. In the absence of detrusor contraction, the bladder expands until the elasticity of its walls overcomes the outflow resistance.

4. Autonomic reflexes, probably for the same reasons as stretch and withdrawal reflexes, gradually become hyperactive after loss of descending inputs. In this case, the vesicovesical reflex (see Fig. 18-9) reemerges and is strengthened, so the detrusor contracts automatically at low bladder volumes. However, the external sphincter is also tonically contracted, so the bladder cannot empty completely.

Index